Physiotherapy in Obstetrics and Gynaecology

Physiotherapy in Obstetrics and Gynaecology

Physiotherapy in Obstetrics and Gynaecology

Margaret Polden
Grad Dip Phys, MCSP
Superintendent Obstetric Physiotherapist
Hammersmith Hospital, London

Jill Mantle
BA, Grad Dip, Phys, MCSP, Dip TP
Senior Lecturer, Physiotherapy Division, Institute of Health and Rehabilitation
Polytechnic of East London

Contributions from
Barbara Whiteford and Diana Ireland

BUTTERWORTH
HEINEMANN

Physiotherapy in Obstetrics and Gynaecology

Margaret Polden

Grad Dip Phys, MCSP
Superintendent Obstetric Physiotherapist,
Hammersmith Hospital, London

Jill Mantle

BA, Grad Dip Phys, MCSP, Dip TP
Senior Lecturer, Physiotherapy Division, Institute of Health and Rehabilitation
Polytechnic of East London

Contributions from
Barbara Whiteford and Diana Keating

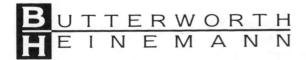

Butterworth-Heinemann
Linacre House, Jordan Hill, Oxford OX2 8DP
A division of Reed Educational and Professional Publishing Ltd

◿ A member of the Reed Elsevier plc group

OXFORD   BOSTON   JOHANNESBURG
MELBOURNE   NEW DELHI   SINGAPORE

First published 1990
Reprinted 1992, 1994, 1997

© Margaret Polden and Jill Mantle 1990

British Library Cataloguing in Publication Data
Polden, Margaret
    Physiotherapy in obstetrics and gynaecology.
    1. Medicine, Physiotherapy
    I. Title II. Mantle, Jill
    615.82

ISBN 0 7506 0016 0

Photoset by Wilmaset Ltd, Birkenhead, Wirral
Printed and bound in Great Britain by
Hartnolls Ltd, Bodmin, Cornwall

Contents

Preface

This book was conceived in a coach travelling between Bristol and Bath, and the first cell divisions occurred in the humid atmosphere of the Roman Baths and the Regency Pump Room. Implantation of the developing morula took place in the offices of Heinemann Medical Books, then in London, and the pregnancy was subsequently confirmed.

The gestation proved to be much longer than originally anticipated, about the length of two elephant's pregnancies, and a period we will certainly never forget! The physical stresses – writer's cramp, aching bottoms and backs – have been great, but in no way did they approach the psychological and emotional traumas to ourselves and our nearest and dearest. We have used every known coping strategy and invented several more to cope with the labour necessary to give birth.

Now, in the postpartum period, we are, like all new mothers, relieved but apprehensive as to how our offspring will be received. We very much hope that it will prove to be a useful and valued contribution to society.

We would like to thank all those who gave their time so freely to answer the numerous queries that arose in our efforts to make sure that information in the book is accurate and up-to-date; our thanks also to Shona Grant, our illustrator, for her patience, Ricky Hoole, Margaret Nokes and Sarah Polden, our long-suffering typists and, most particularly, our dear husbands who have had to endure our raised catecholamine levels over an extended period. They have suffered, like many pregnant fathers, and are undoubtedly hoping that life will now 'get back to normal' – whatever that might mean.

Margaret Polden
Jill Mantle
London, 1990

Foreword

The physiotherapist has been an important member of the maternity team for years, in fact since at least 1912. Then, the physiotherapist Minnie Randall together with the obstetrician J. S. Fairbairn at St. Thomas' Hospital developed special interests in the management of pregnancy, labour and the puerperium. Later the scope was extended to gynaecological cases.

Out of this has grown the Association of Chartered Physiotherapists in Obstetrics and Gynaecology. Its special contribution was recognized in the joint statement by the Royal College of Midwives, the Health Visitors' Association and the Chartered Society of Physiotherapy.

This recognition makes this new book especially timely. The training of a physiotherapist does not necessarily include the role in obstetrics and gynaecology. The book is a definitive statement. It therefore includes chapters on all aspects of the physiotherapist's role in obstetrics and gynaecology, from the basic sciences through to incontinence, a symptom which causes great distress and restriction of life to so many women and one which can so often be helped by the skills of the physiotherapist.

On a personal note I am happy to say that throughout my professional life in obstetrics and gynaecology I was always conscious of the contribution physiotherapists could bring to our work. I was privileged to know and to work with Helen Heardman who did so much to promote preparation for childbirth and the relief of discomfort. The obstetric physiotherapist was always a valued member of the team attending teaching rounds and of course conducting antenatal classes for mothers, and fathers. They have a special role which cannot be properly undertaken by others not trained in their methods.

I am therefore very glad to welcome this book with all the care and effort that has gone into its production, not least in the excellent illustrations and the bibliography which follows each chapter and which makes it an excellent work of reference.

The book has a scope and interest far beyond its authors' intention.

Dame Josephine Barnes, 1990

Introduction

As recently as the late nineteenth century the physiotherapy and midwifery professions shared a common rootstock. In the UK, educating more than just a few privileged women was a new philosophy, and formal and accredited training for occupations thought suitable for women, such as nursing and midwifery, was at best elementary. In addition, professional bodies were only just being formed. Women, who wanted to work outside the home and were inclined to care for people, took whatever training was offered, first in one aspect of caring, then in another.

In 1886, Dame Rosalind Paget, a nursing sister at the London Hospital who was also a midwife, joined the Midwives Institute, which later became the Royal College of Midwives (RCM). In 1902 she was involved in the formation of the Central Midwives Board and appears as number two on their list of members. Also in 1886 Dame Rosalind became interested in a new therapy – Swedish massage. She, and others like her, underwent training and then returned to their hospitals to teach the techniques to their colleagues. However, through her insistence on high standards and her anxiety that properly trained, reputable masseuses should not be confused with those of 'ill repute', she became one of the founding members of the Society of Masseuses and in 1895 became its first Chairman of Council. Over the years the group prospered and developed into the Chartered Society of Physiotherapy (CSP). Dame Rosalind held membership number one.

Miss Minnie Randall OBE, a great physiotherapist of the early part of this century, also had dual nursing and midwifery training before she turned to physiotherapy. She was one of the first to bring the principles of physiotherapy to obstetrics. In 1912, when she was Principal of the School of Massage and Medical Gymnastics at St Thomas' Hospital, London, J. S. Fairbairn, a leading obstetrician who believed in 'preventive obstetrics', asked Miss Randall to devise a system of 'bed exercises' for his postnatal mothers. Because newly delivered women remained in bed for about three weeks at that time, many problems that are rarely seen today were rife. The exercises were designed to aid postnatal physical recovery and to train women to rest through relaxation. Later, Miss Randall turned her attention to antenatal instruction, once again urged on by Mr Fairbairn, who thought that more should be done preventatively to help pregnant women. She was greatly influenced by Dr Kathleen Vaughan who had noticed, while working in Kashmir, that women who had a sedentary, confined and inactive lifestyle frequently had more difficult labours and deliveries than the boatwomen and peasants who led much more active lives. Dr Vaughan felt that heredity was not the only factor that determined the shape of the pelvis and the mobility of its joints and those of the lower spine – the way women used their bodies in their everyday lives also had an important influence on this too. Apart from incorporating squatting into her antenatal programme, as a preparation for labour, Miss Randall introduced many of the pelvic and lumbar spine mobilizing exercises suggested by Dr Vaughan which were based on the movements made by Kashmiri boatwomen. She also encouraged women to adopt different positions of comfort in labour.

Another notable source of influence on Minnie Randall in the 1930s was Dr Grantly Dick-Read who developed his theory of the fear–tension–pain cycle in labour. Fearful women who expected to feel pain became tense as labour began. This led to tension in their minds and, according to Grantly Dick-Read, in their cervices too. This gave rise to more pain which in turn increased their fear. He encouraged his labouring mothers to relax and breathe deeply through their contractions – a system which Miss Randall built into her antenatal classes. In the late 1930s, a dancer turned physiotherapist, Margaret Morris, suggested to Miss Randall that women should actually rehearse labour antenatally in the same way that dancers rehearse for a performance.

It was another physiotherapist, Helen Heardman, who in the 1940s drew together the threads of relaxation, breathing and education for childbirth into antenatal preparatory courses for labour and parenthood. It was she, together with other physiotherapists equally interested in this field, who was responsible for the formation of one of the first Special Interest Groups of the CSP – the Obstetric Association of Chartered Physiotherapists (OACP).

In the forty and more years since then, much has changed in obstetric physiotherapy, midwifery and obstetrics, and many dedicated physiotherapists have added their expertise to the specialty which now includes gynaecology and the treatment of incontinence among its interests. Today, the professional organization for this specialization is known as the Association of Chartered Physiotherapists in Obstetrics and Gynaecology (ACPOG). It is one of the largest clinical interest groups in the CSP and runs validated post-registration courses for physiotherapists wishing to specialize in the field. The association is fortunate to count among its members, both past and present, many women who have reached the top of their profession; who have published books and papers which are widely read, and who are respected, not only by their colleagues, but by the members of the midwifery, health visitor and medical professions too. This mutual respect among individuals has led ACPOG into increasing dialogue and collaboration with the RCM and the Health Visitors' Association

(HVA). Some of the fruits of this were seen recently with the publication of the statement negotiated by ACPOG with the RCM and the HVA, and endorsed by the CSP in April 1987.

Statement by the Royal College of Midwives, the Health Visitors' Association and the Chartered Society of Physiotherapy on working together in psychophysical preparation for childbirth

This statement was submitted to Council by the Association of Chartered Physiotherapists in Obstetrics and Gynaecology through the Planning and Resources Committee and endorsed by Council at its meeting on March 11, 1987. It is now an official document of the Chartered Society.

1. Midwives, health visitors and obstetric physiotherapists take part in providing education in preparation for childbirth and parenthood. This is an important form of preventive medicine and health education, and parents derive maximum benefit where a team approach operates.

2. The role of the midwife is that of the practitioner of normal midwifery, caring for the woman within the hospital and community throughout the continuum of pregnancy, childbirth and the puerperium. She has an important contribution to make in health education, counselling and support. In this context her aim is to facilitate the realization of the woman's needs, discuss expectations and air anxieties. She has the responsibility of monitoring the woman's physical, psychological and social wellbeing and is in a unique position to be able to correlate parent education with midwifery care.

3. The role of the health visitor in this field is to offer advice to the parents-to-be on the many health and social implications of birth and the development of the child. She is in a very special position in the family scene to inform them of the services available and to encourage them to use them. She can also reinforce the advice given by the obstetric physiotherapist and midwife.

4. The role of the obstetric physiotherapist is to help the woman adjust to the physical changes throughout pregnancy and the puerperium so that stress may be minimised. She will assess and treat any skeletal and muscular problems such as backache. She is a skilled teacher of effective relaxation, breathing awareness and positioning and thus helps to prepare the woman for labour. In the post-natal period she will give advice on physical activity, teach post-natal exercises and where necessary give specialised treatments.

5. In order for the services of the team to be of maximum benefit to parents there should be a close liaison between members. Shared learning sessions should take place to help to ensure that techniques and advice are consistent, related to current practice and meet the needs of parents. The midwife, health visitor and obstetric physiotherapist should be in regular contact and operate an effective referral system.

Physiotherapy (1987) **73**, 165

The Health Service in the UK is at a crossroads, and at this moment it is difficult to discern, particularly in obstetrics, what sort of service society will require in the twenty-first century. However, the most pressing need in obstetric and gynaecological physiotherapy must be a thorough, scientific and systematic evaluation of our treatments using respected research methodologies. No physiotherapist wants to waste the time spent on patients by using ineffective therapies. All physiotherapists can contribute to this venture by keeping good records and periodically auditing their own performance e.g. quality of recovery and time taken in relation to a specific condition. These findings could be compared with colleagues' records, and reasons for differences sought. In addition, some physiotherapists need to have time specially allotted to more formal investigation, and a reasonable number must be funded in full-time research. We owe it to ourselves and to our clients and patients to enquire and test; to seek out what is true and best.

Our motivation in writing this book is our deep conviction that thorough and effective physiotherapy is essential in this field, and that physiotherapists should carry out the work rather than attempt to pass their skills on to other professionals. Up to now no fully comprehensive textbook has existed covering all aspects of this work. There are very few specialist tutors for undergraduate physiotherapists, so students often receive a rudimentary introduction to obstetrics and gynaecology, and obstetric placements that give students practical experience are not compulsory and are few in number. Yet newly qualified physiotherapists are expected to work efficiently in obstetrics and gynaecology, often, in many centres, without the supervision of properly qualified seniors.

Over 50% of the population is female, and at the present time there are close to 700000 births per annum in the UK – a figure that probably reflects the most clients in any specialist area. It is interesting to note that physiotherapy departments often accept open referrals of problems to their sports injuries clinics which could be seen as being self-inflicted by self-selected people – yet physiotherapy managers still relegate obstetric and gynaecological practice to the 'bottom of the pile'. Women have to put up with myriad physical discomforts during and after pregnancy. For example, those with backache can consider themselves lucky if their backs are examined antenatally. The trauma that they sustain in labour, through no fault of their own, could be treated and their pain relieved by skilled physiotherapists, yet such women regularly go unattended. Mothers of young families and women approaching the climacteric as well as those well past the menopause often live with back pain that restricts mobility, and with bladder and continence symptoms that cause great distress. A referral to a sympathetic, empathetic physiotherapist who has a proper understanding of such problems and the appropriate therapies could improve their quality of life enormously.

There is no better forum for health education, in its widest sense, than is offered by the contact between the whole obstetrical health-care team and women experiencing pregnancy, labour and the puerperium; and the benefits go on and on, into later years. The knowledge so gained radiates out, like the ripples from a stone tossed into a pool, and influences whole families and the wider community. The physiotherapist has a great deal to offer in this field, particularly in terms of fitness, coping with stress, wise back care and the promotion of continence.

This book is for physiotherapists, and particularly those who fall into the following categories:

- students making their first contact with this field;
- newly qualified physiotherapists on obstetric and gynaecological rotations;
- physiotherapists embarking on this specialist post-registration training;
- physiotherapists who are actively involved in the specialty (as a resource book).

We have tried not to perpetuate information that has been stated and restated in other textbooks without proper testing, and we have been very careful not to dictate prescriptions for treatment, particularly in the field of electrotherapy where, in our view, there is an urgent need for very carefully planned and controlled scientific research to evaluate its efficacy.

In a book of this size we have had to set limits on what is included and the depth in which it is covered; some knowledge is assumed. We have tried to write clearly and simply, with a minimum of jargon, explaining underlying physiology and the reasoning behind certain approaches. We include references for further reading in each aspect of the subject. Cross-references have been used extensively, but, in places, material has been repeated to avoid an irritating break in the reader's train of thought caused by having to turn to another page. We hope that other physiotherapists will be infected by our enthusiasm for the specialty, and will enjoy, as we do, working with our midwifery, health visitor and medical colleagues, for the benefit of women of all ages.

CHAPTER 1

Anatomy

PELVIS

The pelvis provides a protective shield for the important pelvic contents; it also supports the trunk, and constitutes the bony part of the mechanism by which the body weight is transferred to the lower limbs in walking, and to the ischial tuberosities in sitting. The pelvis consists of the two innominate bones and the sacrum with the coccyx; these bones articulate at the symphysis pubis, and at the right and left sacroiliac joints to form a bony ring. They are held together by some of the strongest ligaments in the body (Fig. 1.1). The ring of bone is deeper posteriorly than anteriorly and forms a curved canal. The inlet to this canal is at the level of the sacral promontory and superior aspect of the pubic bones. The outlet is formed by the pubic arch, ischial spines, sacrotuberous ligaments and the coccyx. The enclosed space between the inlet and outlet is called the true pelvis, and the plane of the inlet is at right angles to the plane of the outlet.

The female true pelvis differs from the male in being shallower, having straighter sides, a wider angle between the pubic rami at the symphysis and a proportionately larger pelvic outlet. The ideal or gynaecoid pelvis is recognized by its well-rounded oval inlet and similarly uncluttered outlet (Fig. 1.2c).

The inlet has its longest dimension from side to side, whereas at the outlet the longest dimension is anteroposteriorly (Table 1.1). The fetal skull is longest in its anteroposterior dimension. Most commonly in labour the head enters the inlet of the maternal pelvis transversely placed (i.e. long axis to long axis), rotates in mid-cavity and leaves by the outlet with its longest dimension lying anteroposteriorly.

Some other possible pelvic shapes are shown in Fig. 1.2. Difficulties can be experienced in childbirth from such adverse features as protuberant ischial spines, a heart-shaped inlet produced by an invasive sacral prominence, or an asymmetrical pelvis (e.g. as a result of rickets or trauma). It is also possible for the inlet or outlet to be too small to allow the fetal head to pass through (cephalopelvic disproportion).

The wedge-shaped sacrum is virtually suspended between the innominates by the exceptionally tough interosseous and posterior sacroiliac ligaments which, in the cadaver, detach themselves from their periosteal junction rather than tear when the bones are forcibly

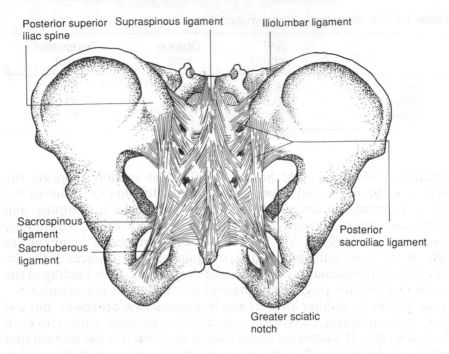

Posterior superior iliac spine

Supraspinous ligament

Iliolumbar ligament

Sacrospinous ligament

Sacrotuberous ligament

Posterior sacroiliac ligament

Greater sciatic notch

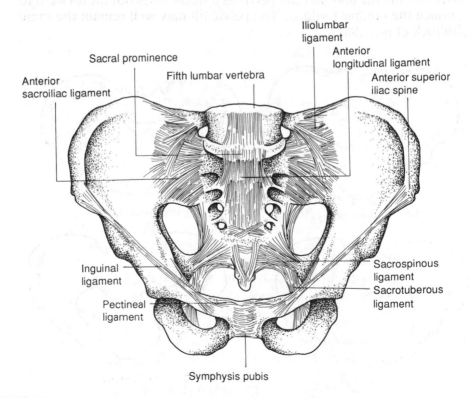

Sacral prominence

Fifth lumbar vertebra

Iliolumbar ligament

Anterior longitudinal ligament

Anterior superior iliac spine

Anterior sacroiliac ligament

Inguinal ligament

Pectineal ligament

Sacrospinous ligament

Sacrotuberous ligament

Symphysis pubis

Figure 1.1 The pelvis: (a) posterior view, (b) anterior view.

Table 1.1 The diameters of the gynaecoid true pelvis

	A/P (cm)	Oblique (cm)	Transverse (cm)
Inlet	28	30.5	33
Midcavity	30.5	30.5	30.5
Outlet	33	30.5	28

separated (Meckel, 1816; Sashin, 1930). The sacrum supports the weight of the trunk and upper limbs; usually loading of it pushes the sacral prominence down and forward, producing a complex and individual series of changes, rotating the sacrum about a generally transverse axis (Fig. 1.3). This causes the connecting ligaments to tighten, so drawing the undulating, irregular articular sufaces of the ilia into firmer approximation with those of the sacrum. Thus loading of the sacral prominence (e.g. in pregnancy) is often – but not invariably – accompanied by lumbar lordosis and its associated adaptations, hip and knee flexion, thoracic kyphosis and cervical extension with a forward thrusting chin. It should be noted that in this case it is the sacrum that moves on the ilia and that the pelvis as a whole does not tilt forward to produce the lumbar lordosis. The pelvic tilt may well remain the same (Bullock et al., 1987).

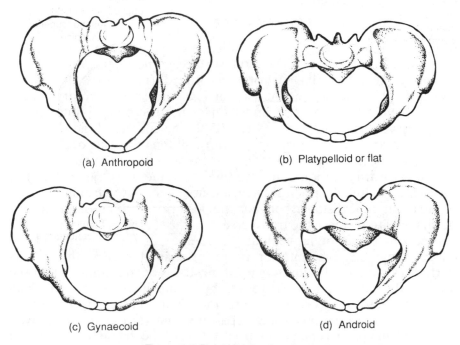

(a) Anthropoid

(b) Platypelloid or flat

(c) Gynaecoid

(d) Android

Figure 1.2 Pelvic inlet – four types.

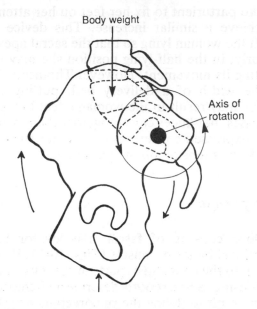

Figure 1.3 Rotation of sacrum under loading.

The range of movement at the two sacroiliac joints and the symphysis is normally small, and may not be exactly similar at each joint. As a result of the generalized increased joint laxity in pregnancy it has been claimed that movement in these joints may increase by as much as two and a half times. Certainly an increase in width of the symphysis pubis from 4 mm to 9 mm is documented (Abramson et al., 1934). It has been suggested that where hypermobility, permissive configuration of opposing uneven iliac and sacral surfaces, and appropriate stress coincide, one or both ilia may rotate backwards (i.e. the sacrum rotates forward) or forwards on the sacrum (i.e. the sacrum rotates backwards), resulting in tension and pain at the sacroiliac joints and/or symphysis pubis. However uncomfortable this increased mobility may be in pregnancy, the benefit in parturition of the bony ring of the pelvis having some 'give' is obvious. There is no doubt that the possibility of greater forward rotation and 'shuffling' movements (Grieve, 1981) of the sacrum on the ilia provides a means at delivery by which inclination of the ilia and the distance between the posterior portions of the ilia can be changed to increase the transverse diameter of the pelvic outlet. The consequent posterior movement of the apex of the sacrum and the coccyx lengthens the anterior posterior diameter also; this occurs particularly in the full squatting position. It has been estimated that the area of the outlet can be increased by as much as 28% in this way (Russell, 1969). In squatting, the femora apply pressure to the ischial and pubic rami thus producing separation outward at the symphysis pubis and an upward and backward rotation of the ilia on the sacrum. It has been suggested that the old practice in the second stage of labour of encouraging the parturient to fix her feet on her attendants' hips may sometimes achieve a similar increase. This device would be most successful with the woman lying so that the sacral apex and coccyx can move posteriorly; in the half-lying position she may be sitting on her tail, thus limiting its movement. However Thomson (1988) noted that because of the width of a delivery bed, putting her feet on the attendants' hips may result in the woman's feet being far wider apart and, in some cases, her knees closer together than in normal squatting. Thomson also expressed concern as to whether such a position could place extra sideways tension on the perineum.

THE PELVIC FLOOR

The pelvic floor consists of fascia, the levator ani muscles and reinforcing perineal bands of muscle (Figs. 1.4, 1.5). Different names have been given to the constituent parts of the levator ani muscles, and this can be confusing. Some reports describe an ischiococcygeal portion posteriorly, and omit to define the puborectalis muscle and the fibres skirting the urethra and vagina and inserting into the perineal body. Others call these latter fibres the periurethral muscle of the pelvic floor (Gosling et al., 1981). The labelling of Fig. 1.4 has been carefully chosen for the insight it gives to function. If strong, the levator ani muscle, which is enveloped in fascia on both surfaces, forms an efficient

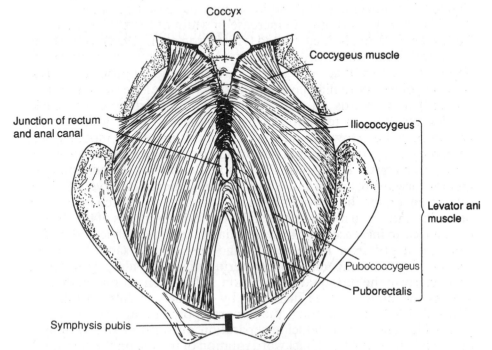

Figure 1.4 The pelvic floor.

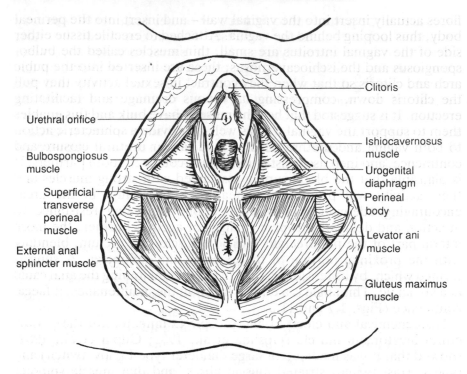

Figure 1.5 Superficial muscles of the perineum.

muscular sling (Fig. 1.6) which supports and helps maintain the pelvic viscera in position. In addition, the most medial fibres of the puborectalis portions of levator ani run either side of the vagina – some say a few

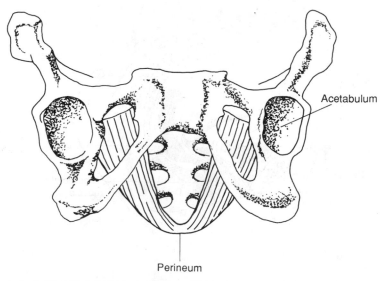

Figure 1.6 The supportive effect of the levator ani muscles.

fibres actually insert into the vaginal wall – and insert into the perineal body, thus looping behind the vagina. Attached to erectile tissue either side of the vaginal introitus are small, thin muscles called the bulbo-spongiosus and the ischiocavernosus; these are inserted into the pubic arch and clitoris so that when they contract in sexual activity they pull the clitoris down, compressing its venous drainage and facilitating erection. It is suggested that healthy muscles have bulk and this enables them to support the vaginal wall as well as provide a sphincteric action to both vagina and urethra which would favour urethral closure and continence, and increase satisfaction in intercourse for both partners. It is plausible that the blood supply associated with strong muscles and their activity will promote the health of epithelium in the area, encouraging adequate vaginal lubrication, increasing resistance to infection and delaying atrophic changes of ageing. Further, the more lateral part of the puborectalis muscle encircles the rectum, blending with the proximal portion of the external anal sphincter. A sling is formed which, by its tension, results in the rectum joining the anal canal at a 90° angle. This angle is a critical factor in the maintenance of faecal continence (Figs. 1.7 and 11.3).

Histochemical and electron microscopic examination of the periur-ethral levator ani muscle (Gosling et al., 1981; Gilpin et al., 1989) showed that it was made up of large diameter type I (slow twitch) and type II (fast twitch) striated muscle fibres, and that muscle spindles were found. Type I fibres are highly fatigue resistant and consequently can produce contraction over long periods although the power of the contraction tends to be of a relatively low order. Muscle activity may be recorded by E.M.G. from the levator ani muscle 'at rest' and even in

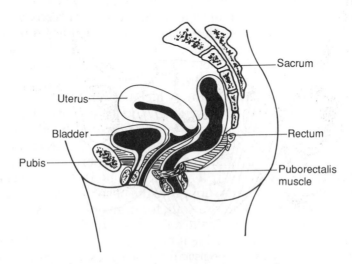

Figure 1.7 The sling formed by the puborectalis muscle.

sleep, presumably the type I fibres are responsible for this. By contrast type II fibres are highly fatiguable but produce a high order of power on contraction. All these facts support the contention that the levator ani muscle is a skeletal muscle adapted to maintain tone over prolonged periods and equipped to resist sudden rises in intra-abdominal pressure, as for example on coughing, sneezing or running. At such times fast twitch fibres may be recruited reflexly if needed to brace the floor and contribute to urethral closure. It is known that there are two subgroups of fast twitch fibres IIa and b, where IIa are relatively more fatigue resistant but produce slightly less power than IIb. However at the present state of knowledge the possible relevance of this for the physiotherapist is not clear. Table 1.2 shows the percentage of type II fibres found by Gilpin et al., (1989) in the pubococcygeus muscle.

Table 1.2 The percentage of type II fibres found in pubococcygeus muscle

	Type II fibres (%)	
	Anterior pubococcygeus	Posterior pubococcygeus
Asymptomatic women	33	24
Symptomatic women	39	10

The levator ani is a voluntary muscle and is supplied by the perineal branch of the pudendal nerve (S2–S4). The urogenital diaphragm – sometimes called the pelvic diaphragm or triangular ligament – lies superficial (inferior) to the levator ani muscle and fills the space anteriorly between the descending pubic rami. It consists of two layers; the urethra and vagina pass through it, and it is reinforced by the deep transverse perineal muscles. These apparently insignificant muscles lie between the layers of the urogenital diaphragm posterior to the vagina and urethra, and connect the ischial rami to the perineal body, which it is suggested they help to stabilize. The perineal body is a central coneshaped fibromuscular structure which lies just in front of the anus (Fig. 1.5). The cone is about 4.5 cm high and its base, which forms part of the perineum, is 4 cm approximately in diameter. In addition to the deep perineal muscles, some fibres of the levator ani muscles insert into it, as already described, and the superficial perineal muscles also radiate to the pelvis from it. The perineal body is of considerable importance because it affords support to the posterior wall of the vagina and thus indirectly to the anterior wall, for in an upright posture one lies against the other. This explains the concern obstetricians and midwives have for the welfare of the perineal body in labour, particularly in the second stage. At delivery the pelvic floor provides a gutter to guide the fetal head towards and down the birth canal.

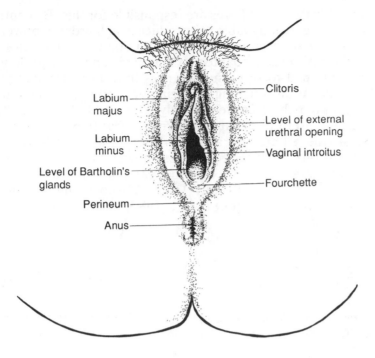

Labium majus

Clitoris

Labium minus

Level of external urethral opening

Vaginal introitus

Level of Bartholin's glands

Fourchette

Perineum

Anus

Figure 1.8 External genital organs.

THE PERINEUM

The external genitalia are shown in Fig. 1.8. Either side of the entry to the vagina (introitus) are the Bartholin's glands, which are activated mainly in sexual arousal to produce mucoid secretions; they are normally about the size of a pea. The skin and structures of the perineum are supplied by the pudendal nerve (S2–S4).

THE ABDOMINAL MUSCLES

The anterior and lateral abdominal wall is formed by the abdominal muscles (Fig. 1.9). The deepest of the group is the transversus abdominis muscle and this is covered by the internal and external oblique muscles. From each side these three muscles insert into a broad aponeurosis which connects with its fellow at the linea alba. This tendinous raphe, which is wider above the umbilicus than below, is formed by decussating aponeurotic fibres. The aponeurosis is reinforced by the two rectus abdominis muscles which run in sheaths formed in the aponeurosis on either side of the linea alba. Of particular relevance is the fact that the sheaths are elastic longitudinally and less so transversely. Each rectus abdominis muscle has three transverse fibrous intersections which are firmly attached to the anterior wall of

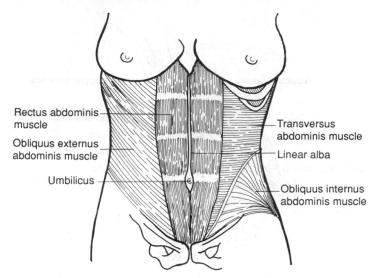

Figure 1.9 Abdominal muscles dissected to show deeper muscles on the right.

the enclosing sheath. The lowest intersection is about the level of the umbilicus, and the sheaths are deficient posteriorly in the lowest portion.

The oblique and transversus muscles are innervated by the lower six thoracic nerves, the iliohypogastric and ilioinguinal nerves. The recti are innervated by the lower six thoracic nerves. The abdominal muscles are vascularized by the superior epigastric vessels from above (branches of the internal thoracic or mammary vessels) and the inferior epigastric vessels from below (branches of the external iliac artery and vein).

THE BREAST

The female breast (Fig. 1.10) consists of fat and glandular tissue, overlying the pectoralis major muscle. It is roughly circular, but a small tail of tissue extends up and laterally to the axilla. The breasts undergo two bursts of hormonally mediated growth, one in puberty, the second in pregnancy. In addition, many women notice fullness and tenderness directly related to stages in the menstrual cycle.

In the breast are 15–20 secreting lobes, each with its own duct, and opening on to the nipple area. Just proximal to each opening there is a widened portion in the duct (lactiferous sinus) which, when milk is being produced, acts as a temporary reservoir. The nipple is composed of erectile tissue and is surrounded by loose pigmented skin – the areola. Nipples are normally slightly raised but in some women they are flat or even inverted. A baby may experience difficulty suckling from inverted nipples.

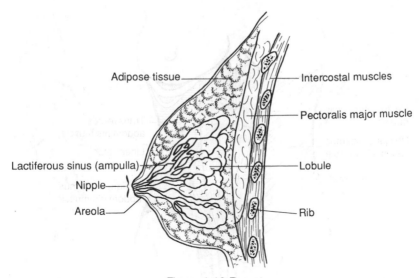

Adipose tissue —

Intercostal muscles

Pectoralis major muscle

Lactiferous sinus (ampulla) —

Lobule

Nipple —

Areola —

Rib

Figure 1.10 Breast.

The blood supply to the breast is via the axillary, internal thoracic and the second to fourth intercostal arteries; the breast is drained by accompanying veins. The lymphatic drainage is of some importance because of the possible development of carcinoma in breast tissue and its subsequent dissemination via the lymphatic system. There is an anastomosing network of channels, the majority of which drain to the anterior axillary nodes, but the medial part of the tissue is drained to the internal thoracic nodes. The nerve supply is from the anterior and lateral cutaneous branches of the fourth to sixth thoracic nerves.

THE REPRODUCTIVE TRACT

The female genital tract (Fig. 1.11) consists of highly specialized organs whose structure is elegantly functional: two ovaries, the fallopian tubes, the uterus and the vagina.

Ovaries

The ovaries produce ova, and also secrete oestrogens and progesterone under the direction of the anterior pituitary gland. In the cortex of these two pinkish-grey structures, the size and shape of almonds, lie thousands of primary follicles, each consisting of an immature ova and a single layer of stroma cells. At birth the ovaries contain about 2 million follicles; by seven years of age there has been some wastage and weeding out of imperfect cells to reduce this number to about 300 000, a process that continues throughout life. From puberty through the

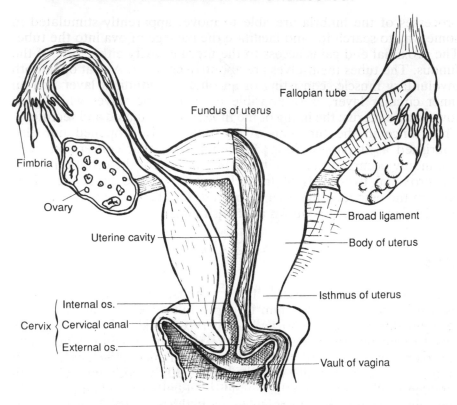

Figure 1.11 The reproductive tract – left half in cross-section.

reproductive years, a number of follicles develop but only one follicle usually ripens fully every month. The ovum in this follicle develops in size and in maturity and the stroma cells differentiate to be able to secrete oestrogens and progesterone in increasing amounts. At ovulation the ovum is ejected from the surface of the ovary, the follicle collapses and undergoes a further phase of development to become a corpus luteum, which is yellow in appearance. It continues to produce oestrogens and progesterone and, if fertilization of the ovum does not occur, then shrivels in about 10 days. If pregnancy occurs the corpus luteum enlarges and continues to be active for 3–4 months; it probably then degenerates. Thus, over the years the initially smooth ovarian surface becomes increasingly wrinkled and puckered, and in a woman in her late 40s there are just a few hundred follicles left at most.

Fallopian tubes

The two fallopian or uterine tubes connect the ovaries with the uterus. The outer end of the tube is funnel-shaped and fimbriated; one fimbria is longer than the others and is attached to the ovary. The tentacle-like processes of the fimbria are able to move, apparently stimulated in some way to search for and facilitate the passage of ova into the tube. The proximal end gains access to the uterine cavity either side of the fundus. The tubes themselves are about 10 cm long. A coat of smooth involuntary muscle, consisting of an outer longitudinal layer and an inner circular layer, is responsible for peristaltic waves which pass towards the uterus; the lining of the tubes is both ciliated and secretory. Thus, once in the tube, an ovum is not only propelled but also nourished as it passes along. It seems likely that conception most commonly occurs in the vicinity of the junction of the distal third and the proximal two-thirds of the relevant tube. The tubal secretions contain the essential ingredients to condition the sperm and ovum for fertilization, a process known as capacitation.

Uterus

The uterus (womb) consists of the fundus, the body, the isthmus (which is no more than 5 mm in depth but develops into the lower segment during pregnancy) and the cervix (neck). The uterus is the shape of an inverted pear and in the nulliparous adult it measures approximately 9 cm long, 6 cm wide and 4 cm thick; it weighs about 50 grams. It is a potentially hollow organ with a thick muscular wall (myometrium) lined with lush, highly vascular endothelium (endometrium), whose thickness varies with the menstrual cycle but is approximately 1.5 mm. This mucous membrane is shed at each menstruation, and consists of columnar epithelium, connective tissue and many tube-like uterine glands. After implantation of the ovum, the endometrium is called the decidua because it is shed following delivery. It is a rich source of prostaglandins. The muscle fibres of the myometrium are smooth and involuntary, swathing the fundus and body and encircling the isthmus (Fig. 1.12). They are supported on a collagenous connective-tissue base. The body of the uterus lies against the superior surface of the bladder and moves as the bladder fills and empties. Congenital malformations of the uterus, resulting for example in the uterus being in two separate halves to a greater or lesser extent (bicornuate uterus), sometimes become evident only in pregnancy or labour.

The cervix or neck of the womb forms a fusiform or spindle-shaped canal at the junction of the main body of the uterus with the vagina. It consists chiefly of fibrous, collagenous and elastic connective tissue, but contains some circularly disposed muscle fibres (10%) in the proximal part or internal os. The distal two-thirds protrudes into and forms the vault of the vagina – the lowest portion is called the external os. The canal is lined with columnar epithelium which produces mucoid secretions. At the external os there is a change to squamous epithelium which is continuous with the lining of the vagina. The mucoid secretions

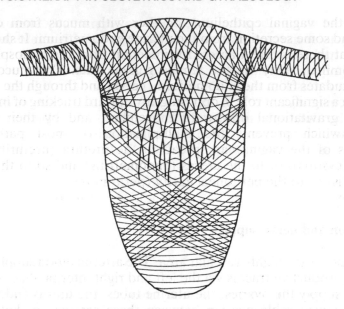

Figure 1.12 Diagrammatic representation of the muscle fibres of the uterus.

from the cervix moisten the lower part of the genital tract, and their downward movement, together with the constrictive nature of the cervix, acts as a deterrent to rising infection. Following conception and before the pregnancy test becomes positive, there are dramatic changes in vascularity, and consequently in the colour and texture of the cervix, and this can be used in the diagnosis of pregnancy. Until recently the cervix was credited with a largely passive role in childbearing, simply being dilated in labour in response to uterine forces. However, it is now recognized that a very active 'ripening' process occurs.

Vagina

The vagina is about 7.5 cm long and passes upwards and backwards towards the rectum from its opening on the perineum, most commonly in a direction that meets the longest axis of the uterus at about 90° (Fig. 1.7). The vagina connects with the uterus via the cervix, which projects into its vault. The vagina is a highly elastic channel capable of considerable distension. Within its wall is a layer of smooth muscle, the fibres of which are placed both longitudinally and circularly, and the lining is of stratified squamous epithelium. The vagina is positioned posteriorly to the urethra and the base of the bladder, and anteriorly to the rectum. The urethra is embedded in the anterior vaginal wall and is therefore vulnerable to trauma during childbirth, pelvic surgery and even occasionally during sexual intercourse. There are no glands in the vagina so the vaginal moisture is composed of transudate which seeps through the vaginal epithelium together with mucus from cervical glands and some secretion from the uterine endometrium. It should be noted that there is direct access for infection from the atmosphere to the abdominal cavity via the female genital tract. The mucoid and serous exudates from the endometrium, cervix and through the vaginal wall have a significant role in opposing any upward tracking of infection by their gravitational downward movement, and by their acidity (pH 4), which prevents the multiplication of most pathogens. Infections of the vagina can spread to the urethra (urethritis) and bladder (cystitis), or to the uterus (endometritis) and so to the tubes (salpingitis) or to the peritoneal cavity (peritonitis).

Circulation and nerve supply

The true pelvis is a highly vascular area. The arterial blood supply to the female reproductive tract is via the left and right internal iliac arteries; branches supply the ovaries, the uterine tubes, the uterus and vagina. There is considerable overlap between these arteries so that where bleeding occurs it may well be considerable and difficult to control. The uterine arteries develop greatly in pregnancy to serve the enlarging uterus and placenta. There is a highly developed lymphatic system with many nodes within the pelvic cavity, apparently providing a good defence to infection but unfortunately facilitating the spread of carcinoma. The veins return blood via the internal iliac vessels and so to the inferior vena cava. The uterine muscle is innervated by the autonomic nervous system via the pelvic plexuses, and both parasympathetic (S2–S4) and sympathetic (T10–L1) efferents are found. Sensory nerve endings are more numerous in the cervix and in the lower uterine segment than in the rest of the uterus, and pain impulses such as those arising from labour are relayed via the hypogastric plexus to enter the spinal cord through the posterior roots of T10–L1. Sensation from the perineum is conveyed via the pudendal nerve to the spinal cord (S2–S4).

Suspensory ligaments

The female genital tract is loosely suspended across the midline of the true pelvis, enfolded within the double layer of the slack, flimsy broad ligament which is attached either side to the lateral inner surface of the pelvis. The ovaries are attached to the posterior layer of this ligament, and to the posterior aspect of the uterus by a fibromuscular cord. The uterine round ligaments are attached anteriorly to either side of the fundus of the uterus; they are lax, and pass forward via the deep inguinal ring and the inguinal canal to insert into the subcutaneous tissue of the labia majora. The round ligaments help to keep the uterus

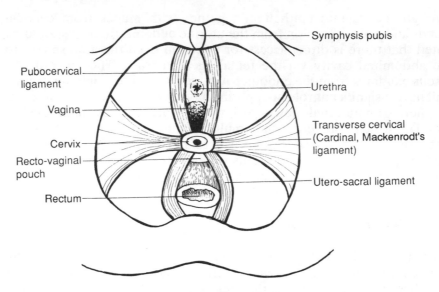

Figure 1.13 The ligamental supports of the cervix.

anteverted and anteflexed (see also p. 300). However, both the broad and round ligaments permit considerable movement of the uterus, tubes and ovaries before becoming taut, allowing adaptation to the constantly changing volumes of bladder and rectum. Further, it is probable that hormonal influence enables them to increase in elasticity to adapt to the changing size of the pregnant uterus as it gradually rises to become a temporary abdominal organ.

The lower fringe of the connective tissue of the broad ligament condenses to form the more substantial transverse cervical ligaments – also known as the cardinal and Mackenrodt's ligaments – connecting the cervix to the lateral walls of the pelvis (Fig. 1.13). Two bands of connective tissue – the pubocervical fascia – pass anteriorly either side of the neck of the bladder anchoring the cervix to the posterior surface of each pubis. In addition, two moderately strong fibromuscular bands of fascia – the uterosacral ligaments – connect the cervix and the upper part of the vagina to the lower portion of the sacrum. Both the transcervical and uterosacral ligaments contain some smooth muscle fibres and elastic fibres. Thus the cervix is suspended and located by 'guy ropes' on the four aspects, and these risk being traumatized in labour. This support is supplemented by the lifting support of the pelvic floor which forms the base of the pelvic cavity.

THE URINARY TRACT

The urinary system comprises two kidneys which excrete urine, two ureters which conduct urine to the bladder where it is stored, and the urethra which channels urine to the outside of the body.

The kidney

The kidney is the size of the owner's fist and of a shape so typical that it is used as a descriptive term. The indentation on its medial aspect is called the hilum, and here the ureter and renal vein leave and the renal artery enters. The kidneys have a huge blood supply via two branches directly from the aorta, and returning to the inferior vena cava. The kidneys are placed posteriorly in the loin associated with the first lumbar vertebra; the left kidney is a little higher than the right because of the wedge-shaped liver superiorly. The kidney consists of a fibrous capsule, a cortex, medulla, and major and minor calyces or collecting ducts which channel urine into the pelvis of the kidney and so to the ureter.

The ureter

Each ureter is about 25 cm long and is a hollow muscular canal about the diameter of a small drinking straw, and lined with transitional epithelium as is the whole urinary tract. Contraction in peristaltic waves of the smooth muscle in the wall of the ureter assists urine down to the bladder – even when a person is supine. As the ureter enters the pelvis it lies in front of the sacroiliac joint, separated from it by the bifurcation of the common iliac artery. At the level of the internal os, it is 1 cm from the cervix and passes through the transverse cervical ligaments. The ureter enters the thick muscular wall of the bladder obliquely at each of the upper corners of the trigone of the bladder; this arrangement results in closure of these two orifices and the prevention of reflux of urine when the bladder contracts.

The bladder

The bladder is a hollow sac of smooth muscle corporately called the detrusor muscle, whose fibres are arranged in a complex meshwork. When the detrusor muscle is relaxed the bladder acts as a reservoir, when it contracts it becomes a pump; it is lined with transitional epithelium and the outer surface is covered with connective tissue composed of collagen and elastic fibres. The muscle fibres, which lie in all directions are in an ideal arrangement to reduce the lumen of the bladder in all directions when they contract in unison; there is no specific polarity as there is with the uterus. The bladder is roughly boat-shaped when empty, and lies directly behind the pubic symphysis (see Fig. 1.7). It becomes oval and rounded as it fills and rises out of the true pelvis and into the abdomen. The posterior part of the superior surface is related to the anteflexed uterus. A little further posteriorly the bladder is related to the cervix and vagina, and here a triangular,

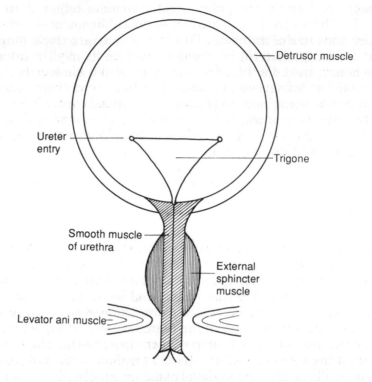

Figure 1.14 Diagrammatic representation of the bladder in the female.

flattened portion is called the trigone (Fig. 1.14); the apex of the triangle points downward and the base is uppermost. The trigone area is thicker than the rest of the bladder, and the internal lining is very smooth and particularly richly innervated. The ureters enter at the two corners of the base and the urethra leaves at the apex of the trigone. The bladder is connected to the urethra by way of the bladder neck, and the trigone contributes to its funnel shape. In this zone the detrusor muscle fibres are progressively replaced by elastic and collagen fibres and by urethral smooth muscle fibres, all of which are arranged obliquely and longitudinally to the urethra in such a way that when the muscle component is relaxed the bladder outlet is passively drawn together, closed and watertight. When the muscle component contracts the bladder neck opens. The angle made posteriorly between the bladder and the urethra is called the urethrovesicular angle; it is usually about 100° and appears to be an important factor in the maintenance of continence. The medial fibres of both puborectalis sections of the levator ani muscle blend with the fascia surround the urethra and vagina. They pull the vagina and urethra forward when they contract, favouring this angle.

The bladder is loosely held in position by ligaments; it is joined to the anterolateral fascia of the pelvis by the fibroareolar lateral ligaments of the bladder. Anteriorly the pubovesical ligaments tether it to the pubes, and a fibrous cord – the median umbilical ligament – connects the bladder apex to the umbilicus. Posteriorly there are thickenings in the pelvic fascia attached to the bladder which also carry the internal iliac vessels supplying the bladder. The wall of the bladder is richly supplied with stretch receptors, and impulses from these pass in afferent nerves to the micturition centre in the spinal cord, S2–S4. The motor innervation of the detrusor muscle is by parasympathetic fibres in the pelvic splanchnic nerves (S2–S4). In addition there is also sympathetic innervation (T11–L3).

The urethra

The urethra is a fibromuscular tube of variable length, but usually about 4 cm long, and is embedded in the anterior wall of the vagina and lies behind the symphysis pubis. It is the connection between the bladder and the anterior opening on the perineum, and its function is to convey and control urine. It should be noted that the shortness of the female urethra makes urinary infections more likely and the fitting of incontinence devices more problematical in women than in men. The urethra is lined with transitional epithelium. Its intermediate layer is of smooth muscle whose fibres are longitudinally and obliquely placed. In the middle section of the urethral length, and external to the smooth muscle in the urethral wall, is a circularly disposed band of type I (slow twitch) striated muscle fibres; this band is thicker anteriorly than posteriorly where it lies against the vagina. This striated muscle structure, called the external sphincter, contains no muscle spindles, and the individual fibres are very narrow, about one-third of the diameter of the usual slow-twitch skeletal muscle fibres (Gosling et al., 1981). The external sphincter applies closure pressure on the urethra and is important in the maintenance of continence. It appears that, like the levator ani muscle, there is electrical activity within the sphincter even in sleep.

The blood supply to the urethra is via branches of the internal iliac arteries, and drainage is via the venous plexuses in that region to the internal iliac veins. It was long held that the striated muscle of the external sphincter, sometimes called the rhabdosphincter, was supplied by somatic efferent fibres via the pudendal nerves, but it now seems possible that it is supplied via the pelvic splanchnic nerves (S2–S4), travelling with the fine, easily damaged parasympathetic fibres to the smooth muscle of the urethra (Hilton, 1989). However, there is still controversy as to whether the actual motor supply to the sphincter is somatic or autonomic, or both. Because the fibres are striated, a somatic nerve supply is most logical. There is also sympathetic innervation to the smooth muscle of the urethra.

THE ANORECTAL REGION

The descending colon is about 25 cm long and passes down inside the left lateral aspect of the trunk to enter the pelvis posterior to the anterior superior iliac spine. At the pelvic inlet it is continuous with the sigmoid colon, a 25-cm long loop of gut which passes medially and posteriorly to the anterior aspect of the sacrum. From the level of the third sacral vertebra it is called the rectum; for about 13 cm, it follows the curve of the sacrum and coccyx posterior to the vagina. On piercing the pelvic floor it is continuous with the anal canal. At the junction of the rectum and the anal canal, the puborectalis portion of the levator ani muscle forms a sling which pulls the junction anteriorly to create the anorectal angle (see Figs. 1.7, 11.3). The peritoneum reflects across from the upper two-thirds of the rectum to the uterus, dropping a little between the two structures to produce the pouch of Douglas. The anal canal is about 4 cm long and joins the rectum with the anus; it is kept firmly closed by the pull of the puborectalis muscle and the external anal sphincter.

The rectum has a muscle wall composed of a layer of longitudinal fibres outside a layer of circularly disposed smooth muscle. There is a lining of mucous membrane which falls into three very specific transverse folds, two on the left wall and one on the right. In the anal canal the muscular wall is similar but the circular layer is thicker in the upper part and is called the internal sphincter; this is enclosed and augmented by the external sphincter. The structure of the muscular external sphincter is in three parts: a deep, circular band of striated muscle around the proximal end of the canal which blends with the striated puborectalis fibres; a superficial circular band at the lower end of the canal; and in between are bands which pass from coccyx to perineal body either side of the canal. The lining of the upper half of the anal canal is of columnar epithelium, which lies in vertical folds called anal columns. By contrast, the lining of the lower half of the canal is of squamous epithelium which is continuous with the skin surrounding the anus. Just behind the anus and below the coccyx is a mass of fibrous tissue called the anococcygeal body.

The blood supply to both the rectum and the anal canal is via the rectal vessels. The nerve supply to the rectum and the smooth muscle of the upper half of the anal canal is via the inferior hypogastric plexuses, and responds only to stretch. It was thought at one time that there were sensory stretch receptors in the lining, and that these relayed the sensation of fullness to consciousness. It is now known that the stretch receptors within the levator ani muscle are stimulated by change in volume and pressure of the distending rectum (Parks, 1980). The nerve supply to the lining of the lower half of the canal and the external anal sphincter is from the pudendal nerve and the perineal branch of the fourth sacral nerve. Thus this area responds to pain, temperature, touch and pressure.

References

Abramson D., Roberts S.M., Wilson P.D. (1934). Relaxation of the pelvic joints in pregnancy. *Surg. Gynaecol. Obstet.*, **58**, 595.

Bullock J., Jull G., Bullock M. et al. (1987). The relationship of low back pain to postural changes during pregnancy. *Austr. J. Physiotherapy*, **33**, 10.

Gilpin S.A., Gosling J.A., Smith A.R.B., Warrell D.W. (1989). The pathogenesis of genitourinary prolapse and stress incontinence of urine. A histological and histochemical study. *J. Obstet. Gynaec.*, **96**, 15–23.

Gosling J.A., Dixon J.S., Caitchley H.O.D., Thompson S. (1981). A comparative study of the human external sphincter and periurethral levator ani muscles. *Brit. J. Urol.*, **53**, 35–41.

Grieve G.P. (1981). Common Vertebral Joint Problems, p. 53. Edinburgh: Churchill Livingstone.

Hilton P. (1989). Mechanisms of urinary continence. *Abstracts of First International Congress on the Pelvic Floor*, Cannes, p. 17–21.

Meckel J.F. (1816). *Handbuch der Menschlichen Anatomie*, vol. 2. 2nd edn. Berlin: Halle.

Parks A.G. (1980). Faecal incontinence. *Incontinence and its Management*, (Mandelstam D., Ed.) London: Croom Helm.

Russell J.G.B. (1969). Moulding of the pelvic outlet. *J. Obst. Gynaecol. Br. Commonwealth*, **76**, 817–826.

Sashin D. (1930). A critical analysis of the anatomy and pathological changes of the sacro-iliac joints. *J. Bone Jt Surg.*, **12**, 891.

Thomson A.M. (1988). Management of the woman in normal second stage of labour: a review. *Midwifery*, **4**, 77–85.

Further reading

Barnes J., Chamberlain G. (1988). *Lecture Notes on Gynaecology*, 6th edn. Oxford: Blackwell.

Gosling J.A. (1979). The structure of the bladder and urethra in relation to function. *Urol. Clin. N. America*, **6**, 31.

Gosling J.A., Harris P.F., Humpherson J.R. et al. (1985). *Atlas of Human Anatomy*. Edinburgh: Churchill Livingstone.

Govan A.D.T., Hodge C., Callander R. (1989). *Gynaecology Illustrated*, 4th edn. Edinburgh: Churchill Livingstone.

Lee D. (1989) *The Pelvic Girdle*. Edinburgh: Churchill Livingstone.

McGuire E. (1979). Urethral sphincter mechanisms. *Urol. Clin. N. America*, **6**, 39.

Schiff Boissonnault J., Kotarinos R.K. (1988). Diastasis recti. *Obstetric and Gynaecologic Physical Therapy* (Wilder E., ed.). Edinburgh: Churchill Livingstone.

Snell R.S. (1986). *Clinical Anatomy for Medical Students*, 3rd edn. Boston: Little, Brown.

CHAPTER 2

Physiology of Pregnancy

MENSTRUATION

A diagrammatic representation of the events and hormonal control of the menstrual cycle is shown in Figs. 2.1 and 2.2. A normal, regular menstrual cycle pattern is sensitive to changes in body health and environment; it can certainly be disturbed by disease, and also by such life changes as extreme shock or stress, excessive activity and severe loss of weight. For example, anorexic women and girls suffer from amenorrhoea related to their overall decreasing body mass. It is thought that this results from changes in the hormonal balance. Endocrinologists have suggested that the hormonal control of the human body is like a major orchestra, a large number of instrumentalists working together to perform a great orchestral work. As knowledge increases, so does the concept of the size of the orchestra and the complexity of the work being played. Although much has yet to be fully understood, this appears to be particularly true of the menstrual cycle, pregnancy, labour and the puerperium, where changes within the reproductive system are supported by a continuum of secondary adjustments, some of which are in other systems.

One set of changes associated with the menstrual cycle, which seems to be generally little known, concerns the normal cyclic changes in vaginal secretions. Indeed there are women who, in ignorance, fear that they signify some pathology. Following menstruation, women usually experience several 'dry days' when there is little or no obvious secretion within the vagina. The first noticeable mucus is scant but opaque, white, thick and sticky. After one or more days the mucus begins to thin, is still cloudy but feels progressively more slippery. By about the seventh or eighth postmenstrual day the mucus is watery, clear, more profuse and very slippery. Women may have an impression of being wet. This state is associated with ovulation and thus the peak of fertility. Over the remaining days, prior to the next menstruation, the mucus quickly becomes thicker, opaque and more sticky, and then there are several further dry days. This sequence gives the woman the information she needs about her own fertility, and can even be the basis

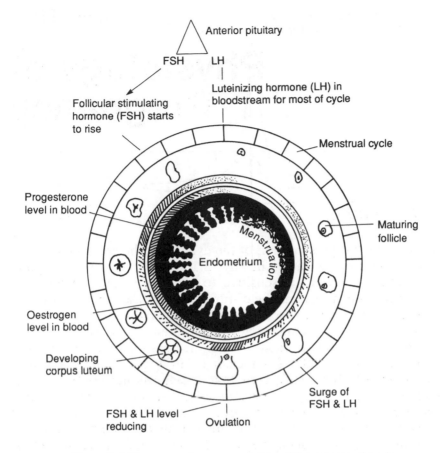

Figure 2.1 Diagrammatic representation of the menstrual cycle.

for natural, non-invasive family planning. In addition, sexual arousal increases secretions to the vagina and also from the Bartholin's glands.

PREGNANCY AND FETAL DEVELOPMENT

Following fertilization the ovum begins to divide, and over the next 6–8 days the group of cells is nourished by secretions from the fallopian tube as it is propelled along towards and into the uterine cavity. From possibly the day of conception the outer layer (trophoblast) of this increasing group of cells (morula) produces human chorionic gona-dotrophin (HCG) to prevent menstruation and involution of the corpus luteum in the ovary. For 6–8 weeks the corpus luteum is the principal producer of the hormones progesterone, several oestrogens and relaxin. If the morula is to survive, implantation must occur in order to develop a more permanent nutritional supply line and additional hormone production. The outer cells become lined with a second layer,

LH – Luteinizing hormone levels
FSH – Follicular stimulating hormone levels

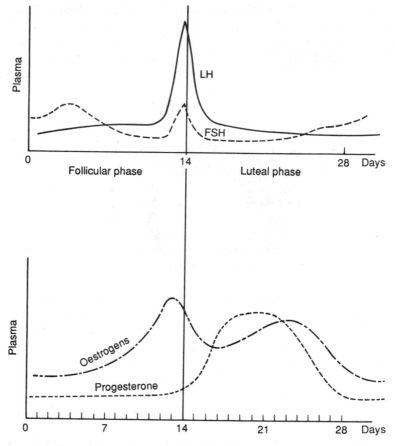

Figure 2.2 Hormone secretion in relation to the menstrual cycle.

and together these two layers are called the chorion. The spherical ball of cells is now called a blastocyst; it is hollow, with an inner mass of cells to one side which will develop into the embryo. The chorion divides to produce a myriad little tongue-like processes or villi all over the outer surface of the blastocyst. These burrow into the uterine endometrium, or decidua as it is also known in pregnancy. It is these chorionic villi that can be sampled between 8–10 weeks to detect inherited disease (see p. 91). The villi actually penetrate the decidual blood sinusoids, and maternal blood washes over them. The blastocyst is thus embedded within the decidua; however, as it grows it protrudes into the uterine cavity, stretching the covering surface of decidua. The villi atrophy over this portion, but not where the blastocyst remains in contact with the inner part of the decidua. The innermost site develops into the placenta from about the sixth week.

The disc-shaped placenta grows through pregnancy, and at term measures about 20 cm in diameter, is 3 cm thick and weighs about 500–700 g – approximately one-sixth of the baby's weight. It maintains the fetal circulation, which is entirely separate from that of the mother, and it is responsible for the vital exchange functions of respiration, absorption of nutrition and excretion; it is both lungs and gut to the fetus. The placenta also becomes a major hormone-producing structure in pregnancy, producing progestogens and oestrogens. By raising the maternal levels of these hormones, menstruation continues to be inhibited. Early in pregnancy the placenta also produces HCG, which reaches a peak around 8–10 weeks and then declines by 18 weeks to a much lower level which is maintained until after delivery. HCG has been implicated in 'morning sickness'. It has been suggested that the corpus luteum may remain active throughout pregnancy as a source of relaxin, but Bigazzi et al. (1980) and Bryant Greenwood and Greenwood (1982) report human decidua as another production site.

It used to be thought that the placenta acted as a barrier to substances in the maternal blood that could be detrimental to the fetus, e.g. viruses and drugs (including nicotine and alcohol). This is now known not to be the case, and a simple principle to follow is that if a substance is in the maternal blood then it is also in the fetal blood. Further, because the fetal liver is immature, metabolism of drugs hardly occurs, so there may be an accumulation over time of a particular drug bound to plasma proteins. This is why great care must be taken in the prescription of medicinal drugs for pregnant women.

A human pregnancy is calculated as usually lasting about 40 weeks or 280 days. If the date on which the last menstrual flow commenced is known, the estimated date of delivery (EDD) can be calculated by adding 7 days to the date and then adding 9 months; for example:

date of commencement of last menstrual flow = 8 January
8 January + 7 days = 15 January
15 January + 9 months = 15 October
EDD = 15 October

Alternatively, add 7 days to the date of the last menstrual flow and then deduct 3 calendar months. Pregnancy is divided for the purpose of description and discussion into three 3-month periods or trimesters: it culminates in labour and the delivery of the fetus and placenta, and is followed by the puerperium, a period of 6–8 weeks during which time the remaining changes of pregnancy revert.

For the first 8 weeks it is usual to call the developing baby an embryo; thereafter to delivery it is called the fetus. The fetus grows within a thin semitransparent sac (the amnion), is bathed in amniotic fluid and is attached to the placenta by the umbilical cord. The fluid is secreted by the placenta, amnion and cord. The fetus drinks it and excretes it as urine; it is said to be replaced every three hours. It is of interest that where fetal kidneys are absent or the urethra is blocked there is less fluid than normal (oligohydramnios), and where the fetus has atresia of the oesophagus there may be increased fluid (polyhydramnios). The volume of fluid normally increases throughout pregnancy to its maximum of about a litre at around 38 weeks of gestation. It contains a variety of substances including proteins, sugars, oestrogens, progesterone, prostaglandins and cells from fetal skin. This is the fluid withdrawn at amniocentesis. Table 2.1 gives a basic outline of fetal growth.

Table 2.1 Basic pattern of fetal growth

Weeks	Detail	Length (cm)	Weight (g)
3	Embryo has primitive circulation	0.2	
4	Head, trunk, tail differentiated	0.7	
6	Limb buds growing	1.5	
8	Now called a fetus; has eyelids, ears, external genitalia	4	
12	Fingers, toes, nails, bones, cartilage forming	9	
16	Moving quite strongly	16	
20	Hair erupting, vernix depositing	21	500
28	Essential development complete	35	1250
36	Greatly increasing in bulk	43	2500
40	Term	50	3500

A baby is said to be 'full term' at a gestational age of 37 or more weeks, providing it weighs more than 2500 g. Survival is good over 34 weeks and is poor under 28 weeks, although survival following birth at 23 weeks' gestation has now been achieved. The poor outcome of the shorter gestational age baby is due to the lungs and respiratory centre not being fully developed, little or no immunity to infection, immaturity of the liver leading to clotting defects, and feeding difficulties.

For international statistics a baby is said to be premature if it weighs less than 2500 g at birth. This is an unsatisfactory definition and has led to the use of 'preterm' where a baby's gestational age is less than 37 weeks. Where the weight is less than normally would be expected for the gestational age the terms 'growth retarded', 'small for dates' or 'dysmature' may be used. With increasingly successful sophisticated care in special care baby units, the abortion laws require regular review.

THE PHYSICAL AND PHYSIOLOGICAL CHANGES OF PREGNANCY

The changes of pregnancy are chiefly the direct result of the interaction of four factors: the hormonally mediated changes in collagen and involuntary muscle; the increased total blood volume with increased blood flow to the uterus and the kidneys; the growth of the fetus resulting in consequent enlargement and displacement of the uterus; and finally the increase in body weight and adaptive changes in the centre of gravity and posture. The demands that these changes must make upon a woman should never be underestimated.

Endocrine system

The changes of pregnancy are orchestrated by hormones and much concerning their action and interaction has yet to be elucidated. However, progesterone, oestrogens and relaxin seem to be the most important for the physiotherapist.

Progesterone is produced first by the corpus luteum, then by the placenta. The output of the corpus luteum reaches a maximum of about 30 mg per 24 hours at about 10 weeks of pregnancy and thereafter declines. The placenta begins an increasing production from about 10 weeks which at first supplements that from the corpus luteum and then completely takes over the role. The amount produced rises steeply from about 75 mg per 24 hours at 20 weeks to 250–300 mg per 24 hours at 40 weeks. Three progestogens are produced in the placenta but the chief one is progesterone.

Oestrogens are produced first by the corpus luteum; as with progesterone, this supply is gradually taken over by the placenta, reaching an output of about 5 mg per 24 hours at 20 weeks and 50 mg per 24 hours at 40 weeks. Several oestrogens are produced in the placenta; one of these (oestriol) is produced in considerable quantities and excreted in the maternal urine. The amount excreted in this way in 24 hours was formerly used as a measure of fetal well-being. Biophysical assessment, e.g. fetal growth by ultrasonography, has replaced this biochemical test. There is evidence to show that the maternal and fetal adrenal glands and the fetal liver also contribute towards oestrogen synthesis in pregnancy (Fransden, 1963). Relaxin is thought to be synthesized in the corpus luteum and later in the decidua (Zarrow and McClintock, 1966; Bigazzi et al., 1980; Bryant Greenwood and Greenwood, 1981; Yki-Jarvinen et al., 1983). Research suggests that it is produced as early as 2 weeks of gestation, is at its highest levels in the first trimester and then drops by 20% (O'Byrne et al., 1978; Weiss, 1984) to remain steady until delivery.

Effects of progesterone

1. Reduction in tone of smooth muscle:
   food may stay longer in stomach, nausea, peristaltic activity
   reduced, water absorption in colon increased, constipation,
   uterine tone reduced, uterine activity damped down,

bladder tone reduced, tone also in ureters, urine stasis,
blood vessel tone reduced, diastolic pressure lower, dilation of
veins.
2. Increase in temperature (0.5 °C).
3. Reduction in alveolar and arterial P_{CO_2} tension, hyperventilation.
4. Development of the breasts' alveolar and glandular milk-producing
cells.
5. Increased storage of fat.

Effects of oestrogens

1. Increase in growth of uterus and breast ducts.
2. Increasing levels of prolactin to prepare breasts for lactation;
oestrogens may assist maternal calcium metabolism.
3. May prime receptor sites for relaxin, e.g. pelvic joints, joint
capsules, cervix.
4. Increased water retention, may cause sodium to be retained.
5. Higher levels result in increased vaginal glycogen, predisposing to
thrush.

Effects of relaxin

1. Gradual replacement of collagen in target tissues (e.g. pelvic joints,
joint capsules, cervix) with a remodelled modified form that has
greater extensibility and pliability. Collagen synthesis is greater than
collagen degradation and there is an increased water content, so
there is an increase in volume.
2. Inhibition of myometrial activity during pregnancy.
3. May have a role in the remarkable ability of the uterus to distend
and in the production of the necessary additional supportive
connective tissue for the growing muscle fibres.
4. May have a role in cervical ripening.
5. May have a role in mammary growth.

Reproductive system

Amenorrhoea is one of the first signs of pregnancy for most women,
although it is not uncommon to experience a slight bleed, for 1–2 days,
at the time at which menstruation would be expected if conception had
not very recently occurred. Within a few days of conception the cervix,
if viewed with a speculum, will be seen to have changed in colour from
pink to a bluish shade. From a firmly closed structure which increases in
depth early in pregnancy, the cervix changes by a gradual but accelerating process, which in the final weeks involves the softening, greater

distensibility, effacement and ultimately dilation (collectively called ripening) of the cervix. It has been described as changing from feeling firm like the cartilage of the nose, to feeling soft like the lips. These changes can be felt on digital examination and are produced by the endocrine-controlled restructuring of collagen and other tissues. As pregnancy progresses a plug of thick mucus forms in the cervical canal, sealing the uterus. The Bishop score (Table 2.2) is the accepted method of calculating the degree of ripeness of the cervix before labour. Nine points or more is considered favourable.

Table 2.2 Bishop score of cervical changes

Score	Length	Dilation	Consistency	Position	Level of presenting parts
0	3 cm	Closed	Hard	Posterior	>3 cm above ischial spines
1	2 cm	1–2 cm	Intermediate	Intermediate	2–3 cm above spines
2	1 cm	3–4 cm	Soft	Anterior	<2 cm above spines
3	Fully effaced	5 cm	—	—	Below spines

Bimanual palpation – one hand on the abdominal wall and two fingers in the vagina – can detect changes within the uterus (Hegar's sign); in early pregnancy it will feel enlarged and soft. The growing uterus rises out of the pelvis to become an abdominal organ at about 12 weeks' gestation, increasingly displacing the intestines and coming to be in direct contact with the abdominal wall. The average fundal height related to gestation is shown in Fig. 2.3. It can be seen that in the final 2–3 weeks the fundal height drops; this is particularly noticed by the primigravida. The fetal head by this times comes to be in the pelvic inlet and is said to be engaged. The uterus increases in size dramatically and so does its blood supply (Fig. 2.4). The weight of the uterine tissue itself increases from about 50 g to 1000 g at term. The muscle fibres of the fundus and body are exceptional in their ability to increase in length and thickness throughout pregnancy to accommodate the growing fetus; it has even been suggested that new fibres may develop. The collagenous tissue, on and by which the muscle fibres are supported, increases in area and also in elasticity through pregnancy under hormonal influence. It has been said that in the nulliparous woman the uterus would hold about a quarter of a teaspoon of fluid while the gravid uterus at term would contain ten pints. As pregnancy progresses the isthmus develops to become the lower uterine segment, and by term it accounts for approximately the lower 10 cm of the uterus above the cervix. The musculature is not highly developed in this area and

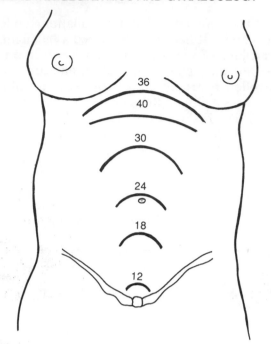

Figure 2.3 Fundal heights in relation to gestation in weeks.

towards term it becomes soft and stretchy, allowing the fetus to sink lower in the uterus and into the true pelvis.

The muscle fibres of the uterus increase in activity, and coordinated contraction of the uterus can be detected by about 20 weeks' gestation. Bursts of irregular, short, usually painless contractions become progressively more evident and systematic. They are called Braxton Hicks contractions; they facilitate the blood flow through the placental site and play a part in the development of the lower uterine segment. At some stage regular and increasingly painful contractions establish and labour is said to have begun; however, in the meantime some women experience considerable sequences of contractions of variable length (20 seconds to 4 minutes), the intensity of which may or may not be painful. Terms such as 'false labour' or 'pre-labour' are used for this; it is more common in the multigravid woman.

There has been a recent increase in research interest in the effects of exercise on the pregnant woman and on the fetus, whether continuing or starting an exercise regimen. Maternal hyperventilation resulting from maternal activity – particularly that using large muscle groups – reflects an increased demand for oxygen, and risks the possibility of blood flow being shunted from the uterus to the active skeletal muscles. This should be borne in mind by obstetric physiotherapists when advising women. It supports the view that it is wise for women to be advised to reduce their workload later in pregnancy when fetal demand is at its greatest.

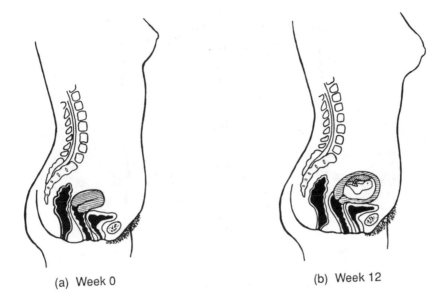

(a) Week 0

(b) Week 12

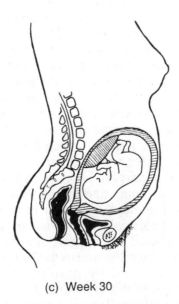

(c) Week 30

Figure 2.4 Diagrammatic representations of the physical changes of pregnancy.

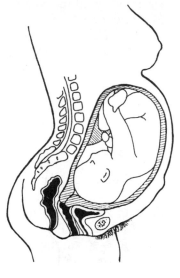

(d) Week 37

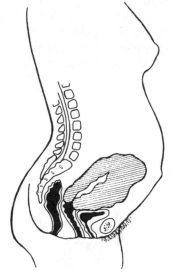

(e) Postpartum day 1

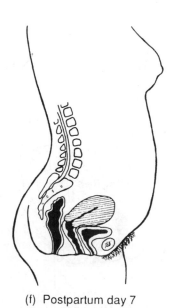

(f) Postpartum day 7

Figure 2.4 (continued)

The fetal heart can be heard using a Sonic-aid from about 14 weeks' gestation, and by stethoscope at about 24–26 weeks. Fetal movements are usually felt by the multigravida somewhere between 16–18 weeks and by the primigravida between 18–20 weeks. This sensation is sometimes called 'quickening'. The outline of the fetus can be palpated from about 24 weeks' gestation.

Cardiovascular system

The blood volume increases by 40% or more to cope with the increasing requirements of the uterine wall servicing the placenta and the other demands placed on the body, e.g. weight gain – both supplying the greater bulk and moving it. There is a greater increase in plasma than in red cells, consequently the haemoglobin level falls to about 80%. This effect is variously called dilution anaemia or physiological anaemia of pregnancy, and is one cause of women experiencing tiredness and malaise from quite early in pregnancy.

Progesterone acts on the smooth muscle of blood vessel walls to produce slight hypotonia, and causes a small rise in body temperature; therefore pregnant women generally have a good peripheral circulation and do not feel the cold. The heart increases in size and accommodates more blood, so the stroke volume rises and the cardiac output increases by 30–50%; there is a progressive small increase in heart rate through pregnancy. These changes begin to occur quite early, and it must be appreciated by physiotherapists involved in training programmes that a standard amount of exercise will produce a greater increase in cardiac output in pregnant women than in non-pregnant ones. This situation is further compounded as a woman gains bulk and weight. Blood pressure may even fall a little through the second trimester of pregnancy, so women may easily feel faint from prolonged standing. Care must be taken when getting up from a lying position. In the third trimester the weight of the fetus may compress the aorta and inferior vena cava against the lumbar spine when the woman is lying supine, causing dizziness and even unconsciousness; this is called the pregnancy hypotensive syndrome. The infallible remedy is to turn the woman on to her side. Vigorous activity or other sympathetic stimulation will result in a redistribution of the cardiac output to the working muscles and away from the abdominal organs – including the placenta. With the upsurge of interest in antenatal exercise in water it is important for the physiotherapist to take account of the physiological effects of immersion, the differences in muscle groups being used and the effects of change in body position on the cardiovascular system. In general it is known that the stroke volume increases but the heart rate and blood pressure show a small decline in water. The response of pregnant women seems to be similar to that in the non-pregnant state (McMurray et al., 1988). However, exercise in heat should be avoided because of the possible teratogenic effect of a raised core temperature, in the early weeks.

Slight vascular hypotonia, downward pressure of the enlarging uterus, weight gain, raised intra-abdominal pressure, and progesterone and relaxin-mediated changes in collagen all predispose to varicose veins, particularly in the legs, and to gravitational oedema. Varicosities of the vulva and anus (haemorrhoids, piles) may also occur. Oestrogens may be responsible for fluid retention generally in the body tissues. Some women can no longer wear hard contact lenses because their eye shape changes.

As a result of the increased peripheral circulation and hormonal stimulation, the mucous membranes (e.g. nasal, vaginal) become more active and lush. This can result in symptoms such as 'stuffy' nose and increased vaginal discharge. Consequently prolongation of coughs and colds may be experienced, also nose bleeds and vaginal thrush.

Respiratory system

The increased circulating progesterone levels of pregnancy further sensitize the respiratory centre in the medulla to carbon dioxide; this and the increasing demand for oxygen act as mild stimulants to ventilation. The resting respiratory rate goes up a little, from about 15 to about 18 breaths per minute, and there is a lowering by some 25% of the maternal blood carbon dioxide tension, consequently women notice breathlessness on activity. Tidal volume increases gradually by up to 40%, and alveolar ventilation also rises. The vital capacity seems to stay much as it was, so it is the expiratory reserve that is reduced. By the third trimester in many pregnant women the enlarging uterus increasingly impedes the descent of the diaphragm. Towards term it may actually displace the diasphragm upwards, often by 4 cm or more. The displacement is most significant where the fetus is large and/or the abdominal component of the maternal torso is short. The upward pressure of the fetus also affects the ribs causing them to flare (see p. 155). Maternal lower costal girth is increased, often by as much as 10–15 cm, as is the subcostal angle. Because of this the respiratory excursion is limited at the lung bases and greater movement is observed in the mid-costal and apical regions, and women frequently experience considerable breathlessness on even modest exertion towards the end of the pregnancy.

It seems probable that the hormone relaxin softens the costochondral junctions and renders them more mobile. Women complain of costal margin pain or rib ache, and of the fetus kicking the diaphragm and ribs; some have evidence of bruising and of disruption of costochondral joints.

Breasts

As early as 3–4 weeks of pregnancy unusual tenderness and tingling may be experienced in the breasts and soon enlargement begins, thought to be stimulated by the rising level of oestrogens, progesterone and relaxin. This growth continues through pregnancy and results in an increase of total breast weight of some 400–800 g. There is an increase in blood supply – veins may become visible on the chest – and in the number, size and complexity of the ducts. At about 8 weeks sebaceous glands in the pigmented area around the nipples become enlarged and more active, appearing as nodules (Montgomery's tubercles). The sebum secreted assists the nipple to become softer and more pliable. By 12 weeks of pregnancy the nipples and an area around them (the primary and secondary areolae) become more pigmented, and remain so for as much as 12 months after parturition. This pigmentation is thought to be due to the stimulation of melanin production by the anterior pituitary. As early as the 12th week a little serous fluid may be expressed from the nipples and by about the 16th week colostrum can be expressed. Human milk 'comes in' about the third or fourth postpartum day. Nipple stimulation results in the release of oxytocin from the posterior pituitary. This can be used in labour to increase uterine contraction and assist dilation of the cervix. It has been suggested that it could even be used to encourage labour to start.

Skin

The pigmentation of the areolae already mentioned is more pronounced in brunettes, and pigmentation is also seen in the linea alba, the vulva and in the face. Blotches which sometimes occur on the forehead and cheeks are called chloasma or the 'mask of pregnancy'. Striae or 'stretch marks' can develop over buttocks, abdomen and breasts and may become pigmented. These striae are a consequence of rupture of the dermis, the overlying epidermis is stretched and the resulting scar is therefore visible and permanent. Striae are caused by the need for skin to stretch rapidly over the enlarging body but may be aggravated by the hormonally mediated softening of collagen and by unnecessary weight gain. Some individuals appear to be more prone to striae than others so a genetic predisposition has been suggested. Certainly the application of oils with or without massage is unlikely to be effective in prevention or cure; however they may ease the sensation of tight and stretching skin.

There is an increase in blood flow to the skin which increases the activity of sebaceous and sweat glands, and so increases evaporation. Pregnant women may be expected to drink more to compensate. Fat is laid down particularly on the thighs, upper arms, abdomen and buttocks, and is said to be a store which is subsequently called on in breastfeeding, providing a woman does not 'eat for two' in the puerperium.

Gastrointestinal system

Nausea and vomiting, thought now to be the response of some to HCG, is not necessarily restricted to the early morning, nor does it always cease by the 16th week. It can be aggravated by certain foods – even by their odours – and by iron tablets, and inappropriately managed in severe cases (hyperemesis gravidarum) can lead to maternal dehydration, malnutrition and weight loss. Gross et al. (1989) showed a higher risk for fetal growth retardation and possible fetal anomalies amongst sufferers with weight loss. The gut musculature becomes slightly hypotonic and the motility is decreased. The inevitable sequelae of this are prolongation of gastric emptying time and a slower passage of food. Delay in the large bowel results in increased absorption of water and a consequent predisposition to constipation because the faeces are dry and hard. The reduced speed of oesophageal peristalsis, a hormonally mediated slackness of the cardiac sphincter, displacement of the stomach and an increased intra-abdominal pressure as pregnancy progresses, all favour the gastric reflux or 'heartburn' of which so many women complain. There is softening and hyperaemia of the gums, and bleeding may occur from quite minor trauma. Salivation may be increased.

It has been estimated that a pregnancy involves an energy expenditure of about 1000 kJ (239 kcal) per day (Hytten and Leitch, 1971; Durnin, 1989); however, since most women reduce or adapt their activity because of fatigue or the restrictions of their increased size and weight, and also because metabolism becomes more efficient (Van Raaij et al., 1987), it is rarely necessary in the UK to increase intake, but only to encourage a well-balanced diet with plenty of fibre. The average weight gain is between 10 and 12 kg (Hytten and Chamberlain, 1980) and is distributed as shown in Fig. 2.5.

Nervous system

Mood lability, anxiety, insomnia, nightmares, food fads and aversions, slight reductions in cognitive ability and amnesia are all well-substantiated and common accompaniments of pregnancy. How these alterations in emotional, cognitive and sensual function are brought about is not known, but they are presumably hormonally mediated phenomena.

Water retention quite frequently causes unusual pressure on nerves, particularly those passing through canals formed of inelastic material like bone and fibrous tissue (e.g. the carpal tunnel), with resulting neuropraxia. Occasionally pregnant women complain of symptoms

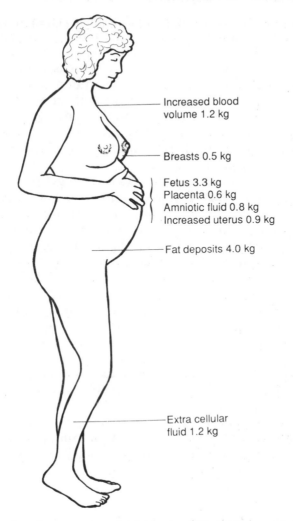

Increased blood
volume 1.2 kg

Breasts 0.5 kg

Fetus 3.3 kg
Placenta 0.6 kg
Amniotic fluid 0.8 kg
Increased uterus 0.9 kg

Fat deposits 4.0 kg

Extra cellular
fluid 1.2 kg

Figure 2.5 To show how an average weight gain of 10–12 kilograms is distributed.

indicating traction on nerves which can be due to increased weight, for example water retention in the arm increasing its weight and producing depression of the shoulder, and paraesthesia in the hand.

Urinary system

The presence of human chorionic gonadotrophin in the urine early in pregnancy forms the basis of the pregnancy test; the level falls after 12 weeks of pregnancy. Throughout pregnancy there is an increase in blood supply to the urinary tract in order to cope with the additional demands of the fetus for waste disposal. There is an increase in size and weight of the kidneys, and dilation of the renal pelvis. The musculature of the ureters is slightly hypotonic so the ureters are a little dilated, and also seem to elongate to circumvent the enlarging uterus; the possible result of these factors is pooling and stagnation of urine, and a predisposition to urinary tract infections. There is an increased urinary output, and small changes in tubular resorption caused by the pregnancy may result in excretion of significant amounts of sugar and protein. Diabetes may be first diagnosed in pregnancy because pregnancy is one of the factors that may precipitate its onset in women genetically predisposed to the condition. This usually regresses after delivery (gestational diabetes).

As the pregnancy progresses the bladder changes position to become an intra-abdominal organ, is pressed upon and even displaced by the increasingly large and heavy uterus. Thus the urethrovesicular angle may be altered and the intra-abdominal pressure raised; the smooth muscle of the urethra may become slightly hypotonic, and it seems possible that supportive collagen components in and to the tract and pelvic floor may become more lax and elastic. What is certain is that many women complain of frequency in early pregnancy, which has often resolved by the time they come to the booking clinic. This may be due to an early rise in urinary output (Francis, 1960a) and to subsequent adjustments to this. Later in pregnancy, particularly towards term, there may be urge and stress incontinence. The latter is said to occur in 50% of primigravida and the majority of multipara (Francis, 1960b). This led Francis (1960b) to suggest that it was pregnancy rather than parturition that caused subsequent incontinence problems in women. However, it is now well established that delivery can damage the urethral closure mechanism (Snooks et al., 1984). The cause of changes in continence in pregnancy is more likely to be multifactorial, as discussed above.

Musculoskeletal system

The influences of pregnancy on the musculoskeletal system are the ones that involve the physiotherapist most directly; first, to attempt to prevent disorders arising and then, where problems do arise, to treat them.

There is a generalized increase in joint laxity, and so in joint range, which is hormonally mediated. Oestrogens, progesterone, endogenous cortisols and particularly relaxin seem to be responsible for this. Research (Calguneri et al., 1982) has shown a greater increase in joint range, and therefore in the degree of laxity, in a second pregnancy than the first, but that subsequent pregnancies produce no greater degree. Generally joint laxity regresses post partum to near its pre-pregnancy state, but this may take up to six months. Histological animal studies suggest that the laxity is made possible by a gradual breakdown of collagen in the target tissue and its replacement with a remodelled modified form which has a higher water content and which has greater pliability and extensibility. The volume of the remodelled tissue is greater. Relaxin receptor sites have been reported in a variety of tissues, e.g. rat uterus, mouse symphysis pubis fibrocartilage, guinea-pig cervix and human skin (MacLennan, 1981).

During pregnancy it is usually necessary for a woman to adapt her posture to compensate for her changing centre of gravity. How a woman does this will be individual and will depend on many factors, e.g. muscle strength, joint range, fatigue and role models. Physiother-apists are in no doubt that for most women the lumbar and thoracic curves are increased. Until recently it was thought that the greater lumbar lordosis was due to an increase in the pelvic tilt; however, work by Bullock et al. (1987) brings this into question. What is certain is that about 50% of pregnant women experience back pain (see p. 134). The increased body weight must result in more pressure through the spine, and increased torsional strains on joints. Women become clumsier and are inclined to trip and fall. These factors, together with joint laxity and fatigue, particularly in the first and third trimester, must make pregnant women more prone to injury. Brisk walking has all the benefits and fewer of the risks of running, and exercising excessively or to the point of fatigue does no good to mother or fetus.

The changing centre of gravity is chiefly made necessary by the distending abdomen. How the abdominal wall adapts to the required degree of distension is worth considering. The muscle fibres permit stretch, but the collagen components – the aponeurosis, fibrous sheaths and intersections, and the linea alba – probably undergo hormonally mediated structural change to provide the necessary temporary extra extensibility. The girth of a woman or the distance from xiphisternum to symphysis pubis can be used as a guide to fetal growth. The distance between the two rectus abdominis muscles can be seen to widen throughout a pregnancy and the linea alba may even split under the strain (diastasis recti). It is of interest that Booth et al. (1980) showed some altered function in the abdominal muscles of pregnant women, in that the muscles were recruited in movements in which they do not usually participate.

Other muscles have increasing loads to lift and, if not encouraged to gain strength by daily use, may on an occasion be overwhelmed. For example, unless a woman makes a habit early in pregnancy of using her hips and knees when bending down to pick things up, weight gain may render it impossible until after parturition.

In the third trimester there is increased water retention which may result in a varying degree of oedema of ankles and feet in most women, reducing joint range. The oedema can also cause pressure on nerves, as in carpal tunnel syndrome where oedema in the arms and hands causes paraesthesia and muscle weakness affecting terminal portions of the median and ulnar nerve distributions (see p. 151).

With so much active growth and adaptation occurring within and supported by the body, the healthier a woman is before pregnancy the better. Obstetric physiotherapists are the health professionals best equipped to assess and advise on a woman's physical health before, during and between pregnancies. They are also well able to judge the effects of particular occupations and sports, and the wisdom of continuing them through pregnancy both in general and for a specific individual.

COMPLICATIONS OF PREGNANCY

Ectopic pregnancy

The fertilized ovum occasionally implants outside the uterus, most commonly in the fallopian tube at the ampulla or the isthmus – the junction of the tube with the uterus. The ovum burrows into the blood vessels of the tubal musculature; there being no decidua, this can cause surrounding necrosis. As the pregnancy develops distension of the tube results in pain, and if left untreated eventual rupture of the tube or bleeding leads in some patients to shock and even maternal collapse. Ideally the situation is first confirmed by laparoscopy and then surgically cleared, either removing part or all of the tube, or repairing the tube.

Pre-eclamptic toxaemia and eclampsia

Pre-eclamptic toxaemia (PET) is the most common and potentially serious complication of pregnancy for both mother and fetus. Estimates put the incidence at 10% of all pregnancies. It is more common amongst the least privileged, primigravid women and in twin pregnancies. The cause is unknown, and the patient may be unaware and uncomplaining. For many years the cardinal signs of this syndrome were considered to be raised and rising blood pressure, oedema and proteinuria. However, oedema is a normal feature of pregnancy, so more recently PET has been defined by a threshold diastolic pressure of 90 mmHg, with proteinuria serving to distinguish severe cases from mild ones (Nelson, 1955). Redman and Jefferies (1988) have suggested that a combination of a high maximum diastolic pressure with a large increase from the early pregnancy baseline is an even better criterion for identifying the 'at risk' group. This is not to say that all new complaints of puffy hands and face, as well as swollen ankles, malaise, vomiting, headaches or of seeing flashing lights, should not be investigated at once. The obstetric physiotherapist is a member of the caring team who must share in the careful monitoring of pregnant women. It is better to take the blood pressure and find it normal than to miss a substantial rise, although wisdom is needed not to cause unnecessary alarm.

In cases of severe pre-eclampsia the HELLP syndrome (haemolysis, elevated liver enzymes and low platelet count) may rarely occur with progressive liver function deterioration arrested only by delivery (Goldberg et al., 1989). Untreated PET may progress to eclampsia, a rare life-threatening state complicating fewer than 1 in 1000 deliveries (Redman, 1988), characterized by epileptic-like fits which, combined with high blood pressure, can result in kidney damage cerebral haemorrhage, cardiac arrest and maternal death. The fetus may also die from such problems as asphyxia or placental separation as a result of the fits. Early diagonosis is vital, and termination of pregnancy – usually by delivery – will alleviate the condition, although postpartum eclampsia occasionally occurs. Alternatively bed rest, sedatives and diuretics may contain the situation long enough to allow a pregnancy to continue to a more auspicious gestational stage.

Antepartum haemorrhage

Antepartum haemorrhage (APH) is another serious complication, defined as bleeding from the placental site at any stage from 28 weeks' gestation to the birth. Bleeding can occur and be contained within the site (concealed), but more often it escapes *per vaginam*. Where the placenta has embedded low on the uterine wall, close to or even across the isthmus and cervix (placenta praevia) it is easy to understand how increasingly intense contractions of the uterine muscle might tear fringe vessels. However, the reason why in other cases the placenta totally or partially detaches (placental abruption, see p. 72) is not well understood.

Placenta praevia

Normally the placenta implants and develops high up on the uterine wall. However, occasionally implantation occurs lower down, close to or over the cervix. There are four degrees:

Type I. The major part of the placenta is in the upper uterine segment, and vaginal delivery is possible.

Type II. Part of the placenta is in the lower uterine segment near the internal os; vaginal delivery is possible, particularly if the placenta is anterior.

Type III. The placenta is over the internal os but to one side; vaginal delivery should not be allowed.

Type IV. The placenta is sited centrally over the internal os; vaginal delivery should not be allowed.

Placenta praevia should be diagnosed ultrasonically in pregnancy. Types I and II may improve during pregnancy, the placenta being moved upwards to a safer level as the lower uterine segment develops.

Intrauterine growth retardation

Fetal growth retardation is the result of impaired placental function. This condition is poorly understood, but can be due to pre-eclamptic toxaemia, hypertension, small placental separations, infarctions, failure of the placenta to develop or premature reduction in its function. Fetal growth may be accurately assessed by serial ultrasound measurement of the biparietal diameter of the fetal skull and abdominal width. Maternal abdominal girth and maternal weight gain are some guide.

Intrauterine death

Even apparently light-hearted comments by pregnant women that fetal movements have substantially reduced or appear to have ceased should be taken seriously, for a fetus can become sick and even die *in utero*. An obstetric physiotherapist should arrange immediate referral to a midwife or doctor, and steps should be taken to monitor the fetal heart. Placental insufficiency and eclampsia can cause fetal death, but often the cause is obscure.

Diabetes mellitus

Patients with diabetes mellitus need careful supervision, as even a well-controlled diabetic may become unstable in pregnancy. In addition the risk of perinatal death remains relatively high for the offspring of diabetic mothers; the incidence of pre-eclampsia, of fetal abnormalities and of intrauterine death are higher. Babies of diabetic mothers tend to be large (macrosomic), weighing more than 3.5 kg, possibly because the high maternal sugar level stimulates fetal insulin production and this in turn favours growth and fat deposition in the fetus. However, some of the babies are very small due to placental dysfunction. Diabetic mothers are often admitted to hospital early (30 weeks) for careful surveillance, and then for early induction for those who are most stable, or for elective caesarean section at 37–38 weeks for those who are not.

Multiple pregnancies

There is increased strain upon the mother with multiple pregnancies, and as might be expected an increased likelihood of the occurrence of the other complications of pregnancy. In addition, possibly due to the proportionately larger content of the uterus at each stage in gestation, there is a predisposition to premature labour.

Less common complications

Polyhydramnios

Polyhydramnios is the presence of an abnormally large quantity of amniotic fluid so that the uterus is tense and distended to a degree inconsistent with the gestation dates, and it may be impossible to palpate the fetus. It may be an indication of fetal abnormality e.g. oesophageal atresia, open neural tube defect, it may be associated with multiple pregnancy and diabetes mellitus.

Oligohydramnios

Oligohydramnios is a rare condition where the liquor amnii is much reduced and milky. It appears to be associated with abnormalities in the urinary tract, such as renal agenesis (Potter's syndrome). It is said to cause fetal abnormalities (e.g. talipes, torticollis) due to the lack of space for movement. The baby's skin is very dry and leathery.

Fibroids

Fibroids of the uterus (see p. 296) are more common in older and in Afro-Caribbean women. Acute abdominal pain may be caused by degenerative changes resulting from altered blood supply or from pressure and tension as the uterus hypertrophies and stretches.

Unstable lie, transverse lie

Towards term, if the longitudinal axis of the fetus is repeatedly changing within the uterus, it is said to be unstable. This occurs almost exclusively in grand multiparae i.e. those with four or more viable past pregnancies, but is also associated with polyhydramnios, fibroids, fetal abnormality and lax abdominal muscles. Occasionally the fetus comes to rest more permanently transversely across the pelvic inlet (transverse lie). In these cases, elective caesarean section is frequently considered as being safest for the fetus.

Associated pathology

Although it is ideal for a mother to be thoroughly healthy prior to and during pregnancy, women with diabetes mellitus, asthma, cystic fibrosis, hemiplegia, rheumatoid arthritis, systemic lupus erythematosus, multiple sclerosis, uterine fibroids or tumours of various sites, and following heart or kidney transplants, have been successfully delivered of healthy children. Society is becoming increasingly prepared to provide the additional support necessary to enable those with disabling conditions to achieve and enjoy parenthood. Patients with rheumatoid arthritis and multiple sclerosis tend to go into remission during pregnancy, but may well suffer exacerbations after delivery.

Subjective evidence suggests that being pregnant does not protect women from contracting most of the diseases suffered by their peer group.

References

Bigazzi M., Nardi E., Bruni P. et al. (1980) Relaxin in human decidua, J. Clin. Endocrino. Metab., **51(4)**, 939–41.

Booth D., Chennelle M., Jones D. et al. (1980). Assessment of abdominal muscle exercises in non-pregnant, pregnant and post partum subjects using electromyography. *A. J. of Phys.* **26(5)**, 177.

Bryant Greenwood G.D., Greenwood F.C. (1982). *Relaxin as a new hormone Endocr. Rev.*, **3(1)**, 62–90.

Bullock J., Jull G., Bullock M. (1987). The relationship of low back pain to postural changes during pregnancy. *Austr. J. Physiother.*, **33**, 10–17.

Calguneri M., Bird H.A., Wright V. (1982). Changes in joint laxity occurring during pregnancy. *Ann. Rheum. Dis.*, **41**, 126–128.

Durnin J.V. (1989). Energy requirements of pregnancy. *Lancet*, **ii**, 895–900.

Francis W. (1960a). Disturbances of bladder function in relation to pregnancy. *J. Obst. Gynaecol. Br. Empire*, **67**, 353–366.

Francis W. (1960b). The onset of stress incontinence. *J. Obst. Gynaecol. Br. Empire*, **67**, 899–903.

Fransden V.A. (1963). *The Excretion of Oestriol in Normal Human Pregnancy*. Copenhagen: Munksgaard.

Goldberg I., Hod M., Katz I. et al., (1989). Severe preeclampsia and transient HELLP syndrome. *J. Obstet. Gynaecol.* **9**, 299–300.

Gross S., Librach C., Cecutti A. (1989). Maternal weight loss associated with hyperemesis gravidarum: a predictor of fetal outcome. *Am. J. Obstet. Gynecol.* **160**, 906–909.

Hytten F.E., Leitch I. (1971). *The Physiology of Human Pregnancy*. Oxford: Blackwell.

Hytten F.E., Chamberlain G., eds. (1980). *Clinical Physiology in Obstetrics*. Oxford: Blackwell.

MacLennan A.H. (1981). Relaxin – a review. *Aust. NZ J. Obst. Gynaecol.* **21**, 195–202.

McMurray R.G., Katz V.L., Berry M.J., Cefalo R.C.V. (1988). Cardiovascular responses of pregnant women during aerobic exercises in water; a longitudinal study. *Int. J. Sports Med.* **9**, 443–447.

Nelson T.R. (1955). A clinical study of preeclampsia. *J. Obst. Gynaecol. Br. Empire*, **62**, 48–57.

O'Byrne E., Carriere B., Sorensen L. et al. (1978). Plasma immunoreactive relaxin levels in pregnant and non-pregnant women. *J. Clin. Endocrinol. Metab.*, **47**, 1106.

Redman C.W.G. (1988). Eclampsia still kills. *Br. Med. J.*, **296**, 1209–1210.

Redman C.W.G., Jefferies M. (1988). Revised definition of pre-eclampsia. *Lancet*, **i**, 809–812.

Snooks S.J., Swash M., Setchell M. et al. (1984). Injury to innervation of the pelvic floor sphincter musculature in childbirth. *Lancet*, **ii**, 546–550.

Van Raaij J.M.A., Vermaat-Miedema S.H., Schouk C.M., et al. (1987). Energy requirements of pregnancy in the Netherlands. *Lancet*, **ii**, 953–955.

Weiss G. (1984). Relaxin. *Ann. Rev. Physiol.*, **46**, 42.

Yki-Jarvinen H., Wahlstrom T., Seppala M. (1983). Immunohistochemical demonstration of relaxin in the genital tract of pregnant and non pregnant women. *J. Clin. Endocrinol*, **57(3)**, 451–4.

Zarrow M.X., McClintock J.A. (1966). Localisation of 131-I-labelled antibody to relaxin. *J. Endocr.*, **36**, 377–387.

Further reading

Artal R., Wiswell R., Drinkwater B.C. (1991). *Exercise in Pregnancy*. 2nd edn. Baltimore: Williams & Wilkins.

Garry M., Govan A., Hodge C., Callander R. (1980). *Obstetrics Illustrated*. Edinburgh: Churchill Livingstone.

Wilder E., ed. (1988). *Obstetric and Gynaecologic Physical Therapy*, Clinics in Physical Therapy **20**. Edinburgh: Churchill Livingstone.

Useful addresses
Pre-Eclamptic Toxaemia Society
33 Keswick Avenue
Hullbridge, Essex SS5 6JL.

CHAPTER 3

Physical and Physiological Changes of Labour and the Puerperium

Normally, after about 40 weeks of gestation, the fetus is expelled from the uterus. The physiological processes by which this is achieved are collectively called labour, although they are a continuum with pregnancy. For the purpose of description only, labour has been divided into three stages.

THE STAGES OF LABOUR

First stage

Regular uterine muscle contractions establish and become progressively longer, stronger and closer together. For most women these contractions are painful and many require some form of analgesia. Commonly (95%) the fetus presents head down to the cervix within the uterus, and the uterine contractions exert an intermittent upward pull on the lower segment of the uterus and cervix, while at the same time applying downward pressure on the fetus. This combination opens the cervix, pushing the fetus against it and through it (Fig. 3.1). It has been compared to pulling a polo-neck sweater over the head. In addition the uterine cavity becomes progressively smaller. The first stage is said to be complete when the cervix has reached a dilatation – about 10 cm diameter – that allows the fetal head through, so that it is able to proceed down the vagina; it is almost always the longest stage.

Second stage

There is often a noticeable change in the tempo of contractions; they may become more widely spaced and even a little shorter, while still remaining intense. This continued action of the uterine muscle further

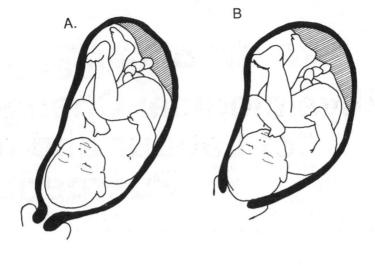

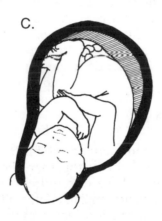

Figure 3.1 Dilatation of the cervix.

reduces the size of the uterus and expels the fetus from it into the vagina. This process is accompanied in most women by a compelling urge to bear down. The diaphragm and the abdominal muscles are brought into action to help push the fetus out. The pelvic floor distends under the pressure, the puborectalis and pubococcygeus muscles are parted and pushed aside and outward, the soft tissues of the perineum extend to form a canal which gutters forwards from the coccyx. This canal protrudes and is directed anteriorly. It takes time for the perineum to stretch sufficiently to allow the fetus through, and delivery of the fetus may be accelerated by performing an episiotomy. The second stage is normally much shorter than the first stage and ends with the birth of the baby.

Third stage

The third stage is the passing of the placenta once it has detached from the uterine wall. It is usually the shortest phase.

Signs that the start of labour may be imminent

1.   A 'show'. This is the release vaginally of the small quantity of thick, slimy mucus which accumulated in the cervix and acted as a barrier during the pregnancy to upward-moving infection. Ripening of the cervix and increased uterine muscle activity results in it being released sooner or later; the mucus may be blood-streaked. Except where there is any measurable loss of fresh blood, women are advised to note the event but take no other special action.

2.   'Ruptured membranes' or the 'breaking of the waters'. This is a rupture of the amniotic sac resulting in a sudden or gradual loss of amniotic fluid. It may be difficult for a woman to discriminate between gradual, slight amniotic fluid loss, and loss of urine due to stress or urge incontinence. Where the fetus presents head first in labour, and the head is beginning to fit snugly into the lower segment and cervix, a small bulging portion of the sac filled with fluid may be in front of the head (the forewaters), and it is essentially cut off from the remainder (the hindwaters). Thus when it is suspected that the membranes have ruptured, the amount lost may be some guide to the position of the fetal head. Where the head is high and not well applied to the cervix a larger amount would be expected to be lost than when the head is firmly applied. A gradual dripping would suggest a small puncture in either the fore or hindwaters. Women are advised to report suspected loss of amniotic fluid, particularly if it is considerable, because it is possible for the umbilical cord to prolapse downwards through the ruptured sac and already dilating cervix, ahead of the presenting part where this is not well engaged. If this is the case then subsequent uterine contractions will plunge the fetus downwards and might compress the cord. Should this happen the resulting vascular occlusion could compromise the fetus and lead to distress or death. It should be remembered that amniotic fluid production will continue until delivery so that, even when large amounts are lost, further dripping will occur.

3. Contractions. Uterine muscle contraction of the fundus and body become increasingly apparent and settle into a regular, continuing and increasingly intense and painful pattern. Once this is occurring, labour is said to be established.

These three signs are commonly presented in the literature and in parentcraft classes as heralds of labour. There is, however, wide individual variation, for example a 'show' and 'ruptured membranes' may occur well in advance of or during labour, and intermittent sequences of strong, painful contractions can be experienced without labour becoming established (Braxton Hicks contractions). Therefore the only really reliable signs that labour is established are regular, painful and continuing contractions, and a progressively dilating cervix.

THE PROCESS OF NORMAL LABOUR

It must be remembered that labour is only part of an ongoing physiological process starting at conception and completed some weeks after the baby is born. What actually initiates the onset of labour is not fully understood, but it is almost certainly triggered by a combination of factors; the following have been suggested.

1. A rise in the oxytocin level. The physical size and pressure of the growing fetus on the ripening cervix may stimulate a neurogenic reflex which causes the posterior pituitary to release more oxytocin. In addition, or alternatively, the maturing fetus may produce increasing amounts of oxytocin which cross the placenta. Oxytocin is known to cause the uterine muscle to contract.

2. Prostaglandin production. The uterine wall has the potential, like many other tissues, to produce prostaglandins. These are fatty acids which in 1930 were first found in semen and shown to cause smooth muscle to contract. They have a short life because they are rapidly metabolized, and therefore have local effects. It is known that oestrogens could trigger the release of myometrial prostaglandins. It is also known that the disruption of decidual cells, such as occurs when the amniotic sac is artificially ruptured, would cause prostaglandin release. It has been suggested that stretching of the uterine wall by the growing, kicking fetus has a similar effect. The prostaglandins in semen may be the explanation for the circumstantial evidence that intercourse appears to stimulate the start of labour in some cases.

3. Fetal adrenal hormones. Studies in animals (Currie et al., 1973, Liggins, 1974) have shown a rapid increase in the production of fetal cortisols a few days before the onset of labour. These high concentrations act at the placenta to reduce the secretion of progesterone and increase the secretion of oestrogens. A marked rise in oestradiol is associated with a prostaglandin being produced in the placenta. It is suggested by some (Shearman, 1986) that a similar set of changes must be operative to enable the human fetus to control the onset of labour.

Late in pregnancy and continuing in early labour, the lower part of the uterus – the isthmus – responds to the contraction of the muscle of the fundus and body by stretching and thinning to form the lower uterine segment. It is thought that uterine contractions are normally initiated around the openings to the fallopian tubes, spread to the fundus and then down the body of the uterus. Ideally there is a gradient pattern in these contractions, with the fundus dominant and the lower uterine segment less active; this is called normal uterine polarity.

The early signs, symptoms and circumstances are highly individual to each labour but contractions usually settle into a regular pattern. Often, initially, these are short in length (about 30 seconds) and some distance apart (15–20 minutes), but progressively become longer, stronger and closer together until they are about 1–1.5 minutes in length and occur every 2–5 minutes. Occasionally women only notice the longer, stronger contractions.

Further tension on the lower uterine segment causes the cervix to be 'taken up' or effaced, so eventually there is no cervical canal as such, because it becomes part of the containing uterine wall. It is then gradually opened or dilated. Thus ultimately it is effacement and dilatation that releases the plug of mucus or 'show' if it has not occurred earlier. As labour progresses there is an increase in oxytocin release by the posterior pituitary which causes contractions to become stronger, and this output is enhanced and continued by a positive feedback from the dilating cervix and the distending vagina to the hypothalamus and so to the posterior pituitary.

The uterine muscle of the fundus and body acquire in labour the unique ability to retract systematically, by alternately contracting firmly, then relaxing, but to a shorter and thicker length each time. Thus the uterine cavity becomes progressively smaller, the uterine muscular wall increases in thickness from about 6 mm to 25 mm, and the fetus and other uterine contents are expelled.

During contractions the shape of the abdomen may be seen to alter, particularly as they become longer and stronger. The fundus moves forwards so that the long axis of the uterus and the thrust of the muscle are brought into the appropriate line and meet the cervix and the vagina at the best angle (drive angle) to propel the fetus into the vagina. This forward tilt (anteversion) occurs more easily if the woman is upright or lying on her side, for gravity opposes it in the supine position (Figs. 3.2, 6.1). It is of interest that women instinctively tend to lean forward.

The first stage of labour can be subdivided into two phases. *The latent phase* is calculated from the onset of labour to 3 cm of cervical dilatation, and commonly lasts 4–6 hours in the primigravida, although it can be much longer. *The active phase* extends from 3 cm to full dilatation of the cervix; in this phase the contractions are stronger, more frequent and more painful, and the cervix opens more rapidly – about 1 cm per hour in the primigravida and 1.5 cm per hour in multigravidae. Cervical dilatation is measured by palpation and estimation of the diameter of the opening in centimetres, it can be digitally assessed vaginally or rectally, although this latter technique is not used often today. This procedure is kept to a minimum – usually not more

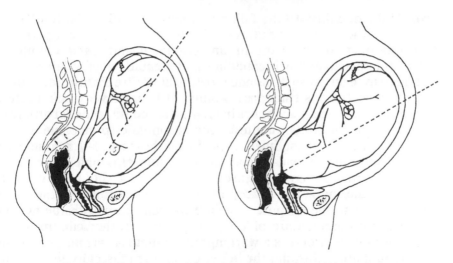

Figure 3.2 To show the forward movement of the drive angle.

frequently than two-hourly – because of the risk of introducing infection and because it is a particularly uncomfortable investigation in labour. The descent can be measured by how much of the fetal head – in fifths – is still palpable above the pelvic brim or is below the ischial spines as palpated vaginally.

The second stage also has two phases: *the phase of descent* in which the fetal head descends on to the perineum, and *the perineal phase* in which the perineum stretches, adaptively remodels to form an extended passage, and allows the head through. It is now appreciated that a prolonged second stage can be dangerous for child and mother, causing fetal distress or maternal pelvic floor neuropathy, so most labour suites have their own criteria for deciding when assistance such as intravenous infusion of oxytocic drugs, episiotomy, vacuum extraction or forceps should be considered to accelerate delivery.

Following delivery, the uterus continues to contract, constricting the placental vascular sinuses and causing the placenta to sheer away from the wall and separate. The contraction and retraction of uterine muscle has the effect of ligating the maternal blood vessels within the placental attachment site and controlling the considerable risk of serious haemorrhage when the placenta eventually detaches. Further contractions and, in most units, an intramuscular injection of ergometrine and oxytocin given after delivery of the head with continuous cord traction, normally result in the delivery of the placenta. It is known that nipple stimulation, e.g. when an infant suckles, causes the posterior pituitary to produce oxytocin. Some midwives utilize this fact by encouraging the newly delivered infant to begin suckling in the third stage of labour to enhance uterine contractions and speed the separation and delivery of the placenta. Some even manually stimulate nipples in the first and second stage where contractions seem to be failing.

THE PAIN OF LABOUR

Pain has been defined as 'an unpleasant sensory and emotional experience associated with actual or potential tissue damage, or described in terms of such damage' (Mersky, 1979). Parturition pain is an experience that is shared by women at every level of civilization (Melzack et al., 1981), and it has been mentioned since the recording of history began. Although cultural, socioeconomic, psychological and emotional aspects must have a place in the intensity of the pain experienced and women's reactions to it, and although current evidence and research have increased understanding about the physical causes and the individual perception of labour discomfort, questions still remain as to the purpose of childbirth pain. Labour is the normal physiological continuation of pregnancy, but in other circumstances pain is usually regarded as a warning that something is malfunctioning or is being damaged within the body. Could the reason for what many women perceive and record as the most intense pain they will ever experience, be simply an alarm system for the protection of the incredibly helpless new young human being?

The body does have its own way of dulling pain; it has been shown that there is a rise of plasma endorphins through pregnancy (Newnham et al., 1983), possibly in preparation for labour. There is a further rise in labour in response to stress; where epidural analgesia is given there is a significant drop in plasma endorphin levels (Abboud et al., 1983, 1984). Women's reactions to labour pain are influenced by their personalities, their previous experiences and also by how they *feel* at the time; women who feel safe and secure as they labour, and who understand what is happening, will almost certainly record lower pain scores than they would if they were fearful and apprehensive. For very many new mothers the first sight of their baby blots out all memories of pain; unfortunately there will also be those who will say, even many years later, that they have never got over it.

Causes of labour pain

The main cause of pain during the first stage of labour is thought to be directly associated with dilatation of the cervix and distension of the lower uterine segment around the descending presenting fetal parts (Fig. 3.1). The sensory nerve supply from these two areas of the uterus is greater than that from the fundus or uterine body (see p. 15). Other suggested causes of first-stage labour pain include ischaemia of the myometrium and cervix, pressure on sensory nerve endings in the uterine body and fundus, inflammatory changes in the uterine muscles, and reflex contraction of the cervix and lower uterine segment due to the 'fear–tension–pain' cycle (Wall and Melzack, 1984); however, these have not been substantiated by research. Brown et al., (1989) compared the pain experienced at two stages of dilatation in the first stage of labour: 2–5 cm and 6–10 cm. As cervical dilatation increased, there were significant increases in self-reported and observed pain. Using words from the McGill pain questionnaire, pain was characterized as 'discomforting' during early dilatation and as 'distressing, horrible, excruciating' as labour progressed.

In common with pain from other viscera, first-stage pain is referred to the dermatomes supplied by the same spinal cord segments (T10–L1) which receive input from the uterus and cervix (Fig. 3.3). As labour progresses and the intensity and frequency of the contractions increase, the pain zones enlarge and become more diffuse (Fig. 3.4). At the end of the first stage of labour some women experience aching, burning and cramping discomfort in the thighs. This is due to stretching of, and pressure on, pain-sensitive structures (uterine and pelvic ligaments and fascia, bladder, urethra and rectum) and pressure on lumbar and sacral nerve roots. Once the cervix is fully dilated the nature and distribution of pain changes. In the second stage and during delivery it will be felt

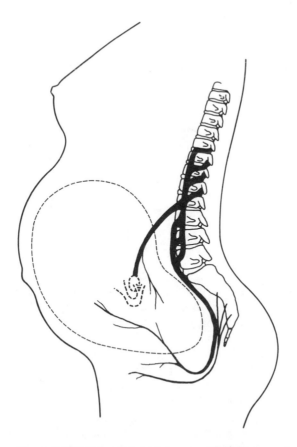

Figure 3.3 The nervous pathways carrying labour pain.

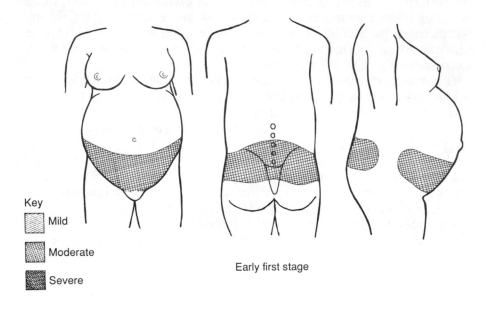

Key

Mild

Moderate

Severe

Early first stage

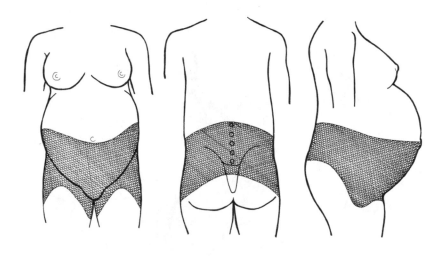

Late – first stage

Figure 3.4 To show the changing pain zones of labour.

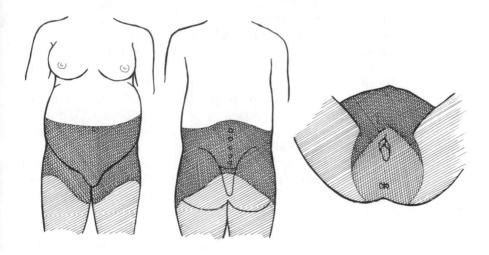

Early second stage

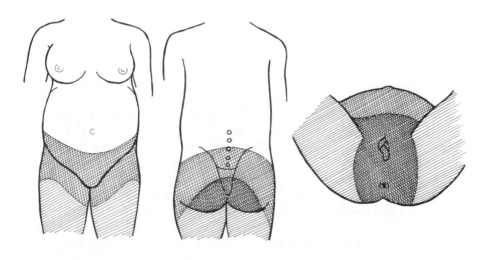

Delivery

Figure 3.4 (continued)

chiefly in the soft tissues of the perineal region (S2–S4) as they stretch, distend and even tear; in addition, pain may be experienced as the pelvic outlet is pushed open by the fetus, affecting the symphysis pubis, sacroiliac and sacrococcygeal joints. An effort has been made to describe the areas of pain distribution as labour progresses (Bonica, 1984), but a tremendous variability should be expected. Some women will experience widespread discomfort, and others will have discrete painful areas.

The intensity of labour pain must never be underestimated by the obstetric team. Using the McGill pain questionnaire, some scores as low as 10 (very mild pain) were recorded by Melzack (Table 3.1), but at the top end of the scale scores as high as 62 (extremely severe pain) were registered (Melzack, 1984). Primiparae tend to experience higher levels of pain than multiparous women, and although those women who have received childbirth training record lower levels of pain than the untrained (Melzack et al., 1981), it is still greater during a first labour than subsequently.

Table 3.1 Pain scores in labour using the McGill questionnaire (possible maximum 80)

Pain scores	Very mild to mild 2–11 and 12–21	Moderate 22–31	Severe 32–41	Extremely severe 42–62
Primiparae (%)	9.2	29.5	37.9	23.4
Multiparae (%)	24.1	29.6	35.2	11.1

Individuals vary greatly in the way they perceive, interpret and respond to pain (Noble, 1983), and a vast range of factors, both physical and emotional, will play their part in the severity of pain felt during labour. Recent research by Wuitchik et al. (1989) investigated the intensity of pain experienced and the women's thoughts – as to whether they were distress-related or not – in three phases of labour. A positive correlation was found between the two parameters – pain and distress-related thoughts – in the latent phase of the first stage of labour, and the subsequent duration of labour. They were also prognostic of obstetric outcome. The inference is drawn that the latent phase is critical and it is suggested that pain and distress-related thoughts could actually contribute to labour inefficiency and poor outcome, e.g. the fetus needing paediatric assistance. If this is so, the implications for childbirth educators and the labour team are important. Childbirth educators have an undoubted responsibility to prepare women realistically and positively for the possibilities that may confront them at the time of birth. Whichever 'coping strategies' are taught, women and their partners must realize that their 'ideal' birth, and the way they wish to handle it, may be unattainable – particularly if it is a first labour or the mother falls into a 'high risk' category. Some women with no preparation find labour entirely manageable; others who attend antenatal classes and acquire pain-relieving skills (relaxation, breathing awareness, massage, movement, positioning, etc.) may find these offer sufficient relief. However, because labour is often still painful even after antenatal training, very many women will need the extra assistance of analgesia and anaesthesia (Melzack et al., 1981; Charles et al., 1978). It may be important for this to be commenced early to avoid distress-related thoughts. It is imperative that the obstetric physiotherapist does not make women, who use *any* of the currently available pain-relieving drugs feel failures because they have not been able to cope with labour without additional help.

NORMAL LABOUR AND DELIVERY

The mechanics of labour

In 38% of cases labour starts with the fetal head in the left occipito-lateral position (LOL), i.e. the fetus is facing the right maternal ilium; a further 24% are in the right occipito-lateral position (ROL). In either case the long axis of the fetal head is on the long axis of the maternal pelvic inlet (see p. 1). Initially the upper part of the head is the presenting portion; however, as labour progresses the head flexes and descends so that the upper and more posterior part of the head (the vertex) leads.

As the descent into the pelvis continues the fetal head rotates through 90° until the face is towards the sacrum and coccyx, and the occiput is below the symphysis pubis. All the diameters in mid-cavity are similar (see p. 3) and this allows a corkscrew action with the body following, ending with the long axis of the fetal head in the long axis of the maternal pelvic outlet. In addition the fetus has to negotiate a 'corner' in its route because the pelvic inlet is at right angles to the outlet.

Further descent produces extension of the fetal neck beneath the symphysis pubis. At delivery the baby's head faces posteriorly, the shoulders are still oblique but turning. As the shoulders descend, their greatest width comes to lie anteroposteriorly in the long axis of the outlet, and the baby's head, which is by now delivered, turns to face the mother's right leg (restitution). The top shoulder slips under the symphysis pubis first, usually quickly followed by the other shoulder and by the rest of the body.

The effect of labour on maternal and fetal physiology

Both the mother and the fetus will experience modest stress even during a perfectly normal and straightforward labour, and levels of adrenaline and noradrenaline (catecholamines) are raised, producing the familiar 'fight or flight' response. In both mother and fetus this will result in the shunting of blood to vital organs such as the heart and lungs, so making more oxygen available, and in the mobilization of energy stores. It must be appreciated, however, that excessive stress is detrimental to both mother and fetus. For example it may result in shunting of blood from the contracting uterus and placenta, leading to slowing of contractions and fetal distress.

The fetus

There is still a great deal that is not fully understood, but it is known that the particular stress of the second stage and delivery on the fetus results in a surge of catecholamines, predominantly noradrenaline, which facilitates normal breathing, and helps the baby maintain body heat and survive adversity – particularly low oxygen conditions – in the first few hours of independent life. Compression of the fetal thorax in both first and second stages squeezes out fluid that normally fills the lungs, but absorption of the remaining lung liquid and the release of sufficient surfactant appears to be dependent on an increase in plasma catecholamines immediately after birth.

The mother

Cardiovascular system. In response to contraction of the large uterine musculature there is a small progressive rise in heart rate which is accelerated by anxiety, pain and dehydration, and cardiac output is increased. Blood pressure may also rise modestly in the first stage but more specifically in the second stage, when it tends to swing up with expulsive pushing and then fall between contractions. The latter is aggravated by prolonged breath-holding with bearing down (the Valsalva manoeuvre), raising the intra-thoracic and intra-abdominal pressure which compresses veins and impedes the return of blood to the heart. The result is a fall in cardiac output and thus in blood pressure.

Respiratory system. The mild hyperventilation of pregnancy becomes more noticeable in labour, when during strong first-stage contractions of uterine muscle both respiratory rate and depth increase in response to the increased oxygen requirement. Some decrease in arterial P_{CO_2} tension appears to be normal, but in severe cases of overbreathing the woman experiences numbness and tingling of the lips and extremities due to the blood becoming relatively alkalotic, leading to calcium ionization which affects nerve conductivity. Maternal alkalosis results in oxygen being more tightly bound to the haemoglobin, and consequently it is given up less easily. Occasionally this will mean that, at the placenta, the fetal circulation may not obtain as much oxygen as it would normally, and this can be compounded by the fact that acute maternal hyperventilation may cause uterine vasoconstriction and reduce placental blood flow. Insufficient oxygen to the fetus may force it to metabolize anaerobically, and this can result in fetal acidosis and distress (see p. 169).

Gastrointestinal system. There is a reduction in peristalsis and absorption, and towards the end of the first stage nausea and vomiting may occur. Eating in labour is therefore discouraged, and drugs taken by mouth will be poorly absorbed.

Temperature. The strong muscle activity results in heat production; there may be a slight rise in temperature, and women feel hot and perspire. However, redistribution of blood often results in the feet being very cold.

The effect of labour on the pelvic floor and perineum

As the fetal head descends it follows the curve of the sacrum and coccyx to reach the pelvic floor. It exerts pressure which dilates the vagina, stretches the perineum, and separates and displaces the levator ani muscles sideways and downwards. The bowel is compressed, and the urethra is stretched as the bladder is pulled up above the symphysis pubis by virtue of its attachment to the cervix and uterus. This makes more space in the pelvis. The stretching, lengthening and consequent thinning of the posterior portion of the pelvic floor and perineum, ahead of the fetus, forms the birth canal, and enables the vaginal opening to be turned and directed more anteriorly. Physiotherapists should note that it is this stretching, bowing and thinning of the pelvic floor, particularly when aggravated by the need for assistance (e.g. forceps) which is thought to be a cause of damage to the innervation of the pelvic floor musculature, shown to be associated with faecal and urinary incontinence post partum (Snooks et al., 1984; Sørensen et al., 1988). It can also cause vascular damage resulting in haematoma, or more general bruising and oedema. Fascia may be overstretched and muscle fibres torn.

The stretching and thinning takes time in the second stage of labour and may result in a tearing of the vaginal opening. It is often a fine judgment, firstly whether fetal and maternal welfare is best served by waiting for the natural stretching to occur or by accelerating the delivery process with an episiotomy, and secondly, whether an episiotomy is needed to avoid an uncontrollable tear, perhaps involving the anal sphincter (see p. 73).

The duration of labour

Each labour is individual, even in the same woman, and there are wide variations in duration, particularly between primigravidae and multigravidae. Statistics seem to indicate that modern obstetric practices – particularly induction, acceleration, sedation, ambulation and the greater use of caesarean section – have resulted in labours on average being shorter now than formerly. In many centres it is general policy to try to ensure that 24 hours is the outside limit for a labour, it being considered more than enough for all parties involved. Nesheim (1988), in a sample of 9703 labours in Norway, found a median duration of 8.2 hours for nulliparae and 5.3 hours for multiparae, whereas Myles (1975) quoted 12 hours (first stage 11 hours, second stage 0.75 hour) and 7 hours (first stage 6.5 hours, second stage 0.25 hour) respectively. Nesheim (1988) showed that induced labours were shorter than those with spontaneous onset – 1.9 hours shorter in nulliparae and 1.4 hours in multiparae – and that tall women had quicker labours than short women. Maternal age did not seem to influence duration, but the weight of the baby, maternal weight gain in pregnancy and the pre-pregnancy weight all correlated positively with longer labours; the implications in health education are clear, that women should be encouraged to achieve an optimum weight for their height pre-conceptually and then control their weight gain during pregnancy. Interestingly, Nesheim (1988) found that while in nulliparae the occipito-posterior positions and failure of the head to flex prolonged labour, breech presentations did not. For multiparae none of these presentations prolonged labour.

Positioning in labour

Considerable research effort has been expended on determining whether there is advantage, as logic would suggest, in the upright positions in labour, e.g. sitting, standing or forward-lean kneeling. Mitre (1974), Mendez Bauer et al. (1975), Flynn et al. (1978) and Caldeyro-Barcia (1979) seem to show a shorter first stage correlating with being upright and ambulant, but McManus and Calder (1978) and Williams et al., (1980) could find no statistical difference whether a labouring woman remained recumbent or was actively encouraged to be upright and move around. It is agreed, however, that the labouring woman's contractions are stronger in the upright position (Flynn et al., 1978; Read, 1981). Positional change also has a positive effect on the efficiency of uterine contractions (Roberts et al., 1983). One hundred years ago, Clark (1891) reported that 'The effectiveness of uterine pains has been increased by change in posture, especially after a patient has maintained for a long time a constrained position.' The other, very important, aspect of this issue is how the women judge being upright and mobile in the first stage of labour. Most of the researchers cited above reported greater maternal satisfaction and comfort where women were free to move and rest as they wished, and Flynn et al. (1978) found the need for analgesia to be significantly reduced for those who were ambulant. Any suggestion that ambulation might compromise the fetus appears to be unfounded for the majority of women with appropriate fetal monitoring, and where proper exclusion criteria are applied, e.g. women at risk for cord prolapse. In addition, from Wuitchik's work (Wuitchik et al., 1989), there is now the inference that good pain control and alleviation of thoughts of distress and fear in the latent phase of first stage may be critical in encouraging an effective shorter labour. Sosa et al. (1980) found that labouring women who were empathetically cared for by a lay female supporter (a *doula*) also had shorter labours.

For the second stage, sitting, standing, kneeling and squatting have advantages over the supine and side-lying positions by resulting in stronger, more efficient contractions (Caldeyro-Barcia, 1979) and more effective use of gravity. In squatting particularly there is also an increase in the size of the pelvic outlet (Russell, 1982) which may be important. Supported squatting (see Fig. 6.4) is helpful for women who find the full squat impossible, uncomfortable or tiring (Pöschl, 1987). Human support with skin contact is often preferred, but special birthing chairs, cushions (Gardosi et al., 1989), stools and beds have been devised. Squatting can hasten the onset of the urge to bear down; while the 'all fours' position, by taking pressure off the cervix, can be used to control this urge (especially if the knee–chest position is adopted, see p. 187), and also eases backache and assists with the anterior rotation of a posterior position (Scruggs, 1982; Grant, 1987).

The third stage usually lasts not more than 30 minutes. The mother is normally so involved with the baby that, if all goes well, she is unaware of the process. The woman intuitively adopts a resting posture with the baby; many midwives prefer the dorsal position for the third stage because the uterus is more easily observed and cord traction, if needed, can be applied more effectively. It is said that there is also less danger in this position of air reaching the blood sinuses in the placental site which could cause an air embolism.

MANAGEMENT OF NORMAL LABOUR

Most maternity units now have written protocols regarding the management of the labouring woman, with set criteria for intervention. These predetermined consensus guidelines have the advantage of overcoming, to some extent, the problems posed by several consultants serving one unit, each with their own management preferences. Such protocols can be of benefit also to midwives where the shift system and staff changes can make continuity of care and communication difficult.

However, it is clear that management of the labouring woman does vary from place to place as evidenced by the variation from one UK health region to another of the caesarean section rate. Extremes of philosophy can be found, by which one unit will routinely monitor women for a short period on admission but only intervene where it is suspected that maternal or fetal well-being are threatened, while another unit will apply a very active management from the start, monitoring continuously and intervening immediately if progress deviates even minutely from a set norm. It has been shown that it is possible for one intervention to lead to the need for another and so on, creating a 'cascade of intervention' (Inch, 1982). Possible sequences are shown in Fig. 3.5.

The start of labour

When a woman decides that labour may be starting she will alert her carers, who will either go to her at home if she has planned a home delivery, or await her at a maternity unit. In either case the midwife will be concerned to establish immediately that both fetus and mother are well, and so will check the fetal heart rate and the maternal temperature, pulse and blood pressure. The midwife will then palpate the lie of the fetus and the presenting part, and palpate and monitor the quality and frequency of any contractions. A vaginal examination determines the state of the cervix and confirms the level of the fetal head. From all these data, in time, it will be possible to determine whether labour is established. Urine will be tested for protein, sugar and ketones.

Recording the progress of labour

In most centres the progress of labour is now recorded on a *partogram* (Fig. 3.6), a combination of charts on which the pattern of uterine contractions, the descent of the presenting part, cervical dilatation and medication, together with measures of maternal well-being such as blood pressure and pulse rate, are graphically recorded against time, and thus are easily evaluated. There is a recognized norm, and this visualization highlights early evidence of labour failing to progress and allows consideration of appropriate action.

Fetal monitoring

Medical and midwifery staff may monitor the fetal heart rate intermittently using a Pinard stethoscope or a simple Sonic-aid. More continuous surveillance requires a fetal heart monitor; this uses an ultrasound transducer on the woman's abdomen, and produces a print-

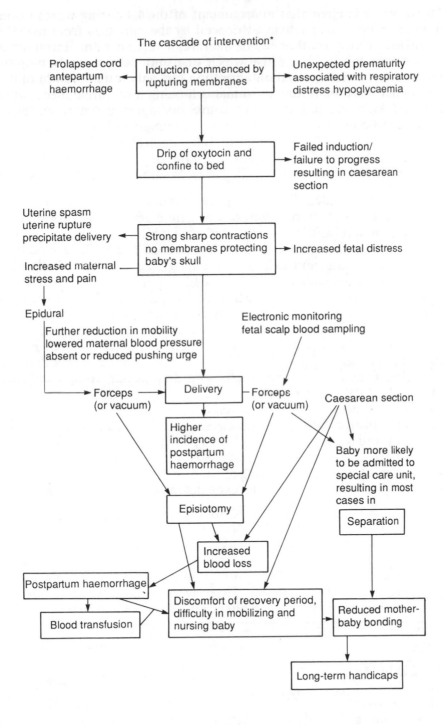

Figure 3.5 The cascade of intervention. Reproduced with permission from Sally Inch (1982), *Birthrights*. Courtesy of Green Print, Publisher, London.

out, as well as signalling the fetal heart rate via a flashing light or an audible bleep. Alternatively the fetal heart rate may be recorded through an electrode attached to the fetal scalp. The same machine, a cardiotocograph (CTG), will also give a print-out of uterine activity by means of a maternal tocograph. For this, a very delicate pressure gauge is strapped externally to the woman's abdomen or, using a modified gauge, may be passed vaginally to monitor contractions more accurately internally.

First stage of labour

Early in labour, unless there are special circumstances, women should be encouraged to continue with rest or gentle activities appropriate to the time of day and consistent with the philosophy of conserving energy. It is a disadvantage to go into labour tired. Once labour is established, eating and drinking are restricted because of the risk (should general anaesthesia be needed) of inhalation of vomit or regurgitated gastric juice. The acidic gastric juice is highly irritant and, if inhaled, causes bronchospasm, dyspnoea, cyanosis and pulmonary oedema (Mendelson's syndrome). Management in the first stage consists chiefly of regular monitoring of fetal and maternal well-being, and relief of fear and pain by – in the first instance – ensuring that the labouring woman has sympathetic and empathetic companionship. Sosa et al. (1980) reported a small study using a supportive lay woman, a *doula*; this showed major perinatal benefits for the supported group, including shorter labours. Women should be encouraged to be as physically and mentally comfortable as possible, moving or staying still as feels best, as discussed previously. So for many women the first stage is passed with periods of walking around, periods of sitting in chairs or beanbags, and periods of resting, even dozing on a sofa or bed. Pleasant

Haemorrhage			Date	Time	Duration		
(a) Before Placenta NIL .		1st Stage began	23-3 90	08 · 00 Hrs	9 Hrs.	00 mins.	
(b) After Placenta 150 mls.		2nd Stage began	23-3-90	17. 00 Hrs	0 "	42 "	
Total 150 mls.		3rd Stage began	23.3-90	17 · 42 Hrs	0 "	06 "	
				TOTAL	9 "	48 "	
Lacerations LABIAL		Repair DOES NOT NEED SUTURING AS.					
Episiotomy No							

Delivered by SR.SUTCLIFFE (S)A.   Conditions of Mother Satisfactory

Placenta Complete   Mode of Delivery C.C.T   Weight 600 gms.

Membranes complete   Cord Clamped 3 vessels.

Conditions of Child Satisfactory   Sex FEMALE Weight 3,740 gms.

If asphyxiated, treatment given Mucous extraction only

Immediate Post Partum Record with complications and treatment Syntometrine 1ml. given I.M.

B.P. 120/80   Pulse 80   Time Recorded 18.45hrs.

Figure 3.6 A partogram.

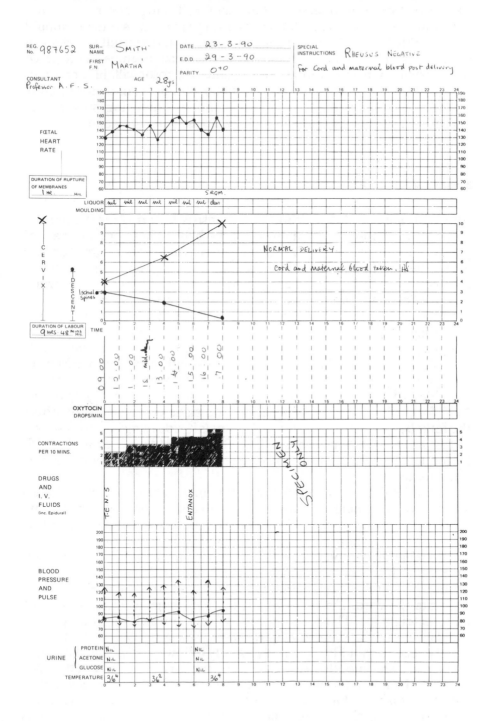

Figure 3.6 (continued)

surroundings (Chapman et al., 1986), music and a warm bath (Lenstrup et al., 1987) or shower may be invaluable. Changes of position are important (Roberts et al., 1983) in assisting progress. A woman should try to empty her bladder every two hours at least, for a full bladder can increase pain and delay progress. If a woman becomes ketotic or dehydrated then intravenous fluids and dextrose will be required. Ideally the decision regarding additional pain relief is one made jointly by the mother and the midwife. Cool flannels for sponging, sucking ice, and massage to the back and abdomen are soothing to some.

Second stage of labour

The management of the second stage consists of caring for the mother and assisting with the safe delivery of the baby. There are a variety of positions in which it is possible for a woman to deliver her baby (see Fig. 6.4). The prime considerations are the baby's safety, the mother's comfort, and which position enables her to respond best to the bearing-down reflex. Difficulties can arise if a midwife finds it impossible to monitor and control the delivery in the position selected by the labouring woman. However, where the conventional reclining posture has been chosen but the mother is not pushing effectively or the urge to bear down is weak, she should be encouraged, even temporarily, to change position, perhaps into some adaptation of squatting if this is possible and safe. It has been suggested for some time that lying on the back for prolonged periods in the second stage could adversely affect the fetus by reducing placental perfusion; left-side lying has been shown to reduce the problem. Johnstone (1987) showed that even a tilt of 15° to the left by using a firm pillow or towels under the right hip was effective in this regard.

As the fetal head descends the perineum distends, the anus dilates and the vagina opens progressively with contractions; however some regression may be seen in between contractions. The midwife controls the head at 'crowning' to allow the vaginal opening gently to complete the extreme distension needed; the mother may be asked at this point to refrain from pushing and to pant instead. The fetal head is encouraged into extension under the pubic arch and the neck explored to locate the cord. Once delivered, the baby's head turns to face the maternal right leg. The head is laterally flexed towards the anus to assist the delivery of the right shoulder, then to the symphysis pubis to ease out the second shoulder; the body usually follows easily. The baby may need nasal and mouth suction to clear the airways but is laid either between the mother's legs or on her abdomen. If active management of the third stage is adopted, an injection of ergometrine and oxytocin is given into the mother's thigh once the head is delivered, and the cord is clamped.

Table 3.2 Apgar a score for neonatal assessment

	0 points	1 point	2 points
Colour	blue, pale	pink body, blue extremities	pink
Respiratory effort	absent	gasping	sharp, cry
Heart rate	absent	less than 100 beats/ min	more than 100 beats/ min
Reflex activity	absent	grimace	cry
Muscle tone	low	some limb flexion	active movement

The accepted method of assessment and recording the baby's condition is by the Apgar score (Table 3.2, see also p. 387)), at 1, 5 and 10 minutes after delivery. A score of less than 7 requires immediate paediatric assistance.

Third stage of labour

Initially the mother usually lies back and holds her baby. Management, which may be passive or active, consists of ensuring the complete separation and safe delivery of the placenta, and monitoring and controlling haemorrhage where necessary.

Passive management allows the natural physiological changes to take their course, and excludes the use of oxytocic drugs. Strong uterine contractions enable the midwife to feel the fundus of the uterus. Initially it will usually be above the umbilicus, and feels bulky because the placenta is there. Once the placenta has separated further contractions assist it to drop into the lower uterine segment, thus enabling the uterus to contract down progressively further, until the placenta is expelled. The mother may be asked to assist with expulsive effort. The midwife may prefer the mother to adopt a standing, kneeling or squatting posture rather than lying back, to utilize gravity and intra-abdominal pressure to help the process.

Active management requires an intramuscular injection of an oxytocic drug after the head is delivered. The midwife places one hand above the symphysis, and when the uterus contracts pressure is applied on the fundus in an *upward* direction toward the umbilicus to prevent the uterus from being drawn down, while the other hand exerts steady downward traction on the cord for 1–2 minutes, then lets go. The sequence may have to be repeated. The chief objective is to avoid inverting the uterus where complete separation has not yet occurred. The mother is usually sitting back with her knees bent, to allow the uterine pressure to be applied. Once delivered, the placenta is weighed and examined for completeness, and the total amount of blood lost is estimated.

COMPLICATIONS OF LABOUR

Failure to progress

The phrase 'failure to progress' is used to indicate that labour has stopped proceeding from phase to phase as expected, and the presenting part is not descending and rotating any further as time passes. There are a variety of possible causes, for example contractions may be insufficiently strong or long, the pelvis may be too small for the size of the fetus (cephalopelvic disproportion) or the cervix may fail to dilate. The experienced midwife will quickly recognize a deviation from normal on the partogram, and most centres now have their own set criteria for appropriate active intervention.

Fetal distress

Uterine contractions are a normal stress to the fetus, compressing it and producing a temporary reduction in the oxygenated blood supply through the placental site. A healthy fetal heart will beat about 100–160 times per minute and individual fluctuations will be small ($\pm$ 10 beats per minute). At best the fetal heart rate is unaffected by the contractions, or there is only a slight deceleration coincident with the peak of contractions (type 1 dip) and the rate then picks up. In the absence of other adverse signs a drop of not more than 40 beats per minute is often acceptable, but fetal hypoxia must be suspected if:

1. the decelerations are by more than 40 beats per minute
2. the time taken for recovery to the higher rate is increasing
3. there is generalized slowing of the heart rate
4. the maximum deceleration occurs after the peak of the contraction (type 2 dip).

Fetal hypoxia is the most common cause of fetal distress and may be due to pressure on the cord, premature separation of the placenta, hypertonia of the uterine muscle or hypertonia of maternal blood vessels. The passing of fetal meconium *per vaginam* may also be a serious sign, indicating the possibility that fetal hypoxia has induced anal sphincter muscle hypotonia. Hypoxia can be confirmed by fetal scalp blood sampling and testing the blood pH value. Normally fetal blood is more acid (pH 7.34) than maternal blood (pH 7.44), but in the presence of hypoxia the pH value falls, e.g. to 7.2.

Maternal distress

The current labour management policy, which aims to restrict labour to 24 hours as a maximum, has reduced the number of women suffering from exhaustion. In a normal labour there is rarely any cause for real anxiety about the mother's physical condition; however, a constant watch is kept. Women do become ketotic more easily under a stress such as that of labour, so urine is regularly checked for protein and ketones. Ketoacidosis is associated with dehydration, and raised heart rate and temperature.

There is, however, maternal emotional distress which some women experience and which is associated with fear, pain and apparent lack of progress. Good antenatal preparation together with continuity of care in labour, sensitive support and companionship, adequate appropriate pain relief, skilled attention to comfort, and regular realistic progress reports and reassurance go a long way towards preventing the labouring woman experiencing excessive emotional distress.

Malpresentation

When the presenting part is other than the vertex, e.g. buttocks, arms or face, it is categorized as a malpresentation. The most common of these, the breech, is discussed here; suggestions for further reading are given at the end of the chapter.

Breech presentation

The presenting part is the buttocks – the 'breeches' end. Approximately 3% of fetuses present buttocks-first at term. In the middle trimester it is much more common, due apparently to there being more room to move at this stage, but the majority eventually turn to become cephalic presentations. A breech presentation is potentially dangerous because of the severe intermittent pressure on the after-coming head from the dominant part of the uterus. In addition the fetal head, which is the largest part, will not have been moulded to the bony birth canal so there could be the risk of cephalopelvic disproportion. There is also some anxiety that the cervix might close on the fetal neck and obstruct the passage of the head; forceps may therefore be used to protect and guide the after-coming head.

Such potential dangers led many centres to prefer to perform elective caesarean sections for all breech presentations. One consequence of this policy was that progressively fewer midwives and junior doctors gained the experience and confidence to conduct a vaginal breech delivery. However, the pendulum now appears to be swinging the other way, for where a breech presentation is apparent, ultrasound and pelvimetry are used, and only if the pelvis and the fetal head appear incompatible or the position of the fetal limbs looks problematical will caesarean section be performed.

There are three types of breech:

1. fully flexed – both legs are flexed and drawn up on the abdomen
2. extended – legs are flexed at the hips but extended at the knees, and the feet are in contact with the baby's shoulders
3. footling – one leg is flexed at hip and knee, the other is extended at hip and knee so that the foot presents first.

Malposition

When the vertex is less than optimally placed there is said to be malposition. The most common malposition is the occipito-posterior, for other possibilities see Further Reading.

Occipito-posterior position

When the fetal head enters the pelvis or turns mid-cavity so that the occiput is toward the maternal sacrum, rather than the maternal symphysis pubis, it is said to be in the occipito-posterior position (OP). Commonly the occiput will be toward the right side of the sacrum (ROP), and less often to the left (LOP). The head will eventually rotate in a majority of cases to present at the pelvic outlet with the head facing posteriorly as previously described. Such labours tend to be longer because the descent of the head and dilatation of the cervix may be slower. Cervical dilatation may, in fact, have to be greater where there is failure of the head to flex sufficiently, because this results in a longer diameter being presented. Severe backache is a frequent problem, probably because of the pressure of the occiput on the sacrum, and epidural anaesthesia may be appropriate. Where rotation becomes obstructed for some reason within the pelvis, it is called a *transverse arrest*.

If the head fails to flex, anterior rotation may not occur. Instead the occiput turns into the hollow of the sacrum, with the face to the symphysis, and the head delivers in this reverse position. This is called *face to pubes* or *persistent occipito-posterior position* (POP). The distension of the perineum is considerably greater with this presentation than with the more usual anterior position, and a large episiotomy may be appropriate. Alternatively the head may become lodged and labour is said to be obstructed; delivery by caesarean section may be needed.

Prolapse or presentation of the cord

For the cord to prolapse into the vagina or to appear at the vulva the amniotic sac must have ruptured (see p. 48), and the presenting part is likely to be high or ill-fitting for some reason, e.g. malpresentation, multiparity. Subsequent pressure on the cord from the head during contractions, traction, or simply the colder environment, outside the amnionic sack may cause the fetal blood supply to be obstructed, so early delivery is imperative. It is possible for the cord to rest alongside and even ahead of the main presenting part within an intact amniotic sac. This is a serious state which can cause fetal distress, and which requires constant vigilance to diagnose.

Incoordinate uterine activity

The ideal pattern of uterine polarity (see p. 49) does not always occur. Disordered uterine action, which is painful yet unproductive, occurs most commonly (96%) in primigravid labours. Hypertonia of the lower segment, alterations in polarity so that fundal dominance is lost, parts of the uterus contracting independently or out of sequence (colicky uterus) and cervical rigidity (cervical dystocia) have been described. This condition prolongs labour and may require active intervention if it does not speedily resolve.

Haemorrhage

Because of the hugely enhanced blood supply to the uterus which has developed through pregnancy, haemorrhage at any stage of labour is extremely serious and emergency steps to expedite delivery must be taken, possibly by caesarean section. Where haemorrhage is uncontrollable a hysterectomy may be necessary. Mercifully this is very rare.

Contracted pelvis and cephalopelvic disproportion

There are some women who have a normally shaped gynaecoid pelvis but it is small – small hands and feet correlate with this. Women with an android pelvis have pelvic walls that converge so that the outlet is narrow and the ischial spines may be very prominent (see p. 3). In women with a flat pelvis the inlet is narrow and difficult for the fetal head to pass through; there are yet others whose pelvis has been affected by trauma or disease. When one of the diameters of the true pelvis (see p. 3) is 1 cm less than in the ideal gynaecoid pelvis, it is called a contracted pelvis. In addition, some babies are large in proportion to their mothers. The pelvis of every woman is assessed during pregnancy, and further measurement made by ultrasound and X-ray if doubts arise as to the feasibility of the fetal head being able to pass through. Where apparently the fetal head is physically unable to go through there is said to be cephalopelvic disproportion (CPD). A decision is usually made toward the end of a pregnancy where there is a potential problem, either to deliver by elective caesarean section, or to allow a 'trial of labour' with or without early induction. However, despite reasonable antenatal care, CPD can arise spontaneously in labour and is a reason for failure to progress.

A 'trial of labour' usually indicates that CPD is suspected, but it is hoped that moulding of the fetal head during labour and the maximum flexibility of the maternal pelvis at that stage may allow a normal vaginal delivery. Very careful monitoring of the descent of the head will soon indicate delay, and caesarean section can be carried out where necessary. Inducing earlier than 40 weeks' gestation will mean the baby is smaller (see Table 2.1, p. 26).

Placental abruption

Occasionally partial or complete separation of the placenta occurs before the birth of the baby. Blood may be retained at the site or drain out through the vagina. Where it is retained it may seep into the myometrium causing marked damage (Coulevaire uterus). Any tendency for placental separation is a critical situation requiring immediate delivery of the baby by the most expeditious means.

Multiple births

Twin pregnancy is the most common to come to delivery; in more than 80% of cases the first baby will present by the vertex, and there is an almost equal chance of the second baby being vertex or breech. There is an increased risk of premature labour due to the bulk of the pregnancy, possibly because uterine muscle has a finite limit of stretch at which labour contractions start and the cervix begins to open.

Where there are more than two babies it is usual for them to be delivered pre-term by elective caesarean section.

Perineal trauma

Labial tears

Labial tears may bleed profusely and may or may not warrant suturing.

Labial haematoma

Stretching of the vagina and labia at delivery may result in rupture of veins. The resulting haematoma can be quite large, causes great pain and may require aspiration.

Perineal tears

Perineal tears occur spontaneously at delivery, or tearing may extend an episiotomy. They are classified according to the structures involved and are almost exclusive to the posterior perineum:

1. first degree involves the skin only, i.e. the fourchette
2. second degree is deeper and affects any or all of the superficial perineal muscles; the tear may extend up both sides or one side of the vaginal wall
3. third degree as above, plus anal sphincter involvement; the tear may extend up the rectal wall
4. fourth degree indicates a very severe third-degree tear.

First and second degree tears will be repaired following infiltration with lignocaine 1% unless there is an epidural block in progress. The repair may be performed by a midwife or doctor. Third and fourth degree tears may require a general anaesthetic and will be performed by an obstetrician or rectal surgeon. There is considerable debate concerning the best suture material (Grant, 1987), and it is important that the thread is not pulled tight, to allow for the inevitable oedema (see p. 247).

Retained placenta and placenta accreta

The placenta may have separated normally from the uterine wall but still needs a little assistance to leave the uterus. Allowing the baby to suckle to stimulate oxytocin production and uterine contraction, or rubbing the abdomen to stimulate contractions and firmly pressing upward on the fundus while applying gentle traction on the cord, is often sufficient (see p. 67) for it to be delivered.

Where separation appears to be incomplete or not occurring at all, manual removal under general anaesthesia will be attempted. In rare instances the placental chorionic villi have invaded the myometrium (placenta accreta) to such an extent that separation is very difficult and may cause life-threatening haemorrhage. In this case a hysterectomy may be the only safe course.

INTERVENTIONS IN LABOUR

To initiate labour and in the first stage

Prostaglandins

If for some reason induction of labour is being considered and the normal ripening of the cervix has not yet occurred, then prostaglandin pessaries or gel applied to the cervix may produce the required effect. Sometimes this is sufficient in itself to encourage the uterus to begin contracting, and labour to commence.

Oxytocin

Synthetic oxytocin via an intravenous drip causes uterine contractions; it works best where the cervix is ripe (favourable) and the membranes have been ruptured. It may also be used to re-establish or accelerate labour at any stage when contractions have weakened or stopped altogether.

Amniotomy

Amniotomy or artificial rupture of membranes (ARM) is sometimes called a surgical induction, and labour can be initiated or accelerated by rupture of the membranes. An amnihook or forceps are used to nick the amniotic sac, as a result of which prostaglandins appear to be released, and contractions may begin or be accelerated.

To assist delivery in the second stage

Episiotomy

Episiotomy involves an incision in the perineum (Fig. 3.7) to enlarge the vaginal opening, and may be mediolateral or median. Local anaesthetic should be used, although a well-distended perineum is said to have little sensation. The objective is usually to speed delivery or avoid excessive stretching or tearing of the surrounding tissues. Episiotomy used in conjunction with forceps or vacuum extraction allows more space for introduction of the instruments into the vagina. The incision is sutured after delivery is complete.

Forceps delivery

Assistance with forceps may be necessary in the second stage:

1. where progress is nil or very slow
2. for fetal distress to speed delivery
3. for maternal distress, exhaustion or where minimum maternal effort is desirable, e.g. in cardiac failure, cystic fibrosis or raised blood pressure.

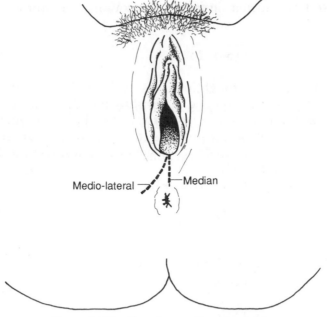

Figure 3.7 To show the position of episiotomy.

Local, pudendal or epidural anaesthesia is required, and the woman will most commonly be placed in the lithotomy position.

Wrigley forceps. These are short, light forceps designed for use when the fetal head is low on the perineum – hence the term 'low forceps'. They have curved blades to receive the head and also have curved shafts to match the curve of the birth canal.

Kielland forceps. These have longer, straighter handles and are used to assist the head at a higher level within the pelvis, e.g. for deep transverse arrest or OP positions, where rotation of the head or even downward traction to encourage rotation is needed – hence the term 'high forceps'. A large episiotomy is required.

Vacuum extraction or ventouse delivery

The indications for vacuum extraction are similar to those for forceps. A suction cup of an appropriate size is introduced into the vagina and applied to the fetal scalp posteriorly. Suction is used to draw the scalp up into the cup. Careful traction can then be given during uterine contractions. At delivery the baby will have a raised, red imprint of the cup on its head (*chignon*) which will persist for some days. This method of giving assistance has taken longer to gain acceptance in the UK than in other parts of the world (Chalmers and Chalmers, 1989). It is regularly used by midwives in many Third World countries.

Caesarean section (see also p. 262)

Delivery of the infant through incisions in the abdominal and uterine wall may be classified as 'elective', indicating that this mode of delivery has been chosen for specific reasons ahead of labour, or 'emergency', where it is decided on safety grounds to terminate labour. It may be carried out under either epidural or general anaesthetic, and at any stage of labour (see p. 202).

Reasons for an elective caesarean section are:

- contracted pelvis or CPD
- diabetes
- eclampsia
- serious illness or injury to the mother
- previous caesarean section
- placenta praevia
- multiple births of more than two babies.
- breech

Reasons for an emergency caesarean section are:

- fetal or maternal distress
- failed trial of forceps
- prolapse of cord
- failure to progress.

There are two types of caesarean section. One is the classical section, consisting of a longitudinal incision in the upper uterine segment, via a paramedian incision. It may be chosen for speed or for other reasons such as fibroids, certain types of placenta praevia (see p. 41) or where the lower segment is very stretched and friable as might be the case following a trial of labour. The other type is the lower segment section; it is the more common today and is favoured by women for its good cosmetic result. A Pfannenstiel (bikini line) incision and a transverse incision into the lower uterine segment are used. These heal well, and do not usually preclude repeated caesarean section for future pregnancies nor subsequent normal vaginal deliveries.

Procedure for lower segment section

An incision is made through skin and subcutaneous tissue in the natural fold just above the pubic hair. Transverse incisions are made in the anterior part of the rectus sheath on each side, the linea alba is divided, and these are blended into one transverse incision which can be stretched manually (the posterior portion of the rectus sheath is deficient at this level). The rectus sheaths are mobilized to expose the rectus muscles, which are then retracted laterally to gain access to the abdominal cavity.

The peritoneum is exposed and is opened with a transverse incision. The bladder is located and retracted away from the lower uterine segment, which is excised transversely and the wound further extended by manual stretching and tearing. This causes less bleeding and avoids the risk of instrumental damage to the fetal head. The head is eased out first, either manually or with Wrigley forceps, and then the body. The cord is clamped and the baby held head down, while suction is used to clear mucus and liquor from the upper respiratory tract.

Active management of the third stage with an intravenous injection of ergometrine into the uterus obtains placental separation, and when this has occurred the placenta can be gently withdrawn. The incision in the uterus is then closed with two layers of sutures, followed by closure of the peritoneum. The two recti are gently approximated and held together by three or four lightly tied sutures. The sheaths of the recti and the skin are then closed. A drain may be inserted.

Postoperative complications

Complications include haemorrhage, abdominal wind causing acute discomfort, wound infection, deep vein thrombosis, pulmonary embolism, abdominal adhesions and pelvic infection. Occasionally women experience urine retention, and it must be appreciated that neurological damage is possible, as is 'nicking' the bladder or ureters, particularly in emergency sections.

THE PUERPERIUM

The puerperium is the final phase in the childbearing continuum, and is the period of 6–8 weeks following delivery in which the woman's genital tract returns to a non-pregnant state. The process by which this occurs is called 'involution', and it commences as soon as the placenta is expelled. Once the placenta separates from the uterus placental hormone production ceases, causing a dramatic decline in maternal blood levels of oestrogens and progesterone, and consequently in the physiological effects of these on maternal respiration, cardiovascular system, digestion and metabolism (see p. 26).

The uterus

By the end of labour the uterus has considerably reduced in size, and this reduction continues by three processes. Firstly, uterine contractions continue after delivery, becoming intermittent. Suckling by the baby at the breast stimulates the posterior pituitary to release more oxytocin, which causes further bursts of uterine contraction. Even the sight, sound or smell of the baby can have this effect, which causes labour-type pain to be felt in the lower abdomen; it may also be referred to the lumbar region. More multiparous women experience this than primiparae, in a ratio of 2:1 (Murray and Holdcroft, 1989); it is described as throbbing, cramping or aching. For some women the pain is considerable – moderate to severe as scored on the McGill pain questionnaire – and is referred to as 'after pains'. Secondly, there is an actual reduction in uterine tissue: retraction of the uterine muscle has the effect of controlling haemorrhage, and also gradually reduces the blood supply to the muscle tissue to a point where the additional muscle and supportive collagen required for pregnancy can no longer be maintained. Consequently a degrading process (autolysis) is set in motion, whereby the excess material is liquefied and absorbed into the blood stream to be excreted via the kidneys. Thirdly, for two to three weeks a parturient woman experiences a diminishing discharge called the lochia, similar to a heavy period, which consists of blood and necrotic decidua. The lochia is alkaline and organisms flourish in it more readily than in the normal vaginal secretions which are acid, so there is an increased risk of infection. Much of the endometrium is regenerated in a fortnight; only the placental site takes longer. In the first few hours after delivery the cervix remains flaccid and open, but then gradually closes.

One sign that the uterus is involuting i.e. returning to a non-pregnant state, will be found in the gradual drop in the fundal height which can be palpated. On the first postpartum day it is usually just above the umbilicus, by six days it is midway between the umbilicus and the symphysis, and by ten days has disappeared down behind the symphysis. However, the parous uterus is always a little bigger than it was when nulliparous, and the parous cervix has a permanently different appearance to a nulliparous one, the opening at the external os being a slit rather than a tiny circle.

The vagina and perineum

In the first few hours women often experience numbness of the perineum whether or not local anaesthesia was used. At first the vagina is very lax and women may notice air held within it, being released when they move, sit down or take a bath. In addition trauma such as labial tears, episiotomy, oedema and haematoma is painful and takes time to heal. There may be pain inhibition of pelvic floor contractions;

actual trauma to the nerve supply to the pelvic floor musculature may manifest itself in difficulty in contracting the pelvic floor and in bowing of the pelvic floor on straining.

There is a noticeable increase in the amount of urine passed in the first few days as the body releases the excess fluid retained in pregnancy. It has a high nitrogen content due to the autolytic process in the uterus; women often complain of frequency. Continence is sometimes disturbed in the puerperium and women experience variously urgency, pain on micturition, stress incontinence, retention of urine and occasionally faecal incontinence. Trauma to the urethra, to supportive ligaments in the pelvis and to the muscle in the area and its nerve supply account for this.

Lactation

The level of prolactin produced by the anterior pituitary rises steadily throughout pregnancy, but its effect on the milk-producing cells of the breast is inhibited by the placental hormones (particularly oestrogen). As the placental hormones decline, a point is reached – usually about the third or fourth postpartum day – when prolactin is free to act and milk production begins. Up until that time the suckling child will obtain colostrum. Milk is produced by glandular cells and stored in the alveoli of the 15–20 lobes of each breast. Suckling, and eventually by a conditioned reflex even the sight, sound or smell of the baby, stimulates the posterior pituitary to release oxytocin which, in addition to its effects on uterine muscle (see p. 78), causes myoepithelial cells around the alveoli to contract. This contraction propels the milk with variable force into the lactiferous sinuses ready for removal by the baby, and is called the 'let down' or milk ejection reflex. Some women feel sharp pains and experience actual spurting out of the milk, while others sense only tingling and find the milk just dripping from their nipples.

It is important for the physiotherapist to understand the physical process by which the baby gains the milk. This is well described in the booklet *Successful Breastfeeding* produced by the Royal College of Midwives (RCM, 1991). In addition to the 'let down' reflex, milk is transferred from the breast by the baby taking the whole nipple and some of the areola well into the mouth so that it lies over the length of the tongue. The baby then squeezes the milk-filled sinuses behind the nipple by compression of the lower jaw and tongue against the upper jaw and hard palate (see p. 10 and p. 227).

Human breast milk is unique, and although an infant does apparently thrive on other available milks, there is no question but that 'breast is best' for babies, with very rare exceptions. It is the recommendation of the RCM (1991) that babies should be exclusively breast-fed until they are at least four months (preferably six months) old. Regrettably, although 64% of women in the UK choose to breast-feed (OPCS,

1985), only 26% are still fully breast-feeding at four months. Myles (1989) documents the subtle and critical differences that make colostrum and then human breast milk so infinitely superior to anything else for babies. Breast milk not only contains the right nutrients in the correct proportions for all aspects of human development, it also contains enzymes to help digest them appropriately, and important anti-infective agents such as macrophages, neutrophils, IgA and lysozyme, as well as anti-allergic factors, to protect the growing child.

Very few women are physically unable to breast-feed if they really want to, and very few babies are best fed by anything other than their mother's milk. The establishment of breast-feeding is therefore one of the most important matters in the early puerperium, and a person prepared to give the unhurried, skilled, consistent help to women to achieve this, ranks very highly in value to both mother and baby. The length of each feed should not be restricted because it has been shown (RCM, 1991) that the calorific content of the later or hind milk is higher than the foremilk.

Management in the puerperium

It is usual to encourage women to rest quietly for the first six hours, even after the most straightforward labour, to allow clotting over the placental site to occur and to give the body time to adapt to the substantial changes that have taken place. Thereafter a pleasant, relaxed, protected environment, whether in a maternity unit or at home, is required, which provides a woman with a little breathing space and any guidance she wants before she takes up full responsibility for her life again. Most women appreciate having their own basic needs supplied for a few days and being free to follow their instincts in feeding and caring for the baby, sleeping and pottering as they feel inclined. Where partners are able to be at home, they find this supportive role can be hugely rewarding and an excellent start to active fathering.

Women vary greatly in the amount and type of help and direct guidance they need. Those who have had a long, traumatic labour, an assisted delivery or a caesarean section will need more help and rest, and primiparae may require more guidance in baby feeding and baby care than multiparae. All women should be given relaxed opportunities to talk and ask questions about the labour, ideally with one of the professionals who attended them.

In the UK there is provision for every mother to be seen daily for the first 10 days in hospital or at home by a midwife, whether or not there are complications. The midwife is concerned to monitor the fundal height, the amount and colour of the lochia and the condition of the perineum, as well as the general physical well-being of the mother and infant. Whether the child is being breast-fed or bottle-fed, it is important to ensure that feeding proceeds satisfactorily and that the baby is thriving. The midwife is also well placed to observe any early evidence of postnatal depression, as well as encouraging the mother and, where necessary, instructing her in child care. When the circumstances require it the midwife may continue in attendance for up to 28 days. Thereafter theoretically the woman is the responsibility of the health visitor.

Complications in the puerperium

Postpartum haemorrhage

All carers of recently delivered women are on the alert for signs of postpartum haemorrhage (PPH), which is defined as a loss of blood following delivery in excess of 560 ml within the first 24 hours. After that time it is termed secondary PPH. The usual cause is uterine atonia; the uterus fails to contract and control the bleeding from the placental site for some reason, e.g. uterine exhaustion. The uterus may also be prevented from contracting down where the placenta has not completely separated or placental fragments remain. If the blood loss is rapid and severe the woman may collapse very quickly; immediate medical aid must be summoned. Where light bleeding continues well into the puerperium or recurs, placental fragments may be suspected and ergotamine tablets prescribed to stimulate further uterine contractions in the hope of dislodging what may well be only a very small tag of placenta.

Venous thrombosis, pulmonary embolism

Superficial and deep venous thrombosis are not common conditions despite the potential risks of trauma, stasis and infection and heightened activity of the body's coagulation system in the puerperium. However, pulmonary embolism continues to be a cause of maternal death. The physiotherapist is an important member of the caring team in monitoring and preventing any such problems.

Gravitational oedema

Many women have experienced gravitational oedema up to delivery and this must be encouraged to disperse post partum. A few women develop oedema of the feet and ankles for the first time after delivery; this is not easily explained except in terms of vascular damage.

Puerperal infection

Puerperal infection usually refers to infections of the genital tract; but pyrexia may be due to infection anywhere in the body, e.g. chest or urinary tract. Endometritis, salpingitis, pelvic cellulitis (parametritis) and even peritonitis are all possible. Such conditions were the scourge of childbearing until this century, and although they are rarely seen now in developed countries, physiotherapists, particularly those working in the Third World, should be aware of them. Treatment is by administration of the appropriate antibiotic.

Vesicovaginal fistula

Although vesicovaginal fistula is rarely seen in the UK, it has become apparent that in less developed countries women delivering without proper assistance may sustain serious tearing of the perineum and even high vaginal tears which are then not sutured. Prolonged second stage or sheer obstruction can result in ischaemia and necrosis, casuing tissue breakdown and a fistula. The result is that from delivery onwards a substantial number of women suffer from incontinence of urine and faeces; they are disabled and ostracized, and are often too poor to pay the high fees required by doctors to effect a repair (Tahzib, 1989).

References

Abboud T.K., Sarkis F., Hung T.T. et al. (1983). Effects of epidural anaesthesia during labour on maternal plasma beta endorphin levels. *Anesthesiology*, **59(1)**, 1–5.

Abboud T.K., Goebelsmann U., Raya J. et al. (1984). Effect of intrathecal morphine during labor on maternal plasma beta-endorphin levels. *A.J. Obstet. Gynecol.*, **149**, 709–710.

Bonica J.J. (1984). *In Textbook of Pain* (Wall P., Melzack R., eds.) p. 380. Edinburgh: Churchill Livingstone.

Brown S.T., Campbell D., Kutz A. (1989). Characteristics of labour pain at two stages of cervical dilation. *Pain*, **38**, 289–295.

Caldeyro-Barcia R. (1979). The influence of maternal position on time of spontaneous rupture of membranes, progress of labour, and fetal head compression. *Birth Fam. J.*, **6**, 7.

Chalmers J.A., Chalmers I. (1989). The obstetric vacuum extractor is the instrument of first choice for operative vaginal delivery. *Brit. J. Obstet. Gynaec.*, **96**, 505–509.

Chapman M.G., Jones M., Springs J.E. et al. (1986). The use of a birthroom: a randomized controlled trial comparing delivery with that in the labour ward. *Brit. J. Obstet. Gynaec.*, **93(2)**, 182–7.

Charles A.G., Norr K.L., Bloch C.R. et al. (1978). Obstetric and psychological effects of psychoprophylactic preparation for childbirth. *Am. J. Obstet. Gynecol.*, **131**, 44–52.

Clark A.P. (1891). The influence of position of the patient in labor in causing uterine inertia and pelvic disturbances. *JAMA*, **16**, 433.

Currie W.B., Wong M.F., Cox R.I. et al. (1973). Hormonal changes in ewes and their fetuses at parturition. *J. Reprod. Fert.*, **32**, 333–334.

Flynn A.M., Kelly J., Hollins G. et al. (1978). Ambulation in labour. *Br. Med. J.*, **2**, 591–593.

Gardosi J., Hutson N., Lynch C.B. (1989). Randomised, controlled trial of squatting in second stage of labour. *Lancet*, **ii**, 74–7.

Grant A., Sleep J., Ashurst H., Spencer J. A. (1989). Dyspareunia associated with the use of glycerol-impregnated catgut to repair perineal trauma. Report of a 3 year folloup study. *Brit J. Obstet. Gynaec.*, **96**, 741–3.

Grant J. (1987). Reassessing second stage. *J. ACPOG*, **6**, 26–30.

Inch S. (1982). *Birthrights*, London: Green Print.

Johnstone F.D., Aboe Imagel M. S., Haruny A. K. (1987). Maternal posture in second stage and fetal acid base status. *Brit. J. Obstet. Gynaec.*, **94**, 753–757.

Lenstrup C., Schartz A., Berget A. et al. (1987). Warm tub bath during delivery. *Acta Obstet. Gynecol. Scand.*, **66**, 709–712.

Liggins G.C. (1974). Parturition in the sheep and the human. *Basic Life Sci.*, **4**, 423–443.

McManus T.J., Calder A.A. (1978). Upright posture and efficiency of labour. *Lancet*, **i**, 72–74.

Melzack R. (1984). The myth of painless childbirth. *Pain*, **19**, 321–337.

Melzack R., Taenzer P., Feldman P., et al. (1981). Labour is still painful after prepared childbirth training. *Can. Med. Ass. J.*, **125**, 357–363.

Mendez Bauer C., Arroyo C., Garcia-Ramos C. et al. (1975). Effects of standing position on spontaneous uterine contractility and other aspects of labor. *J. Perinat. Med.*, **3**, 89–100.

Mersky H. (1979). Pain terms: a list of definitions and notes on usage. *Pain*, **6**, 249–252.

Mitre I. (1974). The influence of maternal position on duration of the active phase of labor. *Int. J. Gynaecol. Obstet.*, **12**, 181.

Murray A., Holdcroft A. (1989). Incidence and intensity of postpartum lower abdominal pain. *Brit. Med. J.*, **289**, 1619.

Myles M. (1975). *Textbook for Midwives*, 9th edn. p.211. Edinburgh: Churchill Livingstone.

Myles M. (1989). *Textbook for Midwives* (Bennett V.R., Brown L.K., eds.) 11th edn., pp. 491–3. Edinburgh: Churchill Livingstone.

Nesheim B. (1988). Duration of labor. *Acta Obstet. Gynecol. Scand.*, **67**, 121–124.

Newnham J.P., Tomlin S., Ratter S.T. et al. (1983). Endogenous opioid peptides in pregnancy. *Brit. J. Obstet. Gynaec.*, **90**, 535–538.

Noble E. (1983). *Childbirth with Insight*, p. 51. Boston: Houghton Mifflin.

OPCS (1985). *Infant Feeding*. Department of Health, HM. Stationery Office.

Pöschl U. (1987). The vertical birthing position of the Trobrianders, Papua New Guinea. *Aust. NZ J. Obst. Gynaecol.*, **27**, 120–125.

RCM (1991). *Successful Breastfeeding*. 2nd edn. Edinburgh: Churchill Livingstone.

Read J.A. (1981). Randomized trial of ambulation versus oxytocin for labor enhancement. *Am. J. Obstet. Gynecol.*, **139**, 669.

Roberts J.E., Mendez-Bauer C., Wodell D.A. (1983). The effects of maternal position on uterine contractility and efficiency. *Birth*, **10**, 243–249.

Russell J.G.B. (1982). The rationale of primitive delivery positions. *Brit. J. Obstet. Gynaec.*, **89**, 712–715.

Scruggs M. (1982). Personal communication, quoted by Grant J. (1987). Reassessing second stage. *J. ACPOG*, **60**, 20–30.

Shearman R.P. (1986). Endocrine changes during pregnancy. In *Integrated Obstetrics and Gynaecology for Postgraduates* (Dewhurst J., ed.). Oxford: Blackwell.

Snooks S.J., Setchell M., Swash M. et al. (1984). Injury to innervation of pelvic floor sphincter musculature in childbirth. *Lancet*, **ii**, 546–550.

Sørensen S.M., Bondesen H., Istre D., Vilmann P. (1988). Perineal rupture following vaginal rupture. *Acta Obstet. Gynecol. Scand.*, **67**, 315–318.

Sosa R. et al. (1980). The effect of a supportive companion on perinatal problems, length of labour and mother–infant interaction. *New Engl. J. Med.*, **303**, 597–600.

Tahzib F. (1989). An initiative on vesico–vaginal fistula. *Lancet*, **i**, 1316–1317.

Wall P.D., Melzack R. (1984). *Textbook of Pain*, p. 378. Edinburgh: Churchill Livingstone.

Williams R.M., Thom M.H., Studd J.W. (1980). A study of the benefits and acceptability of ambulation in spontaneous labour. *Brit. J. Obstet. Gynaec.*, **87**, 122–126.

Wuitchik M., Bakal D., Lipshitz J. (1989). The clinical significance of pain and cognitive activity in latent labor. *Obst. Gynec.*, **73(1)**, 35–42.

Further reading

Chamberlain G., Stewart M. (1987). Walking through labour. *Brit. Med. J.*, **295**, 802.

Lagercrantz H., Slotkin T. (1986). The stress of being born. *Scientific American*, **4**, 100.

Lupe P.J., Gross T.L. (1986). Maternal upright posture and mobility in labor – a review. *Obst. Gynec.*, **67**, 727.

Myles M. (1989). *Textbook for Midwives* (Bennet V.R., Brown L.K., eds.) 11th edn. Edinburgh: Churchill Livingstone.

CHAPTER 4

The Antenatal Period

THE TEAM – WHO IS IN IT?

In spite of the fact that pregnancy is a normal physiological event, usually being experienced by a healthy woman, in the UK the number of professions involved in the caring team continues to proliferate. In the sequence of involvement, this team consists of general practitioners, midwives, obstetric physiotherapists, dieticians, obstetricians, dentists, laboratory technicians, health visitors, ultrasound operators, and paediatricians. Where necessary, other medical consultants, radiographers and social workers may also be part of the team. It is essential that all personnel are aware of the very special needs of pregnant women and respond to them accordingly. Increasingly, some pregnant women turn also to practitioners of alternative therapies or other activities, e.g. yoga, aerobics, swimming, acupuncture or hypnotherapy.

At the opposite end of the spectrum, in less developed countries, most women go through pregnancy and give birth without ever meeting a medical professional. Every year 500 000 women die during pregnancy – 99% of them in developing countries (WHO, 1986; Fry, 1987) – although a quarter to a half of these deaths are due to illegal abortions because these women do not have access to effective family planning services or the safe procedures of termination of pregnancy. The main causes of the rest of these tragic deaths are eclampsia and obstructed labour. Because women in Africa and Asia have larger families (an average of four to six children, compared with fewer than two in Europe), in a developing country the risk of maternal mortality during pregnancy may be as high as 1 in 15; in Britain it is now less than 1 in 10 000 births. For every death, 10–15 women will suffer major impairment to their health; although this is partly due to lack of medical services, many other factors contribute to this shocking problem: poverty and ignorance, religious belief and social customs, discrimination against women in many countries – legally, educationally and nutritionally – coupled with a general shortage of health resources. In addition, for every woman who dies or who is damaged by pregnancy or childbirth, a family is greatly affected too.

Two of the worst consequences of childbirth are anorectal and/or vesicovaginal fistulae (see p. 82). These are often caused by prolonged, obstructed labour, and result in continuous leakage of urine and/or faeces. Women suffering from these horrific conditions, which are particularly endemic in the subSaharan region of Africa (Tahzib, 1989), often become rejected social outcasts. Tragically the restorative surgery which could transform their lives is largely unavailable.

These problems, and the following four aims to begin dealing with them, were set out at a conference on safe motherhood in which the World Health Organization, the World Bank and other United Nations agencies were involved (Mahler, 1987).

1. To provide adequate primary health care and an adequate share of food for girls from infancy to adolescence, and to provide universal family planning to avoid unwanted or high-risk pregnancies.
2. To provide good antenatal care including advice on nutrition, with efficient early detection and referral of those at high risk.
3. To give assistance from a trained person to all women in childbirth, both to those at home and in hospital.
4. To provide effective access to essential obstetric care for all women at high risk, and for emergencies during and after the pregnancy.

Obstetric physiotherapists working in affluent Western countries where women are increasingly demanding a better quality of birth, must never forget their less fortunate sisters for whom simply surviving pregnancy and giving birth to a healthy baby who grows into adulthood may be all that matters.

The aims of modern antenatal care are:

1. To promote and maintain optimal physical and emotional maternal health throughout pregnancy.
2. To recognize and treat correctly medical or obstetrical complications occurring during pregnancy.
3. To detect fetal abnormalities as early as possible.
4. To prepare for and inform both parents about pregnancy, labour, the puerperium and the subsequent care of their baby.
5. The overriding goal is that pregnancy will result in a healthy mother and a healthy infant.

ANTENATAL CARE OPTIONS

Legally a woman is entitled to choose the place of delivery of her baby and the type of care she would prefer. The options available to her are shown in Table 4.1.

Home birth

If a woman decides that she would like to have her baby at home, in the UK she does not need to have the permission of her general prac-

Table 4.1 Antenatal care options in the UK

Place of birth	Type of antenatal care
Home birth	Local GP's surgery, midwive's clinic, midwife at home
General practitioner obstetric unit	Local GP's surgery or midwive's clinic, or home
'DOMINO'	GP's surgery, midwive's clinic or home
Consultant unit	Hospital antenatal clinic or GP and hospital shared care

titioner or an obstetrician. There is a statutory obligation on the part of the local Supervisor of Midwives to provide midwifery care antenatally, during labour and delivery, and postnatally. The mother does not have to provide herself with a doctor – if the midwife feels that medical cover is necessary, it is her duty to provide this (Beech, 1987). Forty years ago in the UK, 50% of all births were at home; twenty years ago 35% were home deliveries; today more than 98% of all births are in hospital (Stanway and Stanway, 1984). Private independent midwives are also available.

General practitioner units

General practitioner obstetric units may exist independently in a district general hospital or may stand alongside a consultant unit. The general practitioner will be responsible for the antenatal, intrapartum and postnatal care of the woman, and will almost certainly make use of antenatal consultant-based diagnostic procedures. General practitioner units are often local, homelike and informal, and are very popular with women – particularly with multigravidae.

Domino

This scheme (DOmiciliary Midwife IN and Out) enables the pregnant woman to be cared for antenatally, delivered and then attended postnatally by the same community-based midwife or team of midwives, thus providing the continuity of care so often lacking in hospital-based obstetrics. The mother calls her midwife to her home when she considers labour to have begun. The midwife accompanies her to hospital, delivers the baby and brings the mother home again 6–7 hours after the birth.

Consultant obstetric units

These larger units are usually based in district or regional centres, although a few still exist as independent entities. They should all have access to up-to-date diagnostic procedures, and be able to call upon staff of many disciplines. Women often complain of an impersonal, fragmented, 'conveyor belt' approach; very few such units seem able to provide continuity of care for all their clients.

There are several other permutations of care available to women. They may opt for 100% hospital-based attention, or they may choose to have 'shared care' with their general practitioners undertaking alternate consultations with the consultant unit, assisted by the community midwives associated with the G.P.'s practice. For most women this will be National Health Service care, but it is possible to arrange private care for any part of the time.

ROUTINE ANTENATAL CARE

Following confirmation of pregnancy by their general practitioner, women, if they decide on a hospital birth, are usually referred to its booking clinic. This normally occurs between 9 and 16 weeks.

Booking visit

As well as recording details of the woman's social, family, medical and past obstetric history – in order to assess her health and attempt to uncover any factor that may adversely affect childbearing – details of the present pregnancy are taken. Note will be made of the woman's height and shoe size, because there is a correlation between these measurements and those of her pelvis. In some centres during this initial visit the mother will be seen by both midwife and obstetrician – but in others the booking clinic is run entirely by midwives.

Subsequent visits

Following the first attendance it is most usual for women to be seen monthly up to 28 weeks' gestation, fortnightly up to 36 weeks, and weekly thereafter. Any anxieties or problems the woman may have should be discussed at each visit. In addition the following are always recorded: blood pressure, urine, weight, presence of oedema, fundal height and 'lie' of the baby, fetal movements and fetal heart rate.

Blood pressure

Although there is an increase in blood volume and cardiac output during pregnancy, this is not normally accompanied by a rise in blood pressure – in fact there may even be a slight drop during the middle trimester, probably due to the hormonally mediated dilatation of blood vessels. Blood pressure is taken at each antenatal visit, and it is important to record a base-line blood pressure early in pregnancy because a rise can be the first sign of a potentially serious complication such as eclampsia.

Urine

Urine is tested at each visit for protein, sugar and ketones; in addition its colour and odour will be noted. It is not routinely tested for infection unless there are other symptoms. Proteinuria may indicate pre-eclamptic toxaemia (PET), sugar the possibility of gestational diabetes, and ketones inadequate glycogen stores (see pp. 40, 42).

Weight

It is inadvisable for a woman to allow her pregnancy weight gain to become excessive – an average of 12.5 kg is advised although it may be more or less. Most centres will weigh women on each antenatal visit; sudden increases in weight will be noted because they may be indications of fluid retention and even PET (see pp. 37, 40).

Oedema

The hands and lower limbs are checked for the presence of oedema, and for other indications of fluid retention and PET (e.g. paraesthesia) (see p. 39).

Fundal height and the 'lie' of the baby

The level of the fundus of the uterus is noted and compared with the gestational stage. Intrauterine growth retardation (IUGR) may be suspected if the fundal height is lower than expected. Multiple pregnancy or polyhydramnios could cause an increase in fundal height. Early in pregnancy the fetus will frequently change position. By 36 weeks more than 95% will be in a cephalic presentation – the remainder will be breech or other variations.

Fetal movements

Although fetal movements are usually noticed by the mother at sometime between 16 and 22 weeks' gestation, the fetus has in fact been moving since 8 weeks. Until the uterus has risen out of the pelvis and is actually in good contact with the anterior abdominal wall, the woman is unaware of movements because the uterus is insensitive to touch. In a second or subsequent pregnancy women will probably notice their baby moving earlier, possibly because they recognize the sensation. As pregnancy advances fetal movements may be used as a measure of the baby's well-being. All women should realize that a decrease or cessation of normal movement for any length of time may have serious implications. The obstetric physiotherapist must be constantly alert to this possibility and pick up even the most mild expression of maternal anxiety. It takes only a few moments of the midwife's or doctor's time to listen for the fetal heart, or it can be monitored using a cardiotocograph (CTG). 'Kick' charts are an easily used monitoring device. The mother makes a note of the first ten movements per day, recording the time and strength. The longer the time span for those ten movements the greater the concern.

Fetal heart rate

Somtimes midwives and doctors will prefer to question the mother as to the fetal movements that she feels, rather than listen to the baby's heart rate, this being a good indicator of fetal well-being. Fathers may like to put an ear against their partner's abdominal wall in order to hear this exciting sound. Alternatively the cardboard tube from a toilet roll can substitute for a stethoscope!

Although the fetal heart can be seen to be functioning as early as 8–10 weeks using ultrasound scanning, it is not usually possible to hear the heart beat before 20 weeks using the Pinard stethoscope. However, it can be picked up earlier using a Sonic-aid. The normal rate will vary between 120 and 160 beats per minute.

OTHER TESTS

Blood tests

Blood tests are used to detect haemoglobin levels, the presence of sexually transmitted disease, blood group and haemoglobinopathies.

Haemoglobin levels

A decrease is normal during pregnancy because of the increased blood plasma volume (see p. 33). It is becoming less common to give iron and folic acid supplements routinely to all women – but those showing signs of anaemia will need this help.

Sexually transmitted disease

The Venereal Disease Research Laboratory (VDRL) slide test has replaced the old Wassermann test for syphilis. Where a woman appears to be at risk of suffering from other sexually transmitted diseases appropriate tests will be carried out. She will be routinely screened for hepatitis B and rubella antibodies, but at the present time this is not the case for HIV, although anonymous testing is being carried out in some centres.

Blood group

The woman's blood grouping will be determined, as will her Rhesus factor.

Haemoglobinopathies

Tests for the haemoglobinopathies, e.g. sickle-cell disease and thalassaemia, may be carried out in women of West Indian, African and Mediterranean origin, where indicated.

Ultrasound scanning

During the past twenty years this valuable diagnostic technique has become increasingly more sophisticated. In the UK most pregnant women will have at least one ultrasonic scan around 18 weeks' gestation. This is used as the basis for gestational dating of the pregnancy, and for detection of certain abnormalities, e.g. spina bifida, anencephaly, heart, kidney, and intestinal defects). Where pregnancies are complicated by problems such as PET and IUGR, or where there is more than one fetus, a series of scans may be carried out.

Chorionic villus sampling

Chorionic villus sampling (CVS) is a fairly new technique which can be carried out vaginally or transabdominally. Fragments of placental chorionic villi are removed and inspected for genetic fetal abnormalities such as Down's syndrome. Although the benefit of this technique is that it can be carried out very early in pregnancy (8–10 weeks), there is a small but definite risk of spontaneous abortion.

Alphafetoprotein measurements

It is possible to measure this major fetal serum protein in the mother's blood around 16–18 weeks of pregnancy. High levels of alphafetoprotein (AFP) alert the caring team to the possibility of neural tube or other defects. Where high levels are found it may be necessary to proceed to ultrasonic scanning and amniocentesis. However, it must be remembered that multiple pregnancy will also produce high levels of AFP.

Amniocentesis

A small amount of amniotic fluid is withdrawn transabdominally, with the assistance of ultrasound monitoring to locate the placenta. Culture of the cells shed by the fetus within this fluid is used to give an indication of genetic abnormalities such as Down's syndrome. Fetal sex can also be determined and will be important where there is a familial history of sex-linked disorders such as haemophilia or Duchenne muscular dystrophy. AFP levels can be much more accurately determined from amniotic fluid, thereby further assisting in the diagnosis of neural tube deficiencies.

The drawbacks of amniocentesis are the long delay before results are available, and – once again – the risk of triggering an abortion.

Later in pregnancy this procedure may be used to detect the degree of Rhesus incompatibility, and the lecithin/sphingomyelin (surfactant) ratio in the amniotic fluid to determine the maturity of the lungs in growth-retarded fetuses.

Pelvimetry

Where cephalopelvic disproportion is suspected or where a breech presentation exists, an ultrasound scan to assess the biparietal diameter together with X-ray pelvimetry (measurement of the pelvic inlet and outlet) will be carried out at 38 weeks' gestation. This will enable the obstetrician to decide whether the fetus is likely to be delivered safely vaginally, or whether delivery should be by elective caesarean section.

Acceptability of antenatal testing

The screening of pregnant women is steadily increasing and becoming more universal. Such a policy means that diagnostic tests and procedures are applied to all, rather than just to the small number of women for whom it is deemed necessary by virtue of specific signs, symptoms and facts. Because of the speed with which the medical profession has adopted procedures such as ultrasound investigations during pregnancy, without randomized controlled trials as to their safety and accuracy, some women prefer *not* to be exposed to them. Their wishes must be respected, for there is no mandatory requirement that they should submit themselves to any or all of these investigations. Furthermore, if a woman is not prepared to consider the termination of her pregnancy there is no point in suggesting CVS, amniocentesis or any other test that may show abnormalities.

PRECONCEPTUAL CARE

Although many babies are still conceived accidentally, more and more hopeful parents-to-be and their medical advisers are becoming aware of the benefits of dealing with health problems and attaining optimal physical and mental well-being prior to pregnancy. Both partners may decide to prepare for conception by giving thought to their diet, alcohol consumption, smoking habits, exercise routines and drug (medicinal or social) intake.

Because every organ system within the mother's body will alter and adjust according to the demands made upon it by the growing fetus (see p. 26), the woman who begins pregnancy feeling fit and comfortable is more likely to be able to cope with the physical and emotional changes during the subsequent nine months. Women who have been taking the contraceptive pill are usually advised to discontinue its use three to six months before the hoped-for pregnancy.

Where such conditions as spina bifida and anencephaly have previously occurred, vitamin supplements may be recommended. Genetic counselling should be available to parents with a family history of diseases likely to be inherited, and complaints such as diabetes, systemic lupus erythematosus, renal or cardiac disorders and hypertension should be treated and an attempt made to stabilize them before conception. Essential drug regimens and their possible teratogenic effects should be considered. In the present social and medical climate it is increasingly accepted that conditions like multiple sclerosis, rheumatoid arthritis, hemiplegia and organ transplantation should not be a bar to motherhood.

Many of today's women are becoming more and more aware of their responsibility in asserting control over their own health and body, and are very open to sound advice preconceptually. Women in the lower socioeconomic groups may be primarily concerned with finance, accommodation and food. Consequently, there may be no desire or enthusiasm for preconceptual planning, physical activities and, later, antenatal classes. Even so, it is still possible for the obstetric physiotherapist to teach the principles of good 'body care' to these women between pregnancies. The postnatal inpatient class is a valuable forum for presenting 'back school' advice, and pelvic floor and abdominal muscle re-education can be suggested. The obstetric physiotherapist should be the member of the postnatal team who, with enthusiasm and knowledge, can create good body awareness during the childbearing years which will benefit mothers and their families throughout life.

In the setting of the well-women clinics which have sprung out of the family planning movement, and as part of the concept of health promotion, the obstetric physiotherapist can play an active role in preparing women for a healthy and happy pregnancy. Some women attempt to become super-fit overnight by means of over-vigorous activity such as aerobics, jogging or weight training. Taken to its extremes this could lead to amenorrhoea. Such over-zealous enthusiasm can be channelled into safer activities by the obstetric physiotherapist; swimming, yoga, cycling and walking for example, are less likely to cause injuries. Assessing and treating back problems before the physiological ligamentous changes begin, and imprinting the concept of good back care, could prove invaluable in the months of pregnancy and later. The obstetric physiotherapist can give advice about urinary disorders, e.g. stress incontinence, urgency or frequency, and begin pelvic floor education or re-education using exercise and possibly electrical therapy. All women, but particularly those who are attending infertility clinics, will benefit from stress-reducing techniques, including relaxation and positive thinking. These can be most helpful when properly taught. Women who are handicapped by physical impairment or pathologies such as multiple sclerosis, rheumatoid arthritis or the effects of a cerebrovascular accident will need the specialized skills and support of the obstetric physiotherapist in preparing themselves for the marathon of pregnancy and motherhood.

EARLY PREGNANCY

'The entire female organism adapts to preserve and nourish the fetus growing within the uterus and with the anabolic metabolism comes a mental tranquillity and somnolent beauty'.

(Llewellyn-Jones, 1969)

This somewhat romantic statement encapsulates the process of pregnancy – practically every system within the pregnant woman's body automatically changes during the nine months. There is also the notion that the fetus is able to manipulate its environment to suit itself!

Once pregnancy is diagnosed and established, physiotherapy should ideally be a continuation and a reinforcement of preconceptual care and involvement. Where this has not been possible an early introduction to good back usage, understanding of stress and its control, and an appreciation of the importance of physical health (with particular reference to strength and endurance) is essential. Activities for the pelvic floor and abdominal muscles, legs and arms can usefully be included.

Different centres will have different ways of introducing appropriate information, and this will depend to a large extent on their clientele. It is most important not to overburden women whether they are primigravid or multigravid. The regimen proposed should take into account individual lifestyles. Those who are engaged in strenuous activity will need to devote more time to rest and stress control; those who are leading a more leisurely life will benefit from a professionally planned programme of exercise.

ANTENATAL CLASSES

In practically every National Health Service centre involved with the care of pregnant women antenatal classes of some sort or another are offered. These may be held in hospitals, but are increasingly held in the community. Wide variation is found around the country in content, presenting personnel and style of teaching. Ideally midwives, obstetric physiotherapists and health visitors should work closely together to provide a comprehensive programme at a time and in a place which is convenient and accessible to the parents as envisaged in the joint statement agreed by the three professions in 1987 (RCM et al., 1987) (see p. xiii).

Antenatal 'preparation for parenthood' classes must be designed to fulfil the *parents' expressed needs*, and should never simply be a forum for professionals to impart the sort of information *they* think their audience requires. In fact the lecturer/student image should be avoided at all costs; antenatal education is most successful when it is parent-centred, with everyone involved contributing fully. It is vital that all aspects of this service are flexible, are regularly reviewed and are evaluated. Rigidity and routine are anachronistic, and are to be condemned. Continuity of professional personnel is as important as their ability and expertise in fulfilling this very special role. The antenatal class is no place for the inexperienced physiotherapist, midwife or health visitor. The precise details of course organization and planning must vary with local needs, and each obstetric physiotherapist should be sensitive to these. Apart from NHS classes, organizations such as the National Childbirth Trust (NCT), the Active Birth movement and occasionally private individuals offer courses in preparation for parenthood.

The earliest antenatal education was primarily concerned with hygiene and nutrition in an attempt to lower maternal and infant mortality rates. Later, teachers began to be concerned with presenting skills to help women prepare for and cope with labour pain. Today, the brief is much wider:

1. Couples should be helped to check and increase their knowledge of the physiological changes of pregnancy, labour and the puerperium.

2. They should be shown ways which may be useful for coping with the physical changes of pregnancy and their associated discomforts.
3. They should be guided towards a realistic understanding of labour and the assembly of a 'tool kit' of coping skills.
4. Couples are encouraged to consider the profound change in lifestyle that parenthood brings, and the emotional maturity necessary to manage their additional responsibilities successfully.
5. They should be encouraged to talk, present their problems, ask questions and helped to obtain satisfying answers.

While the best antenatal classes in the world probably could not prepare expectant couples for the full reality of parenthood, in a recent study on the impact of antenatal classes on knowledge, anxiety and confidence in primiparous women (Hillier and Slade 1989), significant increases in knowledge and confidence in coping with labour and caring for the newborn infant were shown.

'Early bird' classes

More and more centres are offering two sessions directly after the initial booking visit when interest and motivation are often at their highest. Although it is appreciated that some women may miscarry, the support that such a group offers outweighs the disadvantages. Women are encouraged to bring their partners or some other person of their choice. Regrettably, some units are only able to provide one class at this stage, thus substantially reducing the material that can be covered. These classes will probably be shared by physiotherapists with midwives, dicticians, health visitors and, possibly, doctors. Prioritization and quality of presentation are of prime importance for the physiotherapist, and practical participation by all class members is imperative! It is essential that the following subjects be included in the physiotherapist's part of these sessions:

Pregnancy back care

Postural and weight changes, sitting and working positions, bending, lifting and household chores should all be considered (Figs. 4.1–4.5). Ideally no woman should go home without an individual posture check, and easy access to further help if she is experiencing back pain or other physical discomfort is essential (see p. 138).

Pelvic floor and pelvic tilting exercises

A brief explanation of the role of the pelvic floor, using a pelvis, should be followed by the obstetric physiotherapist teaching pelvic floor

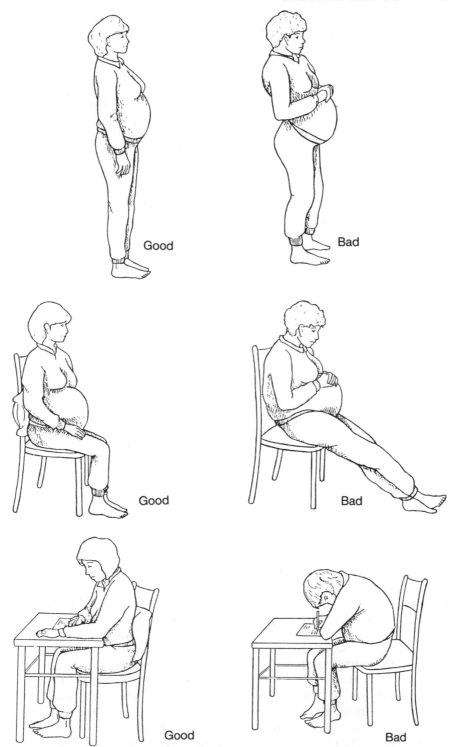

Figure 4.1–3 Back care.

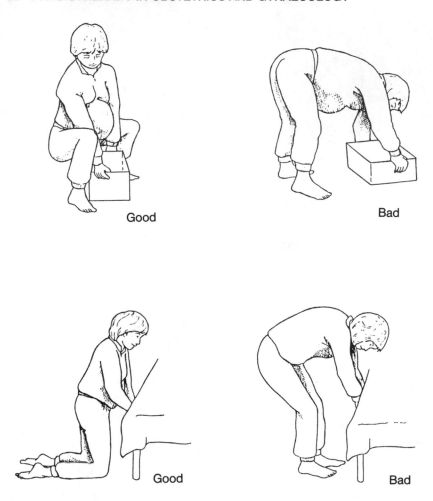

Figure 4.4–5 Back care.

contractions – this can go down well with a mixed audience, especially when it is suggested that the woman can practise the exercise during intercourse! Nielsen (1988) showed that where women learnt and practised pelvic floor contractions during pregnancy, they were better able to use these muscles at eight weeks and eight months post partum than those who had not learnt the skill antenatally. The strength of the pelvic floor muscles was greater postnatally in those who exercised during pregnancy compared with those who did not.

Where the group is large, pelvic tilting can be demonstrated while sitting on the edge of a chair (Fig. 4.6). The group should understand that this exercise can be helpful for maintaining abdominal muscle strength, correcting posture, and easing backache; and that it can be done in standing (Fig. 4.7), crook lying, side lying and prone kneeling (Fig. 4.8) positions as well.

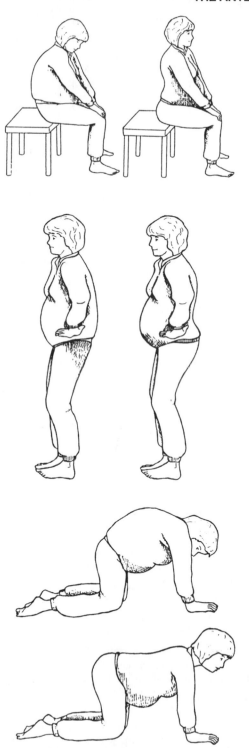

Figure 4.6–8 Pelvic tilting.

ANTE-NATAL RECORD

INVESTIGATIONS	DATE ..	RESULTS
A B O Blood Group*		
Rhesus Blood Group*		
Antibodies*		
WR / KAHN		
X Ray Chest		
Other		

*IMPORTANT NOTE—In the event of a transfusion this record of the blood grouping should always be checked and cross-matching should always be carried out.

HISTORY
Oedema
Headache
Bowels
Micturition
Discharge
Date of quickening

FIRST EXAMINATION	Date	Sig
Height		
Teeth		
Breasts		
Heart		
Lungs		
Varicose veins		
Pelvis		
Cervical smear		

Special observations

EXAMINATION 35/37 week
Date
Head/Brim relationship
Pelvic capacity
Sig

This patient is fit for inhalation analgesia

Date

Signature of Doctor

DATE	WEEKS	WEIGHT	URINE ALB SUGAR	B.P.	HEIGHT FUNDUS	PRESENTA-TION AND POSITION	RELATION OF P.P. TO BRIM	F.H.	OEDEMA	Hb	NEXT VISIT	SIG

NOTES e.g. antibodies, other tests, infections, drugs, immunisation, classes attended, etc.

Printed in the UK for HMSO Dd 80731160 628M 7/87 56715

Figure 4.9 Co-operation record card (Crown Copyright, reproduced with permission of the Controller of Her Majesty's Stationery Office).

CO-OPERATION RECORD CARD FOR MATERNITY PATIENTS

NAME
(Block capitals – surname first)

Address   Tel. No.

AGE   N.H.S. No.

FAMILY DOCTOR   Tel. No.
Address

DOCTOR BOOKED FOR MATERNITY SERVICES   Tel. No.
Address

MIDWIFE   Tel. No.
Address   ALT No.

DOCTORS   Tel. No.
MATERNITY CLINIC

HOSPITAL   OBSTETRICIAN

BOOKED FOR DELIVERY AT   E.D.C.   /   /

RELEVANT FAMILY HISTORY   T.B.   Diabetes
High B.P.   Twins

PAST ILLNESSES, ALLERGIES, BLOOD TRANSFUSIONS, DRUG THERAPY.
CONTRACEPTION

PREVIOUS OBSTETRIC HISTORY
No. confinements before 22 weeks.............after 22 weeks............

NORMAL MENSTRUAL CYCLE   D.L.M.P. (First day)   E.D.C.
Oral Contraception   YES/NO

POST-NATAL EXAMINATION

Sig   Hb

DATE

Urine   B.P.

Symptoms and duration

Breasts and feeding

Abdomen

PUERPERIUM

Pelvic examination

Rubella Vaccination

Treatment and advice

Cervical Smear   Date   /   /

SPECIAL NOTES
(Including recommendations for future pregnancies)

This card when completed should be returned to the family doctor

CONFINEMENT AND PUERPERIUM

CONFINEMENT   Date   Place

PUERPERIUM

MOTHER'S CONDITION ON DISCHARGE   Date   Hb
B.P.   Urine   Nipples
Breasts
Uterus
Perineum

Contraceptive Advice

BABY   Sex   Birth Weight

Condition at Birth

Date of discharge   Weight
Examination
Cong Malformation
Gestational Age
PKH
CDH
Feeding

Exercises for circulation and cramp

An explanation should be given as to how pregnancy can affect leg circulation, and women who have sedentary jobs should especially be encouraged to carry out frequent foot exercises at work. Ankle dorsiflexion and plantar flexion, and foot circling carried out for 30 seconds regularly should be suggested; women should be advised not to cross the knees when sitting, and the technique of stretching in bed with the foot dorsiflexed and not plantar flexed, for preventing and easing calf cramp, should also be shown. Additional suggestions for cramp relief include avoiding long periods of sitting, a pre-bedtime walk, a warm bath, and foot exercises in bed before going to sleep.

Fatigue

Many women pregnant for the first time (and their partners) are appalled by the intense tiredness which they experience in the first trimester. Sometimes this is so severe that they feel totally unable to function when evening arrives. This fatigue is sometimes aggravated by 'evening sickness'. The assurance that this will pass for most of them, and advice on coping strategies and relaxation, are reassuring and helpful.

The effects of stress on body and mind

An attempt should be made to elicit the causes and the effects of stress from the group itself. The Mitchell method of physiological relaxation is ideally suited for teaching informally and can be reinforced by a handout. Other stress coping strategies should be discussed, e.g. music, a warm bath or shower, a walk or exercise, dancing and massage (see p. 105 and p. 195).

Emotional reactions

The session will not be complete without some discussion of the amazing range of possible psychological and emotional responses to the recently confirmed pregnancy experienced by both partners.

Advice on lifestyle

Work, and how long to continue it, adaptations and alterations in lifestyle if necessary, sport and exercise should all be discussed.

Plenty of opportunity should be given for questions and discussion and the co-operation card, which is given to and carried by most women, explained (see Fig. 4.9).

At the end of these 'early bird' sessions, a leaflet reinforcing the main points and illustrating the exercises and positions for relaxation can be a useful *aide-mémoire*; an additional side-effect of pregnancy is a mental slow-down and forgetfulness! The leaflet should include the obstetric physiotherapist's name and a telephone number for contact if necessary.

STRESS AND RELAXATION

The changes in role being experienced by women in the late twentieth century, combined with a materialistic and more mobile society, its search for wealth and possessions and loss of close family support, impose pressure on us all, and especially on young women and their partners embarking on parenthood. Life crises will always take their toll, and pregnancy and becoming a parent for the first time is certainly one of these.

With the growing prevalence of unemployment throughout the world it is not uncommon for the woman in a partnership to be the sole breadwinner as well as the childbearer. Many women during the early weeks of pregnancy experience extreme fatigue and nausea; to this may be added unsympathetic and demanding employers, moving to larger accommodation and anxieties about finance. Supporting women in the antenatal period presents the obstetric physiotherapist with a priceless opportunity to enable them to understand the causes and physiological effects of stress, to become aware of it in themselves and others, and to be able to control, manage and dissipate it, throughout their lives, whenever it threatens to reach harmful levels.

There is a variety of ways in which the subject of stress can be introduced. Women quickly identify with such experiences as going to the dentist, a job interview or an examination, and will have no difficulties in describing their physiological response. Similarly after a moment's thought they can describe the appearance of someone who is angry, grieving, frightened or in pain.

Physiological effects of stress

The body's response to threat, whether physical or mental, real or imagined, is essentially that of 'fight or flight'. The physical manifestations include, increased heart rate, raised blood pressure, rapid respiration or breath holding. Blood is drained from areas of low priority, e.g. the gastrointestinal tract and the skin, and is diverted to skeletal muscle. The mouth dries, the pupils dilate, the liver releases its glycogen store, blood coagulation time decreases, and the spleen discharges additional red blood cells into the circulation. Sometimes the bladder and bowel may be affected, causing frequency and diarrhoea.

There are certain similarities in joint and muscle response whatever the causative stress. A common theme runs through the positions adopted which combine to produce a posture of tension. These include hunched shoulders, flexed elbows and adducted arms, clenched or clutching hands, and flexed head, trunk, hips, knees and ankles. The face contorts to express the relevant emotion. In anger, the chin juts forward; in grief, pain or fear, it is drawn in and down to the chest. The jaws are frequently clenched together. Examples of stress-causing life events and their suggested rating are shown in Table 4.2.

TEACHING NEUROMUSCULAR CONTROL

The Mitchell method of physiological relaxation

This method utilizes knowledge of the typical stress/tension posture and the reciprocal relaxation of muscle – whereby one group relaxes as the opposing group contracts. Thus, stress-induced tension in the muscles that work to create the typical posture may be released by voluntary contraction of the opposing muscle groups. Proprioceptive receptors in joints and muscle tendons record the resulting position of ease, and this is relayed to and registered in the cerebrum.

Laura Mitchell, who developed this beautifully simple and elegant technique (Mitchell, 1987), devised a series of very specific orders which are given to the areas of the body affected by stress: e.g. for hunched shoulders – 'Pull your shoulders towards your feet. STOP. Feel your shoulders are further away from your ears – your neck may feel longer.' Because of the simplicity and the physiological basis of this method it is suitable for all levels of intellect. Physiotherapists would be wise to use the exact instructions prescribed, which have been developed after many years of trial and error.

Contrast method

The contrast method stems from the work of Edmund Jacobson and involves alternately contracting and relaxing muscle groups progressively round the body to develop recognition of the difference between tension and relaxation (Jacobson, 1938). Although this technique has been taught extensively for many years (*Progressive Relaxation* originally appeared in 1938), some people find that it increases a feeling of tension, which makes it of doubtful benefit for those feeling tense and tired.

Table 4.2 Stress caused by change in lifestyle on a scale of 0–100 (Holmes and Rahe, 1967)

Score	Event	Score	Event
100	Death of spouse	29	Son or daughter leaving
73	Divorce		home
65	Marital separation	29	Trouble with in-laws
63	Jail term	28	Outstanding personal
63	Death of close family		achievement
	member	26	Wife begins or stops work
53	Personal injury or illness	26	Begin or end school
50	Marriage	25	Change in living conditions
47	Fired at work	24	Revision of personal habits
45	Marital reconciliation	23	Trouble with boss
45	Retirement	20	Change in work hours or
44	Change in health of family		conditions
	member	20	Change in residence
40	Pregnancy	20	Change in schools
39	Sex difficulties	19	Change in recreation
39	Gain of new family member	19	Change in church activities
39	Business adjustments	18	Change in social activities
38	Change in financial state	17	Mortgage or loan less than
37	Death of close friend		$10 000
36	Change to different line of	16	Change in sleeping habits
	work	15	Change in number of family
35	Change in number of		get-togethers
	arguments with spouse	15	Change in eating habits
31	Mortgage over $10 000	13	Vacation
30	Foreclosure of mortgage or	12	Christmas
	loan	11	Minor violations of the law
29	Change in responsibilities		
	at work		

Suggestion and visualization

Participants are encouraged to imagine a pleasant and warm environment of their own choice – a park, a garden or a hot sunny day on the beach. Suggestions of ease, comfort and relaxation are given. This technique can be successfully used in combination with most of the other methods.

Touch and massage

All physiotherapists will naturally appreciate the physiological potentials of massage in inducing relaxation and relieving pain. Simple touch can communicate a sense of companionship, caring and sharing, particularly when received from a loving partner. Soothing stroking, effleurage or kneading to appropriate areas may be used with good effect when properly taught.

Breathing

Expiration frequently accompanies the spontaneous release of tension – e.g. a sigh of relief. The outward breath is the relaxation phase of the respiratory cycle; this fact can be utilized to enhance the relaxation response. The very rhythm of slow, easy breathing and its predictability is reassuring and calming. Those who may not remember more complex techniques will almost always be able to rely on this approach.

Whichever method is used, thought must be given to the position in which it is taught. Initially the woman should be comfortable and fully supported in lying, side lying or sitting (Fig. 4.10). As she becomes more proficient she should be able to adapt the concepts to less supported postures, even standing. However, the obstetric physiotherapist must be aware that as pregnancy progresses and the weight of the uterus and its contents increases, aortocaval occlusion may occur in the supine position resulting in hypotension and syncope (faintness) see p. 33. If this occurs the woman should be encouraged to roll on to her side. To avoid this occurring in late pregnancy, the use of the fully supine position for long periods should be avoided.

Through the course of antenatal classes, it is hoped that women and their partners will become increasingly able to identify the effects of stress in those around them, and more particularly in themselves. This recognition is an essential part in the development of 'body awareness', and enables women to know when to use the appropriate stress-reducing technique to induce a relaxation response. It should be emphasized that this approach is not limited to pregnancy and labour, but should become a life-long philosophy. The obstetric physiotherapist must not forget that formally taught relaxation techniques, as described above, are *not* the only ways to manage stress. Yoga, biofeedback, movement, music, eating, warm water, and countless other alternative coping strategies, all have a place. People should be guided and encouraged to seek their own individual solutions.

EXERCISE AND PREGNANCY

It has long been suggested that women whose lives were filled with hard active work and who were consequently physically fit tended to have easier labours than those with a more sedentary lifestyle. (Exodus 1:19; Vaughan, 1951). Until this century, however, most women were grateful simply to survive the multiple hazards of pregnancy, labour

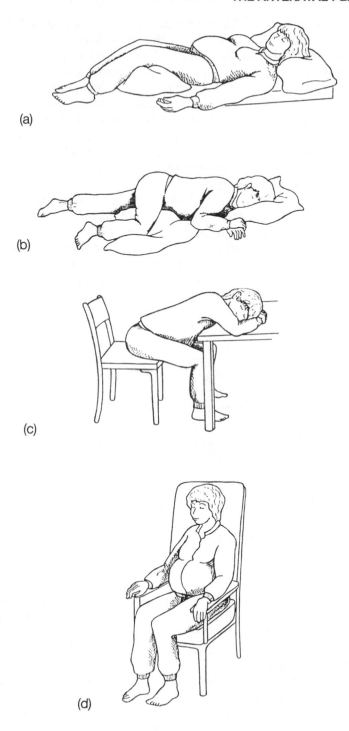

Figure 4.10 Women should be encouraged to practise relaxation in a variety of positions.

and the puerperium; a healthy baby was an additional bonus! With the environmental and medical advances that have led to safer childbirth and a substantial drop in the maternal and fetal mortality rates has come an enormous change in expectations of parturient women. Some, particularly middle-class professionals, approach childbirth as they would a job or an examination – they study, prepare and *train* for it. 'Moderate exercise' has long been a prescription for mothers-to-be, and many different programmes of exercise specifically for pregnancy have been devised (Randall, 1948; Balaskas, 1983; Delyser, 1983; Van Zyl, 1985). Because of the current fitness craze for exercise of all sorts, many women want to continue their chosen sport or activity throughout pregnancy. Others, conscious of being relatively 'unfit' (in the athletic sense of the word), feel that they ought to improve their strength, flexibility, stamina and endurance in preparation for pregnancy and childbirth – or actually during the months after their pregnancy has been confirmed. All these women probably hope that exercise will give them an easier pregnancy and a shorter labour, and enable them to cope more efficiently with the exhausting early days of new mother-hood.

The physiological effects of exercise and sporting activities are well documented (Artal et al., 1991) and affect all the major systems of the body. Although considerable work has been done on the response to exercise in non-pregnant women and girls, there is less information available dealing with the specific effects of exercise on those who are pregnant; but it seems certain that however fit a woman may be, a high level of exertion will have a greater effect on her physiological and endocrine responses if she is pregnant, and will also affect her baby and its environment (Hall and Kaufmann, 1987).

Risks of intensive exercise in pregnancy

The following risks can be fairly confidently stated.

Maternal risks:

1. There is a greater risk of musculoskeletal trauma because of connective tissue laxity. Pregnant women are more accident-prone, because of the substantial change in body weight and shape. This may be compounded by changes in perception and slightly impaired cognitive function.
2. There will be increased demand on a cardiovascular system already altered by pregnancy.
3. Hypoglycaemia may arise.

Fetal risks:

1. Fetal distress could occur during strenuous and prolonged exercise because of the selective redistribution of blood flow away from the splanchnic organs and hence the placenta and towards the working muscles. In the normal healthy woman and during mild and moderate exercise this will only rarely be a problem.
2. Intrauterine growth retardation could result.
3. Fetal malformations, arising from the teratogenic effects of a raised maternal core temperature during the first trimester, are possible.
4. Pre-term labour, with or without delivery, may occur particularly in women unaccustomed to vigorous exercise.

Contraindications

Contraindications to vigorous exercise in pregnancy are listed in Table 4.3. Women in these categories tend to be aware of their limitations; there is no reason, however, why routine antenatal exercises for leg circulation and the pelvic floor, and gentle movements to maintain good posture and back comfort (e.g. pelvic tilting), should not be taught and practised regularly.

Activities that may be contraindicated include competitive and contact sports; and activities such as horse riding, skiing, water-skiing and scuba diving carry far greater risks when a woman is pregnant.

Table 4.3 Contraindications to vigorous exercise in pregnancy

Absolute	Relative
1 Cardiovascular disease	1 Women unused to high levels of exertion
2 Acute infection	2 Blood disorders such as sickle-cell disease and anaemia
3 A history of recurrent spontaneous abortion (miscarriage) or perceived risk of pre-term labour	3 Thyroid disease
4 Multiple pregnancy	4 Diabetes – however, a carefully supervised programme of *gentle* exercising may actually benefit some diabetic patients (Artal et al., 1991)
5 Bleeding or ruptured membranes	5 Extreme maternal overweight or underweight
6 Severe hypertension	6 Breech presentation during the third trimester
7 Suspected IUGR or fetal distress	
8 Thrombophlebitis or pulmonary embolism	

Guidelines for women exercising during pregnancy

1. Jerky, bouncing, ballistic movements and activities should be avoided.
2. Regular exercise sessions – at least three times a week – are safer than intermittent bursts of activity.
3. Careful 'warm-up' should precede vigorous exercise, which must always be followed by a 'cool-down' or gradual decline in activity.
4. Strenuous exercise must be avoided in hot, humid weather, or when the pregnant woman is pyrexial.
5. The maternal heart rate should not exceed 140 beats per minute, and vigorous exercise should not continue for longer than 15 minutes.
6. Fluid must be taken before, during and after exertion to avoid dehydration, and energy intake must be sufficient for the needs of pregnancy plus the exercise.
7. As with women beginning exercise outside pregnancy, it is essential that those accustomed to a sedentary lifestyle should start with low-intensity physical activity – walking, swimming, stationary bicycling or yoga are probably ideal – and they should only increase activity levels gradually according to their own individual tolerance capacity.
8. Exercise should be decided by the limitations imposed by pregnancy – the competitive element must be excluded.

The obstetric physiotherapist will be able to advise and encourage women wishing to continue or begin appropriate physical activity with the consent of their doctors. They should be encouraged to exercise 'little and often', to allow their bodies to dictate the length and strength of their activity, and to decrease the intensity and frequency of suitable exercise in the final stages of pregnancy. However, it must always be appreciated that many women do not wish to participate in group activities – nor are they interested in exercising formally on their own. They should *not* be made to feel guilty. Where it is obvious that a woman's daily workload is minimal, it may be possible to persuade her to walk a reasonable distance regularly, or to use an exercise bicycle. The obstetric physiotherapist, is possibly the best-trained member of the caring team to assess whether the total daily workload of a pregnant woman is too great or too little, and to show her how she may remedy this (Chamberlain, 1984).

Although exercise has undoubted physical and psychological benefits at all times, it has yet to be proved that a particular regimen has any effect on the length or ease of labour and delivery. Recent work, however, is beginning to show that exercise and physical activity, in healthy women with a non-compromised fetus, may actually prevent pre-term delivery (Berkowitz et al., 1983; Jarrett and Spellacy, 1983). Alternatively, the importance of rest and the part it plays in helping to increase birth weight is also being recognized (Manshande et al., 1987).

What is indisputable is the fact that physically fit, athletic women recover more rapidly after the birth than those who spent a less active pregnancy and are athletically unfit.

Swimming and water exercise in pregnancy

Swimming is possibly the perfect pregnancy exercise. Even non-swimmers can benefit from a programme of exercise and relaxation in a pool. The buoyancy of the water supports the mother's increasing body weight, enabling her to continue with the excellent toning and strengthening activity which increases her physical fitness and endurance, as well as promoting her sense of well-being.

The regular swimmer should be encouraged to continue with her normal routine, adapting her strokes and the distance of her swims to her advancing pregnancy; as with all other sports, she should be warned to 'listen to her body' and slow down as necessary. It is recommended that three 20-minute sessions per week are preferable to one hour-long session (Katz, 1985). Women should 'warm up' prior to their main swim, and 'cool down' following it. A session of relaxation aided by the buoyancy of the water can be most therapeutic, particularly in the final trimester. For non-swimmers a programme of suitable exercises can be suggested which should include activities for the legs, arms and trunk, as well as 'water walking' and relaxation. Many swimming pools and leisure centres now provide special sessions for pregnant and postnatal women, but the obstetric physiotherapist who is interested in running this sort of class and who does not have a hydrotherapy qualification will find ample material and suggestions in *Aquarobics* by Glenda Baum and *Swimming Through Your Pregnancy* by Jane Katz (see Further Reading).

Yoga

Yoga is an increasingly popular activity during pregnancy. Although there are many similarities between some yoga positions and exercises traditionally used by physiotherapists, the emphasis placed on stretch and mobility may not be appropriate for all women. It is unwise for health-care professionals to incorporate aspects of this philosophically different approach to their classes without proper training in yoga. Women who express interest in this form of exercise should be directed to properly accredited teachers.

DIET AND WEIGHT GAIN IN PREGNANCY

That 'we are what we eat' is undoubtedly true; but the assertion that pregnant women need to 'eat for two' in terms of quantity is now quite out of date. An antenatal weight gain of 10–12.5 kg (22–28 lb) is recommended for optimal fetal growth (American Academy of Pediatrics, 1983), its approximate distribution can be seen from Fig. 2.5. A mother's height, her weight for height at the start of the pregnancy and her weight gain can all influence the size of her fetus (Truswell, 1985). In general, very overweight women excluded, bigger mothers tend to have heavier babies, and the greater the pregnancy weight gain the heavier the baby (Abrams et al., 1986). The average woman will lose most of the weight she gains during pregnancy, retaining probably 1–1.5 kg (2–3 lb) – but most women are heavier after the birth of the baby than before (one in ten retaining excessive weight), and the more weight over 9 kg (20 lb) that is put on, the more remains (Greene et al., 1988; Samra et al., 1988).

The total energy requirement for pregnancy is calculated to be 335 MJ (80 000 kcal) and it used to be suggested that pregnant women needed an extra 1 MJ (239 kcal) per day (Hytten and Leitch, 1971). However, it is increasingly being recognized that there is a deficit between the energy cost of pregnancy (the amount deposited as new tissues, plus the associated increase in basal metabolic rate) and energy intake (Van Raaij et al., 1987), and that the main mechanisms by which the pregnant body is able to save energy are by adjustments in physical activity, an increase in work efficiency and an adaptation of the metabolic response to food.

The five basic food elements – proteins, fats, carbohydrates, vitamins and minerals – are all necessary to maintain the mother's health during pregnancy, and to help her baby grow and develop normally (Table 4.4).

Because so many people have unbalanced diets – a study in Belfast (McKnight and Merrett, 1987) showed this figure to be 38.7% – it is most important to introduce the subject of eating well in pregnancy at 'early bird' classes, and to refer regularly to healthy eating and pregnancy weight gain during antenatal classes. Women and their partners may need help to realize that a good diet need not be expensive, nor even require much preparation time. It is perfectly possible, by studying what is for sale in shops from week to week and making use of seasonal foods, to eat well and inexpensively. It is useful to know that 'meat and two veg' do not necessarily constitute the best diet; an easily prepared meal of a glass of milk, a sandwich (preferably wholemeal bread) made with meat, fish, eggs or cheese, and salad, plus some fruit, is nutritious, cheap and very quick to prepare – an important fact for the pregnant woman. It is also much better for her unborn baby than a sticky bun, a canned drink and a chocolate bar! Because of current 'food scares' (salmonella in eggs and poultry, and listeriosis – soft cheeses using unpasteurized milk were implicated), it is most important for obstetric physiotherapists to keep up-to-date with the most recent recommendations as to what is and what is not safe to eat during pregnancy. Their clients will want to discuss the latest government guidelines and may well be worried that something they have eaten or drunk could have harmed their baby. A physiotherapist who does not know the answer to such questions must find out or refer the mother to an appropriate professional.

It is probably useful for women to know that latest findings suggest that the metabolic efficiency of lactating women is enhanced, so that they may not need to increase their energy intake to the level suggested by some authorities (Illingworth et al., 1986). This fact could explain why some women complain of putting on weight instead of losing it while they are breast-feeding. It would appear that the metabolic adjustments made by the human body during pregnancy, in order to grow a healthy baby without requiring large extra amounts of food, continue during lactation.

Table 4.4 Basic Food Elements

	Found in	*Needed for*
Proteins	Meat, fish, eggs, pulses, cereals, cheese, milk, wholemeal cereals, nuts, bread	Body building and repair. Only 6 g extra required per day
Fats	Butter, margarine, oil, meat, some fish, nuts, some vegetables (e.g. avocado)	Supplying energy and vitamins – but should not be eaten in excess because they can lead to excessive fat deposits
Carbohydrates	Potatoes, bread, cereals, sugar	Supplying energy, but foods containing sugar must be restricted if excess weight gain is occurring
Vitamins	Found in most foods, particularly in fruit and vegetables	Essential for normal health. Folate (found in liver and kidneys, wholegrain cereals, nuts and legumes) is the only vitamin whose requirements double in pregnancy. Its deficiency has been implicated in the development of neural tube defects
Minerals	Meat, liver, kidneys, chicken, fish, eggs, dark green vegetables, milk (calcium)	Iron, zinc and iodine intake needs to be slightly increased; calcium requirements are doubled during pregnancy
Dietary fibre	Wholegrain cereals, wholemeal bread, fruits, nuts, leafy vegetables	Important because of the tendency for pregnant women to become constipated

Alcohol

The American Surgeon General (Sokol et al., 1989) has suggested that pregnant women should not consume alcohol. Although no such recommendation has been made in the UK, the fact that excessive drinking during pregnancy causes a condition known as fetal alcohol syndrome (Jones et al., 1973) which presents as growth retardation, craniofacial and cardiac defects and mental retardation, and that alcohol has been linked with increased risk of spontaneous abortion, stillbirth, congenital abnormalities and abnormal neurobehavioural development (Sokol, 1983), has led to pregnant women being advised to restrict their alcohol consumption to two or three measures per week (1 measure = 10 g alcohol).

Many women planning pregnancy are now aware that it is advisable to eliminate alcohol from their diet prior to conception, and those who are pregnant increasingly refrain from all but the occasional glass of wine, spirits or beer. This is certainly a subject which should be discussed at 'early bird' classes, when suggestions for non-alcoholic drinks can be made.

It is also most important that women and their partners understand that the alcoholic content of similar drinks varies enormously. Half a pint (quarter litre) of some beers may contain one unit of alcohol, whereas others – lager in particular – may actually hold five units per half pint.

What is a unit/measure of alcohol?

1 single pub measure of spirits
1 small glass of sherry or fortified wine
1 small glass of table wine
1/2 pint (0.28 litre) of ordinary lager, beer or cider
1/4 pint (0.14 litre) of strong lager, beer or cider

From 'Sensible Drinking' Health Education Authority.

Smoking in pregnancy and later

There is strong evidence to show that maternal smoking, and possibly maternal passive smoking, is harmful to the fetus, and that it can affect the pregnancy and the subsequent development and health of children after they are born. It is accepted that there is a direct link between smoking and low birth weight (Meyer and Tonascia, 1977), which can, of course, be a problem in itself. It has been shown (MacArthur and Knox, 1988) that the weights of babies born to women who stopped smoking by 16 weeks' gestation were approximately 215 g greater than the weights of babies born to persistent smokers, and were similar to those of babies born to non-smokers. Even if women gave up later than

16 weeks, their babies weighed more than those of mothers who continued smoking throughout their pregnancy. However, Burton et al. (1989) found that the placentas of women who smoked during pregnancy, and even the placentas of those who gave up smoking during the course of their pregnancies, showed changes that impair gaseous interchange. These changes did not occur in non-smokers nor in women who gave up smoking before they became pregnant. The implications of these findings are clear – women must be encouraged to give up smoking before conception.

Smoking is also associated with fetal hypoxia, intrauterine growth retardation, placental abruption, premature rupture of membranes, miscarriage, premature delivery and low Apgar scores. It has been demonstrated ultrasonically (Pinette et al., 1989) that there is an acceleration of placental maturation, and therefore of premature senescence and calcification leading to poor function in smokers. The problems do not cease with the birth of the baby. A review of literature dealing with the postnatal sequelae of parental smoking during and after delivery (Stevens et al., 1988) shows that perinatal mortality, sudden infant death syndrome (SIDS), lactation, respiratory illness and hospitalizations, hyperkinesis (hyperactivity) and general intellectual ability were all adversely affected by smoking in pregnancy. When children are brought up in families where smoking continues, long-term after-effects have been reported including increased childhood mortality, postnatal growth retardation and chronic respiratory illnesses.

The damaging effects of smoking on the fetus during pregnancy and on infants and children later must be pointed out at 'early bird' classes. It is a difficult habit to stop, but many women will be motivated to do so. The obstetric physiotherapist, who will be meeting clients as early as 10–12 weeks of gestation, is in the ideal position to direct women and their partners to local agencies and self-help groups, who will support them in their decision and advise and help them accordingly.

Medication in pregnancy

Since the thalidomide disaster in the 1960s, when an antiemetic drug given in early pregnancy to women suffering from nausea and vomiting was found to be the cause of severe limb and organ deformities in their babies, it has become obvious that the placenta does not act as a barrier to harmful chemicals. It is important for women who find that they are pregnant, and those likely to become pregnant, to understand that some drugs can damage the developing fetus, and the subject of medication should be mentioned at 'early bird' classes. Even though the most sensitive time for embryonic damage (up to 13–14 weeks) will probably have passed by the time this class takes place, women and their partners need to know that it is not only doctor-prescribed medicines that can damage babies, but also self-prescribed treatments.

The mother's health must be the primary consideration, but where a woman becomes ill in pregnancy or has a pre-existing condition that obliges her to take medication, doctors will always try to use drugs with the least known risk, changing original prescriptions to substances known to be safer. Drugs with major teratogenic effects are rare; but retinoic acid (used to treat severe acne), some cytotoxic drugs and radiochemicals can cause grave damage. Pregnant women whose fetuses have been exposed to these substances are offered terminations. Tetracycline taken in pregnancy is known to cause subsequent discolouration of children's teeth, and many other drugs in common usage can cause damage of various sorts and degrees depending on the stage in the pregnancy that they were taken.

It is important for women to realize that they have a responsibility in this context too; they should always remind their doctor, dentist or pharmacist that they are pregnant whenever medication is prescribed or when they buy 'over the counter' remedies of any kind. Although it is probably safest to avoid unnecessary medication during pregnancy, simple therapies such as paracetamol for headaches or colds and antacids for heartburn are commonly prescribed without ill effect.

Looking ahead to the puerperium, some drugs are contraindicated in breast-feeding women; most drugs, however, only appear in breast milk in quantities small enough not to be harmful to the infant. (See Further Reading.)

Addictive drugs in pregnancy

Although some centres have pockets of drug users, addiction in the UK is not as great as it is in other parts of the world. Many regular drug abusers will have other health problems and probably poor social conditions too; they may not attend regularly for antenatal care so that the fetus is at risk from several sources.

Congenital abnormalities have been reported following the use of the narcotics, LSD and the amphetamines. Placental insufficiency, intra-uterine growth retardation and perinatal mortality are all increased where women use heroin and its derivatives. A major problem is the effect of narcotic drug withdrawal on the fetus and neonate which can prove fatal if not very carefully managed both during pregnancy and the immediate postpartum period. However, the prognosis for the infant of the drug-addicted mother is good if the mother cooperates with antenatal care and drug control (Bolton, 1987).

Multiple pregnancies

Twin pregnancies occur about once in every 100 pregnancies in the UK; the incidence is much higher in West African and Afro-Caribbean women, but lower in other parts of the world such as Japan. Although triplets, quadruplets and quintuplets occur naturally much less frequently, with the advent of some infertility treatments the rate has increased.

Twins may arise from the splitting of one fertilized ovum (monozygotic or uniovular) or from the fertilization of two ova (dizygotic or binovular). There may be a family history of twins, and the tendency for double ovulation will be passed on to other women in the family. The original diagnosis will be made either because of a uterus which appears very much larger than it should for the stage of pregnancy, or by ultrasonic scanning.

Pregnancy discomfort and problems can be intensified, and towards the end of gestation women can be extremely uncomfortable because of increased pressure from the very large uterus. Pre-term labour is a definite possibility, and it is advisable for mothers expecting twins to book in to a course of antenatal classes scheduled to finish rather earlier than would have been necessary for singleton pregnancies.

PLANNING AND RUNNING ANTENATAL PREPARATION FOR LABOUR AND PARENTHOOD CLASSES

When planning new antenatal courses it is imperative for the team to explore the perceived needs of the prospective clientele, for these vary from area to area and from time to time within the same community. Whether urban or rural, populations develop and change, and the ethnic and socioeconomic composition can be dramatically altered. When taking over responsibility for ongoing classes the obstetric physiotherapist will be wise to appraise the situation, and adapt the programme if necessary. Each fresh group of women will be different, and therefore a very flexible approach is essential. The old-fashioned (but in some ways easier) didactic teacher–student relationship should be avoided, and group 'sharing' should be encouraged, with the professional facilitating and assisting all to contribute and gain. From the first class, women should be encouraged to participate in deciding the aims, objectives and content of their particular course.

Class arrangements

Environment

Antenatal classes are frequently held in very unsuitable places – nooks and crannies, basements and windowless 'cupboards'. Ideally the parentcraft accommodation should be purpose-built, carpeted, light and airy, with windows looking, if not on a green and pleasant environment, at least out! It must be conveniently sited for transport and ease of access, and be large enough to include an area for sitting and chatting, drinking tea or coffee, and reading books or magazines from its library. There should be a clear, separate area for exercising and relaxation, and toilets, refreshment and washing facilities and ample storage space must be *en suite*. A homely, welcoming atmosphere can be fostered by attractive curtains, pictures, plants and flowers. All furniture and other equipment, including mats, wedges, bean bags, chairs and pillows should be chosen for their durability, and with ergonomic and safety principles in mind. False economies must be avoided, and everything must be 'easy care' so that hygiene can be easily maintained. Several long mirrors are essential. Notice boards displaying news items of current interest, advertisements of articles for sale and photographs of baby 'graduates' complete the obstetric physiotherapist's dream!

The advantages of an 'early bird' class are generally recognized, and are discussed on p. 96. Commonly the main antenatal course consists of six to eight sessions, and usually begins around 28–30 weeks' gestation. This formula suits women who commence their maternity leave early. However, in the present employment climate many women are remaining at work for as long as possible; in some cases, to term. This poses problems for class organizers concerning both the day of the week (women will become progressively more tired as the week goes by), and the time of day (there may be difficulty in having time off with pay during working hours). Obstetric physiotherapists and their managers must be sensitive to the best interests of their clients, and where necessary offer sessions in what might be considered professionally to be unsocial hours. Ideally groups should consist of 8–16 people, but it should always be possible to integrate latecomers, and women should be encouraged to fit in classes as and when they can.

In some areas it will be possible to run regular courses of eight weekly classes, whereas in other areas it may be better to present a more limited programme over four weeks. Women expecting their first baby may welcome a longer course; those who already have children may appreciate a more condensed programme. While many centres have traditionally concentrated on 'women only' classes, the greater involvement of men in childbearing and rearing has made courses for couples increasingly popular. While there are obvious advantages, the disadvantages must not be overlooked. There may be times when women will be inhibited in their discussion by the presence of men, and vice versa. It may be helpful to split the group at some stage during the session to overcome this. Providing staff for evening sessions is another consideration.

Separate classes for teenagers are being run successfully in some localities where there is a consistently high number of young pregnant women. For the occasional very young girl, individual care may be more appropriate, but in the majority of cases a well-run group can absorb and support pregnant women of any age.

Where there is a substantial ethnic group with language problems and extreme cultural differences, it may well prove beneficial to the women and their carers to make separate arrangements. This is usually only necessary where the women are very sheltered or newly arrived in the country. Carers should take the trouble to inform themselves about and respect religious and cultural differences. However, a community can only be strengthened by its families working together and seeking to understand one another from the start.

From time to time it may be necessary and useful to hold a one-day 'crash course' or 'labour day' for those women and their partners who are unable, for one reason or another, to attend a full course, whatever its length. With the increasing interest in fitness, specific antenatal exercise groups, some of them in water, have been developed. It is a nice question whether or not it is the role of a health service to provide this facility, or whether this is something for which an individual must make her own arrangements. However, it is most certainly in the interests of the health service that the organizers of such classes be appropriately qualified. Where analgesia using transcutaneous nerve stimulation (TNS) is regularly available for women during labour, it may well prove more efficient and cost-effective to run a special session for those who wish to make use of it.

It is recognized that, even in the non-pregnant, an individual's attention span is limited. Sessions of two to two-and-a-half hours allow for plenty of variety in teaching and learning methods, and a break in the middle for refreshment, toileting and informal socializing. Every course plan should be tailored to the locality, and be capable of instant modification! Therefore the following plans must be regarded as 'thought triggers' only, and not as the final word on the subject. For the purpose of description it is assumed that the obstetric physiotherapists will be working with midwives and health visitors, although it is realized that they may well be responsible for the entire programme, particularly if they are working in the private sector. It is also assumed that women will have attended one or more early classes. If this is not the case, earlier topics, such as the cooperation card, should be included.

An eight-week daytime course

Week 1. Introductions – class and class leaders to meet each other. This is the ideal opportunity to elicit immediate problems, worries and special requests.

A discussion on baby equipment, clothing, safety around the home and car seats.

Revision of the physical changes of pregnancy, and the introduction of a suitable, short general programme of exercises to promote comfort, mobility and strength, including (for example) foot movements, pelvic tilting in a variety of positions, knee-bends to 'curtsey' sitting, wall press-ups, pelvic floor contractions, squatting (modified if necessary), 'tailor' sitting and posture correction and back care.

Week 2. A discussion on infant feeding, emphasizing the benefits of breast-feeding.

Relaxation – a discussion on the causes and effects of stress, and coping stategies. Detailed and leisurely instruction and practice, using a variety of positions, of one method of relaxation – e.g. the Mitchell method.

The needs of the group will sometimes be better met by introducing relaxation in the first class instead of the broad programme of exercises, and concentrating on exercise in the second class.

Week 3. A discussion of the first stage of labour: what can happen, what to do and whom to contact.

Coping strategies for:

Early labour: baths, showers, light meals, resting, mobilizing, reading, music, time filling!
Stronger contractions: positions of comfort, relaxation and breathing, abdominal and back massage, the use of baths and birthpools.
Analgesia, including introduction to TNS.

Week 4. Discussion of end of first stage and the second stage of labour, and a visit to the labour ward.

Coping with the end of first stage – how breathing may change, back massage, alternative positions, use of Entonox, dealing with premature pushing urges, pushing, episiotomies.

Week 5. Further discussion of second stage, positions for pushing, delivery of the baby.

Immediate emotional response and early care of the baby.

The first feed and immediate post-delivery exercises.

Week 6. Discussion with a recently delivered mother accompanied by her baby, experience of labour and early postnatal problems and discomforts, and how to cope with them. Comfortable feeding positions and early postnatal exercises. Visit to the postnatal ward.

Week 7. An evening session for women and labour companions. A practical rehearsal of labour, demonstrating and using relaxation, positioning, breathing and massage, second-stage positions and pushing. Discussion on emotional support needs, and physical support in labour and the puerperium. The role of the father. Second visit to labour ward – meet a new baby!

Week 8. Visit from a local health visitor. Discussion of previous week's evening session. Rapid summary of labour, inductions, discussion of caesarean section (epidural or general anaesthetic, see pp. 202, 262), forceps deliveries, postnatal depression and problems. Looking forward – arrangements for class reunion.

Exercise and relaxation should be included where possible during every class and the women must understand their purpose. Antenatal 'aches and pains' should be dealt with in the class as they arise. Where courses have to be shorter, the team and the participating parents must jointly decide on priorities and exclusions.

Regrettably, in some centres financial restraints result in classes being available mainly to primigravidae and only exceptionally to multigravidae. Ideally, any pregnant woman who wants to attend antenatal classes should be free to do so, no matter how many babies she has had. Where courses are available to multigravidae, they are often a condensed or 'refresher' version, but there are great advantages in mixing women of differing parity.

The special needs of multigravidae (which can be met in any class) include talking through previous labour experiences, updating their knowledge of labour management, considering the impending changes in the family, and how to make time for the baby as well as the existing children. Relaxation becomes more important as parity increases. In some respects a multigravid woman will be more self-confident, but age and experience bring other anxieties – she may well feel that her luck is running out: will this baby be normal? What could go wrong in this labour? How will she cope with more than one child? Many of these feelings, problems and their solutions can be fully shared in a group of mixed parity; women can be very supportive of each other.

Although these guidelines may appear rather formal, it must be remembered that the sensitive obstetric physiotherapist will be constantly alert to the day-to-day needs of the individuals in the class, and will be prepared to divert from the original course plan whenever necessary. At the same time the physiotherapist must be able to guide and control discussion. While group discussion can change attitudes and must be encouraged, women and their partners *do* come to antenatal classes to gain information, and may resent the conversation being monopolized by a few vociferous participants. Antenatal educators must not fall into the trap of solely preparing their parents for the 'grand finale' of pregnancy – labour. They must always remember that labour, particularly for the primigravida, is in fact the 'overture' to a totally new lifestyle which will gradually evolve and which may need time for thought and mutual consideration until it becomes acceptable.

Many people, both women and men, have great difficulty when they are expecting their first child in actually appreciating the changes that parenthood can bring. It is extremely important during antenatal classes to look to the future, and to stimulate thought about the

the way the parents will care for their baby, the sort of parents they will be, and how they will reorganize their lifestyle to cope with this major life event.

Antenatal self-help strategies for good maternal postnatal adjustment.

1. Try to make friends with couples who have young children.
2. Reduce housework and its importance.
3. Encourage partners to spend more time at home.
4. Cut down on your social life, but don't give it up entirely.
5. Continue your outside interests, but reduce your responsibilities.
6. Try not to move house less than six months before or six months after the birth.
7. Go to antenatal classes with your partner.
8. Think about organizing someone to babysit occasionally and maybe to help out at home too if possible.

The transition to parenthood

The confirmation of a pregnancy is greeted by a wide range of emotions from women and their partners, joy and satisfaction if the pregnancy is a planned and wanted one; ambivalence, which can turn to acceptance and pleasure, even if it was unplanned; despair and rejection when the pregnancy is unwanted. The 'interesting condition' and 'happy event', which is how pregnancy and birth use to be described in days gone by, may be neither interesting nor happy, if unwanted! Even women and men who have struggled with infertility over the years, undergoing all sorts of physically and psychologically demanding treatments, may, as the wildly hoped-for pregnancy progresses, develop physical and emotional problems. Pitt (1978), in *Feelings about Childbirth*, says that a period of adjustment is needed when even a greatly wanted object, previously unattainable, becomes a reality. Mixed feelings will be present in all expectant parents during and even after pregnancy, and both partners will have fears about what the new baby will do to their relationship and lifestyle. Condon (1985) mentions the significant potential losses many women may sustain as a result of becoming a mother; career (halted or altered), their dyadic marital relationship, their figure, freedom and social activities, among others. Possible threats such as physical damage during the birth, and how they will cope as a parent, will also take their toll. He suggests that depression could be caused by the impending losses, and anxiety by the threats – neither of which is uncommon during pregnancy. However, the major rewards of pregnancy, to offset these, are said to be intimately linked to a sense of love and attachment to the fetus or fantasy child.

Whether classes are for women alone or for both partners, it is important for all those involved in running them to be aware of the wide range of psychological as well as physical discomforts that can be experienced by both men and women. Contrary to popular belief, pregnancy is not automatically a time of increased well-being for expectant parents. In fact, Condon (1987) found that increased psychological well-being during pregnancy was reported by only 10–15% of women, and 5–10% of men. Twenty per cent of men noticed substantial deterioration in emotional well-being, and 10% experienced severe physical symptoms. Women reported a significantly higher prevalence of both psychological and physical symptoms than men; first-time expectant parents experienced *less* physical symptomatology than more experienced ones. The symptoms that were included in this study were:

1. *Psychological*:
   - anxiety
   - depression
   - irritability
   - impaired concentration
   - social withdrawal
   - feeling 'disorganized'
   - feeling 'not in control'
2. *Physical*:
   - energy lack
   - sleep disturbance
   - appetite disturbance
   - decreased sexual drive
   - aches/pains
   - nausea/vomiting

The summary of comparisons of male and female symptomatology, averaging over all the symptoms, gives an interesting insight into the effects of pregnancy on both partners (Table 4.5).

Table 4.5 Comparison of male and female symptomatology in pregnancy (Condon, 1985)

Symptom level	Women (approx. %)	Men (approx. %)
Psychological		
improvement	10–15	5–10
no change	35	70
deterioration	50	20
Physical		
severe or very severe	25	10
moderate	25	15
mild	50	75

Fathers

Although it is the woman's body that conceives, carries and gives birth to the baby, and which is equipped by nature to provide everything in the way of nourishment the infant requires in the first few months of life, parenthood is usually a shared experience. Fathers too go through a sequence of changes as they leave independence or the 'cosy twosome', or face a new addition to an established family. They have gradually to accept the responsibility that the birth of children inevitably brings.

In a few societies ritual *couvade* is practised by men. Special dress, confinement, restriction of activities, avoidance of polluting substances and mock labour are all said to signify magical protection of the mother and infant, symbolic expression of the bond between father and child and the acceptance of fatherhood. As has been seen, many men in our society today also complain of a variety of physical and emotional health problems during their partners' pregnancies and in the early postpartum period as well. It has been suggested that this is an expression of the father's subjective involvement in the pregnancy (Munroe and Munroe, 1971) and also an expression of profound caring for their partner and unborn child (Clinton, 1985). Clinton (1986) mentions some of the risk factors associated with this form of *couvade*; men who experience health problems in the year prior to pregnancy, ethnic minorities, those with previous children, low incomes and with a high affective involvement in the pregnancy are more likely to have problems. Psychological and economic stress could also play a part.

The obstetric physiotherapist must also understand the anxieties expectant fathers may have: 'Will I be able to cope with her distress in labour?'; 'Will I be a good father?'; 'Will I manage to provide for my family if my partner isn't working?'; 'Will this enlarged, moody female ever again become the slim, happy, active girl I used to know?'; 'What is this baby going to do to our social life – we'll be tied down'; 'Will sex *ever* be the same again?'. Liebenberg (1974) mentioned the additional fears that fathers have of 'losing' their spouse to the baby, as well as of 'losing' the new infant to their spouse. These are some of the doubts and fears men have and which they are often unable to express. In the same way that pregnant women benefit from meeting and talking with recently delivered mothers, expectant fathers will gain from the experience of sharing their problems with a father who has 'lived through' this developmental crisis. Some centres now arrange regular evenings for this sort of meeting, often led by an articulate father who can involve the other men.

Antenatal care of the breasts and preparation for breast-feeding

Chloe Fisher, a senior community midwife in Oxford, has described breast-feeding as 'a wonderful, programmed human interaction which gives the mother intense satisfaction, and her baby all it requires to sustain life for many months' (Inch, 1987). Perhaps the best preparation for successful and happy breast-feeding comes long before pregnancy, during childhood in fact. Children who are brought up in an environment where babies are breast-fed will grow up aware that this physiologically normal method of nourishing the newborn can be natural, easy and pleasurable for both mother and baby. Having seen mothers breast-feeding, young women will have confidence in their own bodies being able to provide milk, and their babies knowing how to take it.

A survey to explore the attitudes of teenagers to breast-feeding (Gregg, 1989) was carried out in Liverpool, where only 30–35% of babies were breast-fed. Only 18% of these 14- and 15-year-old girls and boys had been breast-fed themselves, and although 40% of the girls and 28% of the boys had seen relatives breast-feeding, 95% of the girls and 84% of the boys had seen a relative bottle-feeding. The majority of the pupils thought that breast-feeding was healthier than bottle-feeding and more natural, but 60% thought that bottle-feeding was convenient compared to 11% for breast-feeding; 36% thought bottle-feeding was modern compared to 4% for breast-feeding; and 8% of the teenagers – who may only be a few years away from becoming parents themselves – thought that breast-feeding was rude. The majority of these boys and girls felt that breast-feeding should be carried out alone at home and that it was embarrassing to feed anywhere else. In order to prevent these rather rigid attitudes in teenagers, it does seem that education to encourage young parents to embark on breast-feeding must begin in the earliest school years so that the breast is not regarded as a purely sexual object.

It is a matter of grave concern at the present time that twice as many mothers in social class 1 breast-feed their babies (87%) compared with those in social class 5 (43%). Equally, it is disturbing that although 64% of mothers start breast-feeding, only 22% are still doing so at six months (Office of Population Censuses and Surveys, 1985–86; Lancet, 1988).

Antenatal advice on breast care has changed a great deal in recent years, so that it is now limited to a few main points:

1. As soon as mothers are aware of their increasing breast size they will probably feel more comfortable in a good supporting brassière of the correct measurement and cup size. Women with very heavy breasts benefit from wearing a brassière at night. Most of the increase in breast size takes place in the early months of pregnancy, and from the fifth or sixth month the mother will probably be able to wear the nursing brassière which will see her through the first few months of lactation.

   Many young women are accustomed to being 'bra-less' these days and may not like the idea of having to be 'upholstered' during pregnancy and while breast-feeding. If they can understand that the breast is not a self-supporting structure, and that its increased weight could lead to drooping and sagging later in life, most will see the benefit of a good uplift. Some women complain of upper backache if they are very heavy-breasted – for these people a well-made supportive brassière is essential. Simple elbow circling, and thoracic spine flexion and extension, can help relieve this problem.

2. Advice on nipple care during pregnancy used to include 'toughening' them by rubbing with a rough towel, hardening them by applying alcohol and rolling them between the fingers and thumb. Research has shown that none of these techniques is beneficial (RCM, 1991). Today, the main advice given is that women avoid the use of soap on the breasts at the end of pregnancy or while lactating, so that the natural oils produced by Montgomery's tubercles can maintain the suppleness of the areolar and nipple skin.

3. Nipple shapes vary from woman to woman, but the majority will have protractile nipples which can stand out. Where a mother is worried in case she has flat or inverted nipples, reassurance can often be given quite easily – are her nipples obvious through a T-shirt when she is cold, even though they are normally flat? If so, all should be well! Some authorities recommend the wearing of breast shells or shields for an hour or so at first, increasing to several hours a day by the end of pregnancy. Where nipples are inverted it is claimed that nipple protractility will be improved by this – but it often improves spontaneously during the course of pregnancy. The Hoffman technique for the stretching and breaking down of 'adhesions' at the base of flat or inverted nipples may be suggested as a therapy too; placing the index fingers on either side of the nipple and gently stretching the areola in each direction has been claimed to break these down. However, there is no evidence to date that either of these techniques is beneficial (RCM, 1991), and in any event, babies feed from the breast and *not* actually from the nipple.

4. Pregnant women are not usually taught to massage their breasts from the periphery towards the nipple any more, nor is the early expression of colostrum suggested as a routine. For those women who dislike handling or touching their breasts these techniques may help to overcome such problems; seeing a few drops of colostrum can give them confidence that their body is preparing to feed their baby. It can be difficult to express, however, and its non-appearance does not mean that it is not there.

Apart from being informed and advised about the care of their breasts in pregnancy, women who are intending to breast-feed should know that some authorities have shown that putting the baby to the breast very soon following birth, feeding more frequently and not restricting the lengths of feeds can lead to the mother's milk coming in earlier and a prolongation of the time for which breast-feeding continues (De

Chateau and Wiberg, 1977; Salariya et al., 1978; Slaven and Harvey, 1981). Women should be shown the best feeding positions to use antenatally (see p. 240), and because comfort is essential, suggestions for the proper support of the sore perineum and the back should be practised in antenatal classes.

Because the shape of the breast when the nipple is offered is all-important, women must appreciate that it will be more difficult for their baby to be positioned correctly if they are leaning back – their breast will be flatter – rather than leaning forward – the breast assumes a more pointed shape which makes it easier for their baby to 'latch on'. Side lying, as well as leaning forward initially when sitting, can achieve the desired effect.

The obstetric physiotherapist will certainly meet women attending antenatal classes who have decided not to breast-feed their babies. A variety of reasons will have led them to this conclusion. These can include disgust at the whole idea, a previous bad experience, a wish to know *exactly* how much milk their baby is taking, and even partners vetoing breast-feeding because they regard the woman's breasts as their property. It is most important to explore the reasons behind the decision to bottle-feed and to ensure that the women understand all the advantages of breast-feeding, both for themselves and their baby.

References

Abrams F., P.H., R.D., Laros R.K. (two authors are anonymous) (1986). Prepregnancy weight, weight gain, and birth weight. *Am. J. Obstet. Gynecol.*, **154**, 503–509.

American Academy of Pediatrics and American College of Obstetricians and Gynecologists (1983). *Guidelines for Prenatal Care*.

Artal R., Wiswell R.A., Drinkwater B.L. (1991). *Exercise in Pregnancy*. 2nd edn., Baltimore: Williams & Wilkins.

Balaskas J. (1983). *Active Birth*. London: Unwin Paperbacks.

Beech B.L. (1991). *Who's Having Your Baby*? London: Bedford Square Press.

Berkowitz G.S., Kelsey J.L., Holform T.R., Berkowitz R.L. (1983). Physical activity and the risk of spontaneous preterm delivery. *J. Reprod. Med.*, **28**, 581–588.

Bolton P.J. (1987). Drugs of abuse. In *Drugs and Pregnancy: Human Teratogenesis and Related Problems* (Hawkins D.F., ed.). Edinburgh: Churchill Livingstone.

Burton G.J., Palmer M.E., Dalton K.J. (1989). Morphometric differences between the placental vasculature of non-smokers, smokers and ex-smokers. *Brit. J. Obstet. Gynaec.*, **96**, 907–915.

Chamberlain G. (1984). *Pregnant Women at Work*. London: RSM/Macmillan.

Clinton J. (1985). Couvade patterns and predictors (final report). Hyattsville: Division of Nursing, US Department of Health and Human Services (NTIS NO. RONU00977).

Clinton J. (1986). Expectant fathers at risk for couvade. *Nursing Res.*, **35**, 290–295.

Condon J.T. (1985). The parent-foetal relationship, a comparison of male and female parents. *J. Psychosom. Obstet. Gynaecol.*, **4**, 271–284.

Condon J.T. (1987). Psychological and physical symptoms during pregnancy: A comparison of male and female expectant parents. *J. Reprod. Inf. Psychol.*, **5**, 207–219.

DeChateau P., Wiberg B. (1977). Long-term effect on mother-infant behaviour of extra contact during the first hour post-partum. *Acta. Paed. Scand.*, **66**, 137–151.

Delyser F. (1983). *Jane Fonda's Book for Pregnancy, Birth, and Recovery*. London: Penguin Books.

Editorial (1988). Present-day practice in infant feeding. *Lancet*, **i**, 975–976.

Fry J. (1987). Maternal deaths – still a shocking problem. *Update*, 15 Nov.

Greene G.W., Smiciklas-Wright H., Scholl T.O., Karp R.J. (1988). Postpartum weight change: how much of the weight gained in pregnancy will be lost after delivery? *Obst. Gynec.*, **71**, 701–707.

Gregg J.E.M. (1989). Attitudes of teenagers in Liverpool to breast feeding. *Br. Med. J.*, **299**, 147–148.

Hall D.C., Kaufmann D.A. (1987). Effects of aerobic and strength conditioning on pregnancy outcomes. *Am. J. Obstet Gynecol.*, **157**, 1199–1203.

Hillier C.A., Slade P. (1989). The impact of antenatal classes on knowledge, anxiety and confidence in primiparous women. *Journal of Reproductive and Infant Psychology*. **F(1)**, 3–13.

Holmes T.H., Rahe R.H. (1967). The social readjustment rating scale. *J. Psychosom. Res.*, **11**, 213.

Hytten F.E., Leitch I. (1971). *The Physiology of Human Pregnancy*. Oxford: Blackwell.

Illingworth P.J., Jung R.T., Howie P.W. et al. (1986). Diminution in energy expenditure during lactation. *Br. Med. J.*, **292**, 437–441.

Inch S. (1987). Difficulties in breastfeeding: midwives in disarray? *J. Roy. Soc. Med.*, **80**, 53–58.

Jacobson E. (1938). *Progressive Relaxation*. Chicago: University of Chicago Press.

Jarrett J.C., Spellacy W.N. (1983). Jogging in pregnancy; an improved outcome? *Obs. Gynaec.*, **61**, 705–709.

Jones K.L., Smith D.W., Ulleland C.N. et al. (1973). Pattern of malformation in offspring of chronic alcoholic mothers. *Lancet*, **i**, 1267–1271.

Katz J. (1985). *Swimming Through Your Pregnancy*. Wellingborough: Thorsons.

Liebenberg B. (1974). Expectant fathers. In *Psychological Aspects of a First Pregnancy and Early Postnatal Adaptation* (Sherelsky P.M., Yarrow L.J., eds.). New York: Raven Press.

Llewellyn-Jones D. (1969). *Fundamentals of Obstetrics and Gynaecology*. London: Faber.

MacArthur C., Knox E.G. (1988). Smoking in pregnancy – effects of stopping at different stages. *Brit. J. Obstet. Gynaec.*, **95**, 551–555.

McKnight A., Merrett D. (1987). Nutrition in pregnancy – a health education problem. *Practitioner*, **231**, 530–538.

Mahler H. (1987). The safe motherhood initiative: a call to action. *Lancet*, **i**, 668–670.

Manshande J.P., Eeckels R., Manshande-Desmet V., Vlietinck R. (1987). Rest versus heavy work during the last weeks of pregnancy: influence on foetal growth. *Brit. J. Obstet. Gynaec.*, **94**, 1059–1067.

Meyer M.B., Tonascia J.A. (1977). Maternal smoking, pregnancy complications and perinatal mortality. *Am. J. Obstet. Gynecol.*, **128**, 494–502.

Mitchell L. (1987). *Simple Relaxation*, 2nd edn. London: John Murray.

Munroe R.L., Munroe R.H. (1971). Male pregnancy symptoms and cross-sex identity in three societies. *J. Soc. Psych.*, **84**, 11–25.

NWRHA *Sensible Drinking – Here's How*, Manchester: NWRHA.

Nielsen C.A., Sigsgaard I., Olsen M. et al. (1988). Trainability of the pelvic floor. *Acta Obstet. Gynecol. Scand.*, **67**, 437–440.

Pinette M.G., Loftus-Brault K., Nordi D.A., Rodis J.F. (1989). Maternal smoking and accelerated placental maturation. *Obst. Gynec.*, **73**, 379–382.

Pitt B. (1978). *Feelings about Childbirth*. London: Sheldon Press.

Randall M. (1948). *Fearless Childbirth*, pp. 22–35. London: Churchill.

RCM (1991). *Successful Breastfeeding*. 2nd edn. Edinburgh: Churchill Livingstone.

RCM, Health Visitors Association and Chartered Society of Physiotherapy (1987). Working together in psychophysical preparation for childbirth. *Physiotherapy*, **73**, 165.

Salariya E.M., Easton P.M., Cater J.I. (1978). Duration of breastfeeding after early initiation and frequent feeding. *Lancet* **ii**, 1141–1143.

Samra J.S., Tang L.C.H., Obhrai M.S. (1988). Changes in body weight between consecutive pregnancies. *Lancet* **ii**, 1420–1421.

Slaven S., Harvey D. (1981). Unlimited suckling time improves breastfeeding. *Lancet*, **i**, 392–393.

Sokol R.J. (1983). The effects of alcohol on pregnancy outcome. In *Fifth Special Report to the US Congress on Alcohol and Health from the Secretary of Health and Human Services*, pp. 69–82.

Sokol R.J., Marnier S.S., Ager J.W. (1989). The T-ACE questions: practical prenatal detection of risk drinking. *Am. J. Obstet. Gynecol.*, **160**, 863–869.

Stanway A., Stanway P. (1984). *Choices in Childbirth*. London: Pan Books.

Stevens R.J., Becker R.C., Krumpos G.L. et al. (1988). Postnatal sequelae of smoking during and after pregnancy. *J. Reprod. Inf. Psychol.*, **6**, 61–82.

Tahzib F. (1989). An initiative on vesicovaginal fistuala. *Lancet*, 1316–1317.

Truswell A.S. (1985). Nutrition for pregnancy. *Br. Med. J.*, **291**, 263–266.

Van Raaij J.M.A., Vermaar-Miedema S.H., Schouk C.M. et al. (1987). Energy requirements of pregnancy in the Netherlands. *Lancet* **ii**, 953–955.

Van Zyl K. (1985). *Perfectly Pregnant*. London: Granada.

Vaughan K. (1951). *Exercises Before Childbirth*, pp. 9–16, 17–30. London: Faber.

WHO (1986). *Maternal Mortality Rates*, 2nd edn, FHE/86.3. Geneva: World Health Organization.

Further Reading

Artal R., Wiswall R., Drinkwater B.L. (1991). *Exercise in Pregnancy*. 2nd edn., Baltimore: Williams & Wilkins.

Baum G. (1991). *Aquarobics*. London: Arrow Books.

Benson H. (1988). *The Relaxation Response*. Glasgow: Fount Paperbacks.

Enkin M., Keirse M.J.N.C., Chalmers, I. (1990). *A Guide to Effective Care in Pregnancy and Childbirth*. Oxford: Oxford University Press.

Hawkins D.F., ed. (1987). *Drugs and Pregnancy: Human Teratogenesis and Related Problems*. Edinburgh: Churchill Livingstone.

Huch R., Erkkola R. (1990). Pregnancy and exercise – exercise and pregnancy. A short review. *Brit. J. Obstet. Gynaec.*, **97**, 208–14.

Katz, J. (1983). *Swimming Through Your Pregnancy*. Wellingborough: Thorsons.

Kitzinger S. (1977). *Education and Counselling for Childbirth*. London: Baillière Tindall.

Ledward R.S., Hawkins D.F., Stern L. (1990). *Drug Treatment in Obstetrics – A Handbook of Prescribing*. London: Chapman & Hall.

Lewis C. (1986). *Becoming A Father*. Milton Keynes: Open University Press.

Minchin M. (1985). *Breastfeeding Matters*, Victoria, Australia: Alma Publications.

Mitchell L. (1987). *Simple Relaxation*. London: John Murray.

Murphy-Black T., Faulkner A. (1988). *Antenatal Group Skills Training – A Manual of Guidelines*. Chichester: John Wiley.

Noble E. (1980). *Essential Exercises for the Childbearing Year*. London: John Murray.

Oakley A. (1981). *From Here to Maternity*. London: Penguin.

Perkins E.R. (1980). *Education for Childbirth and Parenthood*. London: Croom Helm.

Price F.V. (1990). *Report to the Parents of Triplets, Quads and Quins*. Child Care and Development Group, University of Cambridge.

Prince J., Adams M.E. (1987). *The Psychology of Childbirth*. Edinburgh: Churchill Livingstone.

RCM (1991). *Successful Breastfeeding*. 2nd edn. Edinburgh: Churchill Livingstone.

Williams M., Booth D. (1985). *Antenatal Education*. Edinburgh: Churchill Livingstone.

Wilson P. (1990) *Antenatal Teaching*, London: Faber and Faber.

Useful addresses

Association of Breastfeeding Mothers
131 Mayflower Road
Sydenham
London
SE26 4HZ

Association for Improvements in the Maternity Services (AIMS)
163 Liverpool Road
London
N1 ORF

Association of Chartered Physiotherapists in Obstetrics and Gynaecology
c/o The Chartered Society of Physiotherapy
14 Bedford Row
London
WC1R 4ED

Foresight (Preconceptual Care)
The Old Vicarage
Church Lane
Withey
Godalming
Surrey
GU8 5PN

Health Visitors' Association
50 Southwark St,
London SE1

La Leche League (Breastfeeding)
BM 3424
London
WC1N 3XX

Maternity Alliance
15 Britannia Street
London
WC1X 9JP

Midwives' Information and Resource Service (MIDIRS)
Institute of Child Health
Royal Hospital for Sick Children
St Michael's Hill
Bristol
BS2 8BJ

Miscarriage Association
PO Box 24
Ossett
West Yorkshire
WF4 4TP

National Childbirth Trust
Alexandra House
Oldham Terrace
Acton
London
W3 6NH

The National Council for One-Parent Families
255 Kentish Town Road
London
NW5

Royal College of Midwives
15 Mansfield Street
London
W1M OBE

Society to Support Home Confinement
Lydgate
Lydgate Lane
Wolsingham
Bishop Auckland
Co. Durham
DL13 4HA

CHAPTER 5

Relieving Pregnancy Discomfort

For the vast majority of primigravidae, pregnancy is the first time in their lives that they experience so many different 'aches and pains'. It may also be the very first time that they have to deal with doctors in a hospital setting, and eventually, again possibly for the first time, become in-patients. Perhaps it is because of these factors, and because pregnancy and birth are 'unknown' experiences, that the so-called minor ailments of pregnancy can assume major importance – often out of all proportion to their significance.

The majority of these discomforts can be directly explained by the softening, relaxing effect of pregnancy hormones such as progesterone and relaxin, accompanied by weight gain, fluid retention and postural changes, with the resulting alteration in movement patterns (see Chapter 2, p. 26). The growing uterus and its contents can give rise to significant 'pulling, pressing and pushing' pains; explanations using the Schuchardt charts (showing the changes in the position of the pelvic and abdominal organs as pregnancy progresses) can be invaluable in helping women to understand the 'sharp, stabbing pain down here' or 'the dropping-out feeling' of which so many complain. Frequently, a clear explanation and consequent understanding of the reasons behind these problems – with the reassurance that the birth of the baby will bring complete relief – is sufficient to help the mother-to-be to cope with them. Self-help coping strategies can often be taught so that women are able to treat themselves once a diagnosis has been made. Unfortunately, pregnant women – troubled, say, by backache – are still frequently told 'What do you expect – it's because of your condition, and nothing can be done to help until after your baby is born'.

BACK AND PELVIC GIRDLE PAIN

A great many pregnant women seem to experience back pain or pain associated with their pelvic joints at some stage of their pregnancy (Bullock et al., 1987; Nwuga, 1982); obstetricians, general practitioners and midwives tend to dismiss it as inevitable and unimportant. The intensity and duration of the pain usually fluctuates throughout the pregnancy, and often from one pregnancy to the next in the same woman. There is wide variation in severity between individuals; one person complains of minor, transient stiffness or discomfort, while another is totally disabled. Research indicates that in about 50% of pregnant women pain is of sufficient intensity and duration to affect their lifestyle in some way, and for one-third of these individuals the pain is severe (Mantle et al., 1977, 1981; Nwuga, 1982; Fast et al., 1987; Berg et al., 1988).

The first episode of pain in a pregnancy may occur at any stage, but for the majority it is between the fourth and seventh months (Mantle et al., 1977, 1981; Fast et al., 1987; Bullock et al., 1987). In general, back pain seems to be felt at a lower level by a woman when she is pregnant than when she is not pregnant (Mantle et al., 1981). Mantle et al. (1977) and Fast et al. (1987) found the majority of sufferers have low back pain; for about half of these it radiated into the buttocks and thighs, and occasionally down the legs as sciatica. For many women the back pain is made worse by standing, sitting, forward bending, lifting – particularly when combined with twisting (Berg et al., 1988) – and walking. Some complain, in addition or solely, of pain over or in the symphysis pubis; for a few the thoracic region is affected, rather than the lower back and pelvis. Coccydynia can also be a problem antenatally, although it is uncommon and is often linked with a previous injury.

It is important for those involved in the care of pregnant women to appreciate that surveys (Consumers Association, 1986; Cats, 1986) have shown that at any point in time at least 15–20% of all women of childbearing age will have backache, and a larger percentage still will have had backache in the past nine months – perhaps more than 40% (Scholey and Hair, 1989). Being pregnant does not necessarily protect a woman from the factors – known and unknown – causing backache, and so her carers must not fall into the trap of assuming that a pregnant woman's backache or leg pain is always directly caused by her pregnancy; nor need pregnancy be an adverse or prolonging factor to recovery from back problems. Further, it is worth noting that back pain before pregnancy does not inevitably lead to back pain during pregnancy; some women experience less back pain than usual while pregnant. Changes in spinal loading and posture that prove to be beneficial, and the 'strut' effect of the rising uterus limiting trunk movement, have been suggested as explanations, and of course the natural healing processes must not be forgotten. However, it is generally accepted that fatigue, increased mobility of joints (Calguneri et al., 1982) associated with hormonally induced changes in collagen, the fact that the remodelled collagen has a greater volume causing pressure on pain-sensitive structures, weight gain with increased spinal loading and associated necessary adaptations in posture, and pressure from the growing fetus, are all factors that could account for the significantly higher incidence of back pain in pregnant women compared with that in their non-pregnant peers.

Bullock et al. (1987) showed a significant increase in lumbar and thoracic curves through pregnancy which was still evident at the end of the puerperium. However, they could not substantiate the increase in pelvic inclination propounded by many physiotherapists, nor was there any obvious correlation between the increasing spinal curves and the onset of pain.

It must be borne in mind that hormonal levels begin to change and have their effects from the time of conception; significant weight gain and postural adaptations come later. Fast et al. (1987) has wisely suggested that the aetiology of the pain may vary with each trimester; this is probably true. Even so, it is worth remembering that Mantle et al. (1981) showed that it is possible to reduce the intensity of and even prevent some back pain in pregnancy. The obstetric physotherapist's role is not only to treat where appropriate, but also to be the member of the obstetric team who seeks to understand the problem, who has all the latest information concerning the causes and treatment of back pain, and who leads the team in aiming first at prevention, and where this fails, at containing and mitigating the problem.

PREVENTION OF BACK PAIN

The obstetric physiotherapist has as a prime objective to help prevent her antenatal clients from having any back pain. This will not be possible in all cases, but often further pain may be prevented, or at least its severity and duration may be reduced. A simple knowledge of wise back usage is every woman's right. The basic principles are the same whether a woman is pregnant or not, but if a woman is pregnant it may be necessary to adapt the application of those principles and the advice offered (Mantle, 1988). It is good sense to encourage a woman to be aware of her own body, and to seek to understand and contain any back pain she is experiencing before undertaking a pregnancy, even though there is no clear correlation between back pain before and during pregnancy.

All antenatal classes should include training in body awareness and appropriate back care advice and instruction, with regular reinforcement and correction where necessary. The health care professionals involved in the classes must be prepared to be role models, understanding and using the principles they preach. The antenatal class provides wonderfully cost-effective opportunities to influence the wider community in this and many other health promotional aspects.

The adaptation of back care principles in pregnancy

Lying. Comfortable resting and sleeping positions are imperative. Increasing weight may make the bed sag so that some additional support for the mattress may be necessary; a little pillow or rolled towel in the waist may be helpful. Increasing hip width and the weight of the abdomen often result in the woman rotating her pelvis more when in side lying, in order to rest the top leg and abdomen on the bed. The additional rotation may be enough to cause pain and the dragging weight may be sufficient to strain laxer sacroiliac joints; pillows under the top thigh and knee solve this. In supine lying, women are almost invariably more comfortable with pillows under their thighs, although it may be wise to discourage supine lying for protracted periods later in pregnancy (see p. 106). When turning over, pressing the flexed knees together will help to avoid sacroiliac strain and pain at the symphysis pubis during the manoeuvre. When one or other partner is restless, it may be appropriate to advise separate beds.

Where a woman has to get up several times a night to micturate, it becomes all the more important that she knows the best way to get in and out of bed without jarring her spine. This is done by crooking the knees, rolling on to the side and sitting up sideways by pushing with the arms, while dropping the lower legs over the side of the bed. On returning to bed the process is reversed.

With many women working in demanding jobs, it is necessary to emphasize that adequate rest is of prime importance and that back pain may simply be a body complaining that it is being required physically or mentally to do too much. The obstetric team must also be alert to indications of stressful problems of other kinds, e.g. anxiety about pregnancy, lack of needed support from carers or family, and financial or housing difficulties, for such stress predisposes to fatigue, sleeplessness, strain and accident, and will enhance pain. Complaints of pain may be a cry for attention and help.

Sitting. A chair should fit the user; ideally the seat is the length of the thigh and buttock, and the height of the seat is the distance from heel to knee, so that the hip and thigh are at a right angle. The contours of the chair back should match and support the spinal curves in a good sitting posture. The buttocks should be set right back on the chair seat, and a firm support in the lumbar region has been shown to be extremely important both to prevent and relieve back pain in pregnancy (Mantle et al., 1977, 1981). Women are encouraged to 'sit tall'. A chair should be appropriate in design and shape to the activity to be carried out; however, sitting for extended periods should be discouraged. Frequent changes in activity and position are keys to back pain prevention. Sitting with one or both feet on a low stool is sometimes beneficial. Toward the end of pregnancy it may be more comfortable to sit astride a chair and lean forward on the chair back for support.

Standing and walking. The simplest way to gain good posture, even in pregnancy, is to stand and walk 'tall'. Walking is preferable to standing still for a pregnant woman, for its movement and circulatory effects, and a modest walk is acceptable daily exercise for most people; walking for too long, however, may provoke pain. Within the home and at work, work surfaces should allow the worker to stand upright or sit in a good position. It is stooping, however little, and repetitively rotating the trunk that seem to be factors associated with back pain. Where an extended period of standing is necessary, standing with the front foot placed on a raised support or rocking from foot to foot will moderate the worst effects. Household activities such as those using a broom or vacuum cleaner should be performed as a forward-and-backward movement with as little trunk rotation as possible.

Bending down and lifting. If a pregnant woman is unaware from early pregnancy of the need to bend at the hips and knees rather than in the back when stooping down, it may prove impossible for her to comply later in pregnancy, simply because the quadriceps muscles are not strong enough to raise the increasingly heavy body from the squat position; hence the importance of checking this early, instructing where necessary and reinforcing regularly. It also becomes progressively more difficult to hold loads close to the centre of the body. Heavy lifting should be avoided or shared; the body has its own increased weight to manage, and laxer joints are 'strain prone'. Load carrying (which includes wearing heavy clothes) should be reduced to a minimum; clothing should be light, and shopping carried as two equal loads, rather than as one which forces the body into side flexion. Tiring repetitive bending can sometimes be reduced by judicious repositioning of equipment. Heavy, strenuous, physically – and even very mentally – demanding employment should be discontinued before the woman feels excessively fatigued or strained.

It is worth discussing ergonomic principles in relation to baby care and equipment early in pregnancy, for this encourages constructive use of the backcare knowledge, may prevent uninformed purchase of inappropriate equipment, and promotes innovative solutions to such perennial back-stressing problems as baby bathing and nappy changing. Antenatal clinics and classes can also provide a source of satisfactory second hand articles for loan or purchase. Clinic waiting areas should be used to display eye-catching posters and instructive videos giving information about back care, which can be reinforced in antenatal classes.

Throughout, the obstetric physiotherapist is seeking to develop in women and their carers the ability to recognize in their own bodies the sensations of comfort and well-being, or strain and fatigue. Activities need to be stopped before, not after, they cause pain, and the cause of any back pain should be sought retrospectively in order to avoid it occurring another time.

MANAGEMENT OF BACK AND PELVIC GIRDLE PAIN

The management of a pregnant woman with back and pelvic girdle pain must be a team concern. As with all such pain sufferers, a full assessment is imperative to determine whether and what treatment is indicated, and the fact that a pain sufferer is pregnant is critical to both assessment and treatment. Obstetric physiotherapists and their managers are frequently guilty of failing to ensure time for this process, and advice and treatment are often dispensed without proper assessment. Why should back pain when a woman is pregnant be less important than when she is not pregnant?

Much publicity has been given to sacroiliac dysfunction as a cause of back and pelvic girdle pain. This is particularly true in relation to pregnancy, so that there is a grave danger of jumping to conclusions as to the cause of a particular patient's pain, although there is no doubt that sacroiliac dysfunction will sometimes be found (Berg et al., 1988). Obstetric physiotherapists would be wise to heed Grieve's advice not to examine the sacroiliac joint 'until the lumbar spine, hip and lower limb examinations, including neurological tests, have been completed . . . one should resist the tendency to find what one would like to find.' (Grieve, 1981).

Assessment of the patient

The classic pattern of back pain assessment familiar to physiotherapists may require minor adaptation in pregnant patients and the findings need special interpretation. A body chart or back assessment form will be helpful in recording the findings.

Subjective examination

The patient should be placed in a comfortable and well-supported position for questioning.

1. Details of present pain and other symptoms:
    Location, type, behaviour, duration?
    What aggravates it, what eases it?
    What functional activities are restricted?
    Any numbness, paraesthesiae or weakness?
    Any other symptoms?

The obstetric physiotherapist will be able to recognize costochondral margin pain from flared ribs, 'stitch' pain from tension on the round ligaments, and paraesthesiae and weakness caused by fluid retention, e.g. meralgia paraesthetica, carpal tunnel syndrome. Any indication of pre-eclamptic toxaemia (e.g. oedema, headaches) or of urinary tract infection requires immediate investigation.

It should be borne in mind in relation to the reported severity of pain that a woman's anxiety principally concerns the welfare of the fetus rather than herself (although of course there may be other important worries), and anxiety heightens pain perception. Dramatic improvements have followed informed reassurance of fetal well-being.

2.Mandatory questions concerning the perineum and micturition. Are there any changes in perineal sensation or micturition habits? It is necessary here to discriminate between significant symptoms and the frequency and stress incontinence experienced by some pregnant women, also the pain, hyperalgia or numbness of the perineum which may be associated with piles, haemorrhoids and venous thrombosis of the vulva, often resulting from constipation in pregnancy or from the direct downward weight of the fetus. Back pain may accompany urinary tract infections.

3. Onset and history of this and any previous episodes. The stage of pregnancy at onset is an important factor because, as described earlier, hormonally mediated collagen changes commence early, whereas important abdominal enlargement and weight gain are later manifestations. Severe backache may also be a sign of impending labour.

The woman's own assessment of the cause is always worthy of note. Of particular interest is a similar episode in a previous pregnancy, for there are some women who recognize conception by a recommencement of 'the backache'. Research has shown that there is a greater degree of joint laxity in second pregnancies than in the first (Calguneri et al., 1982), and Mantle et al. (1977) and Nwuga (1982) noted the incidence and severity of back pain increased with parity. Fast et al. (1987) found more disability caused by backache in women with prior pregnancies, and suggested changes in posture or weakness of trunk muscles as explanations. Berg et al. (1988) found that low back pain in a previous pregnancy increased the likelihood of sacroiliac dysfunction in the present pregnancy.

4. General health, occupation and lifestyle. The general condition of the woman, and the total load being shouldered by her both physically and mentally, must be estimated. The philosophy of equality of the sexes, the employment climate whereby the woman may be the sole breadwinner of a partnership, the dispersal geographically of families and the belief – correct in itself – that pregnancy is a normal physiological process, can all lead to pregnant women expecting and being expected to do too much. Individual limitations must be recognized and conceded. Berg et al. (1988) found a strong association between the type of work – particularly lifting and twisting – and the development of low back pain with sacroiliac dysfunction. Dramatic improvements in back pain in pregnancy have been achieved simply by discontinuing employment. In contrast, there is increasing evidence that physically fit women have fewer aches and pains in pregnancy than their unfit sisters (Hall and Kaufmann, 1987).

Objective examination

Care and ingenuity will be needed in choosing a position of stability and comfort for the patient. For example, pregnant women may lose their balance more easily because of their shape, so the standing examination is best carried out with the woman facing a plinth which she can use for support where necessary. Prone lying may be impossible, or may be made possible with pillows. A patient in late pregnancy may feel faint after a while in supine lying because the gravid uterus can interfere with the blood flow in the inferior vena cava and aorta (see p. 106). Tests in lying should therefore be completed speedily. Side lying is generally well tolerated.

It is reasonable to expect that the mobility of all joints will increase marginally as pregnancy progresses (Calguneri et al., 1982), but the 'strut' effect of the uterus will limit trunk movements, and oedema (particularly at the periphery) may reduce joint range, especially in the final trimester.

1. Observation. The patient's functional ability will be observed throughout the assessment, but once the patient is suitably undressed the following can be readily noted with the patient standing:

- shoulder, scapula and iliac crest levels
- waist and hip contours
- buttock fold and knee crease levels
- spinal posture
- leg lengths
- muscle spasm, soft tissue, swelling
- skin colour, reddening, bruising.

These findings can then be compared with those observed as the patient moves, and with the patient in other positions as the examination proceeds. Virtually all patients have bony anomalies of some sort, so asymmetry must be interpreted with caution. For example Lewit et al. (1970), observed the presence of pelvic torsion, such that one anterior superior iliac spine was higher than the other, in 40% of 450 schoolchildren. In the later stages of pregnancy, as the abdomen becomes distended, postural adaptations are the norm, and commonly (but not invariably) lumbar and thoracic curves increase (Bullock et al., 1987). Waist contours and shoulder levels can be misleading as a result of the asymmetrical lie of the fetus.

2. Assessment of function. The physiotherapist seeks to establish which movements are full and pain-free, and which are limited or painful. Where movements are full and pain-free, they should be tested at the limits by passive overpressure. The physiotherapist will try to reproduce the pain complained of, and to detect muscle tightness, spasm or weakness, or altered sensation. Changes produced by movement are observed. It is important to allow settling time in each new position.

(a) Standing (feet a little apart, facing a plinth for balance):
- check range and observe trunk flexion, extension and side flexion for limitation, stiffness, pain;
- ask patient to toe stand six times, first on one leg then the other (S1 and S2);
- test freedom of sacroiliac joint movement by placing the left thumb over the left posterior superior iliac spine (PSIS) and the right thumb over the posterior tubercle of S2; ask the patient to stand on the right leg and flex the left hip and knee – the left PSIS should move down relative to the tubercle of S2; repeat on other side
- observe walking, going up and down steps.

(b) Sitting (thighs and feet supported, arms crossed on chest):
- check range and observe trunk rotation (fixing same side knee), for limitation, stiffness, pain;
- check relative levels of right and left PSIS;
- check for changes in relative levels of each PSIS on trunk flexion: place one thumb over each PSIS, observe changes when patient flexes trunk forwards – a single rising PSIS indicates a fixed sacroiliac joint on the same side (Vorlauf's phenomenon or Piedallu's sign);
- observe apparent thigh lengths, and malleoli levels on knee extension, compare with levels in lying; a shorter leg in sitting compared with lying could be evidence of a forward and downward rotation of the ilium or the sacrum on the same side, or a backward rotation of the ilium on the opposite side, due to displacement of the acetabulum (Derbolowski's test), but it must be remembered that in any case 10% of the population have leg length discrepancies.

(c) Lying:
- observe lie of the pelvis, discover the reason for any tilt, e.g. hypotonic glutei (S1);
- ask patient to lift head and flex neck, give overpressure to check for dural and nerve root signs through the thoracic and lumbar regions;
- check hip and knee movements actively (L1–L3);
- check passive straight leg raise for dural and nerve root signs through lumbar and sacral regions, and to elicit pain from irritable lumbar facet joints;

- test muscle power of psoas (L1–L2), quadriceps (L3), tibialis anterior (L4), extensor hallucis longus (L5) and peronei (S1), test knee jerk (L3) and ankle jerk (S1);
- test sensation, chart abnormalities and interpret to dermatomes;
- check level of malleoli (see note under sitting section);
- palpate Baer's point, found medial to and slightly below the anterior superior iliac spine, seeking unusual tenderness or spasm of iliacus, test knee jerk (L3) and ankle jerk (S1);
- test compression and gapping of ilia;
- test combined hip and sacroiliac joint by placing left heel on right knee and abducting left thigh, and repeat on opposite side;
- apply vertical pressure to symphysis pubis.

(d) Prone lying, side lying, or side lying quarter turned to prone:

- note tone of glutei, observe contour in prone;
- observe changes in bony alignment, deviation, prominence, absence, muscle wasting, spasm, thickening;
- test muscle power of glutei (S1), test hamstrings (S2);
- test ankle jerk (S1) if not done in lying;
- 'stretch test' the femoral nerve (L2–L3) by extending hip and flexing knee.

3. Palpation. In prone lying, side lying or side lying quarter turned to prone:

- skin sweep for signs of local autonomic activity, e.g. heat, perspiration, and for bony abnormality, e.g. prominence, absence, spondylolisthesis;
- palpate and skin roll for soft-tissue 'feel', e.g. wasting, spasm, thickening, abnormal tenderness;
- give central pressure with straight thumbs (grade 1–2 in middle range) to posterior tubercle of each vertebra through appropriate level of spine, if necessary including coccyx; where sacroiliac joint dysfunction is suspected, give sacral apex pressure;
- give unilateral pressure to the transverse process or to the lateral aspect of the posterior tubercle of each vertebra, on the side of no pain or least pain first, through appropriate levels.

4. Record of findings. In a clinical specialty so prone to litigation, it is prudent to be meticulous in record keeping.

5. Interpretation of findings and decisions regarding treatment. Findings must finally be interpreted. It is worth remembering that neurological anomalies may confound the picture, and pain can correspond to dermatomes, myotomes or sclerotomes. Decisions have then to be made as to whether and what treatment is appropriate. It is important to include the patient in this phase in order that her particular circumstances and the problems as perceived by her be addressed.

Reference should also be made to the obstetrician or the general practitioner to ensure that no obstetric consideration is ignored.

If treatment is appropriate, it must be apreciated that the pregnancy will not diminish and may even heighten the normally powerful placebo effect of any treatment given by a thoroughly competent and effective obstetric physiotherapist; up to 35% success can confidently be expected *whatever* treatment is selected! Combinations of modalities have been shown to be more beneficial than a single one (Coxhead et al., 1981) and patients seem to respond best where treatment is instituted early (Sims-Williams et al., 1978). Although it is generally agreed that short-wave diathermy and interferential therapy are contraindicated, other treatments such as rest and relaxation, support, superficial heat, massage, manipulation or mobilization, traction, transcutaneous nerve stimulation (TNS), instruction and advice on posture and back care, and exercise on land or in the water are all worthy of consideration against the assessment findings (Mantle, 1988). Decisions to stop work or change the living and working environment may also have to be taken.

SOME COMMON SYNDROMES AND THEIR TREATMENT

Low back pain

Haldeman and Meyer (1977) listed some 26 causes of low back pain; the age range of pregnant women allows the physiotherapist to discount a few of these causes, but a substantial number remains. The obstetric physiotherapist must be prepared to study these, and to remember that the pregnant woman is not immune to the ills her peers are prone to. Jill Mantle has treated two women who apparently developed slight disc lesions with neurological deficit early in pregnancy, requiring complete bed rest. On the other hand, pregnant women are more accident-prone, the distended abdomen makes some activities more awkward and the psychological effects of pregnancy may cloud judgment on such issues as wise back care. An increased lumbar curve combined with the gradual weight gain may cause facet joints to override and traumatize the joint capsules, or result in structural anomalies becoming troublesome. Weight and fatigue often produce poor posture. An element of joint instability may arise from the combination of extra weight, soft-tissue laxity and increased torsional strain; spondylolisthesis is not impossible.

Treatment

Where the condition is acute, and particularly if there is neurological deficit, bed rest is the treatment of choice. The patient must be clear exactly what she may or may not do, and it is imperative that she is freed from responsibilities in order to rest completely. The obstetric physiotherapist has a key role in assisting the woman to find a selection of positions of ease and in showing her how best to move herself within the imposed restrictions, especially in relation to toileting, washing and eating meals.

Where the situation is less acute, a reduction in overall activity is still wise, e.g. discontinuing employment, and where possible alternatives to activities that exacerbate the pain should be found. Restful sleep is a top priority. Pain and muscle spasm respond well to gentle heat and massage, given in side lying if necessary. Where the assessment has shown facet joint dysfunction, gentle mobilizations may be appropriate; side lying with the spine in the neutral position is ideal for transverse vertebral pressures. Carefully taught pelvic tilting in crook lying can be soothing, and firm support in the lumbar region when sitting is essential. *All* patients need careful and repetitive instruction in all aspects of wise back usage and posture. If the abdominal muscles are lax or if the abdomen is protuberant or pendulous, some form of support may be helpful.

Once the condition begins to ease a graduated exercise plan should be instituted where possible, to regain strength; water is a useful and pleasant medium for this. Where pain continues despite all efforts, TNS has been used successfully and safely as an alternative to other forms of analgesia (Mannheimer, 1985; Mantle, 1988).

Sacroiliac dysfunction

The possible effects of pregnancy on the sacroiliac joint are several. For example, joint laxity may allow enough repetitive new movement at one or both sacroiliac joints to cause pain if combined with sufficient activity. Alternatively, the newly permitted movement could result in the uneven surfaces moving on one another and then becoming stuck, producing a locked rather than a moving joint. This may well be painful in itself and can also cause strain and pain in the opposite side which is called upon to compensate. Both anterior and posterior torsion or rotation of the ilium on the sacrum have been described, but there is disagreement as to which is the more common (DonTigny, 1985). It seems likely, however, that the complex and highly individual configuration of the sacroiliac joint allows for any number of possible directions of shuffling movement. A further possibility is that one joint becomes more mobile than its pair, thus on activity constant strain is placed on the less mobile joint. Obviously any alteration of the position of an ilium affects the position of the acetabulum, and this is the basis of the longer leg found in lying and the shorter leg found in sitting in the case of an ilium that is rotated anteriorly on the sacrum.

Consider the truncal weight taken through the sacral prominence slung between the ilia and being transmitted to the legs via the sacroiliac joints: increased loading should draw the joint surfaces more tightly together, but with laxer ligaments surely it must be possible for the joint to fail. A pregnant woman may become as much as 25 kg heavier, the sacrum is thrust downwards between the ilia in all upright postures, and in walking, each sacroiliac joint alternately transmits the total loading. Certainly sclerosis of the sacroiliac joints – osteitis condensans ilii – is seen on X-ray after childbirth. It usually disappears in a few months but indicates transient stress. Is it any wonder that patients frequently benefit from bed rest?

Changes in orientation or degrees of movement at a sacroiliac joint may affect the symphysis pubis, and may also affect the spine. Fraser (1976) suggested a distinctive right–left pattern of associated spinal pain. For right sacroiliac dysfunction he describes pain at the following sites – left T12, right T8, left T2, right C2–C3, or alternatively left mid-thoracic, right C2–C3. On the other hand, it has been shown that pain from the lumbar spine and occasionally from the hip may be referred to the sacroiliac region, and there is no doubt that disorders of the lumbar spine and sacroiliac joints can coexist. Thus pain experienced over a sacroiliac joint is *not* synonymous with disorder of that joint; other possibilities must be explored and other confirming or refuting signs sought. Piedallu's test in sitting and the sacroiliac fixation test in standing are useful, as are also the gapping and compression of the ilia and the sacral apex pressure test, but the whole picture must be appraised.

Treatment

Very careful assessment is critical. Where joint locking or torsion appear to have occurred a more normal position may be achieved by carefully gapping the joint and so enabling it to return as quickly as possible to a more normal approximation on release. To do this the patient lies supine with the knee of the affected side flexed and the toes hooked under the lateral aspect of the straight knee. (Fig. 5.1). The

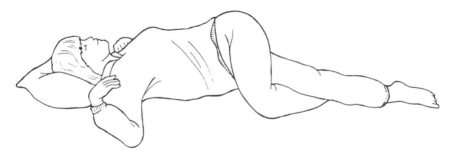

Figure 5.1 A self-help position to relieve sacroiliac pain.

therapist passively takes the flexed knee across the body while holding the shoulder of the affected side against the plinth. Thus tension is applied to the affected sacroiliac joint and any slack is taken up; at the end of range a single, gentle thrust is given. The woman may benefit from repeating this position at home, with or without a gentle rocking movement but minus the thrust. The same objective may be achieved by a less severe manoeuvre described by Fraser (1976) which patients may perform for themselves. It can also be used once or twice a day to encourage the ilium and sacrum to remain in more normal correlation. For the left sacroiliac joint, the patient lies supine and grasps the left flexed knee at the level of the tibial tubercle with the left hand. The left hip is then rotated laterally sufficiently to allow the left calcaneum to be cupped in the right hand. With trunk fully supported and the right leg relaxed and straight, the left knee is gently pulled towards a point just lateral to the left shoulder, and the left heel eased toward the right groin. The pressure is then released and reapplied once or twice. Advocates usually recommend that the movement is then repeated on the other side (Fig. 5.2). Don Tigny (1985) suggests a very similar movement performed with the patient in sitting or standing positon, with the hip and knee of the affected side flexed and the foot up on a chair or bench; in this movement the patient rocks forward to the knee and back. Alternatively, where forward torsion of one ilium on the sacrum is confirmed the affected ilium can be gently oscillated and rotated backward and upward on the sacrum, by forward pressure applied to the ischial tuberosity and backward and upward pressure on the anterior aspect of the ilium with the patient supine and the affected leg flexed at hip and knee.

Alternatively, Cyriax recommended the patient to lie supine on a bed or plinth and cross the leg of the affected side over the other, combining this with sufficient lower trunk rotation to allow the lower leg of the affected side to dangle over the side of the bed and exert traction through the leg and hip to the sacroiliac joint. The patient is instructed to lie in this position and relax as fully as possible for 10–20 minutes, and then to resume activity carefully.

Figure 5.2 Fraser's (1976) self-help manoeuvre for the relief of sacroiliac pain.

Other clinicians have successfully addressed the leg lengthening/ shortening sign by using a sharp longitudinal leg pull, first to the leg on the affected side with the leg slightly abducted, then to the other, with the patient relaxed in supine lying (Golightly, 1982). Sudden traction through the capsule of the hip joint to the ilium can, in some cases, unlock the sacroiliac joint surfaces and so assist with a return to the usual alignment. Patients will sometimes report relief from repeated slow back arching (hyperextension) in standing, with their hands firmly placed either side in the small of the back. Don Tigny (1985) suggests that 'the posterior shift of the line of gravity behind the centre of the acetabula creates a powerful strain in posterior rotation that would help correct an anterior dysfunction (rotation) of the sacroiliac joints.'

Following any of the manoeuvres described above, the application of a sacroiliac support belt or trochanteric belt may increase comfort and help avoid recurrence of the malposition. Where recurrence does occur the therapist will have to decide how often it is wise to manipulate in this way. Repetitive reductions could encourage further joint instability, perhaps even in the longer term. All patients should receive careful advice in order that they understand their problem and know how best to maintain the correction and prevent recurrence. Side lying is usually the most comfortable resting position with a pillow between the knees or forward under the top knee. The knees should be kept together and crooked when turning over in bed. Work involving leaning forward should be avoided, but when essential, placing a foot on a low stool or equivalent controls the anterior rotation of the pelvis to some degree. If the abdominal muscles are weak, and if it is realistic to attempt strengthening exercises, this should be done.

Whether or not there is obvious torsion of an ilium it does seem possible to produce good results simply by encouraging a patient to reduce activity for two or three days and rest on a bed or couch as much as possible. In that the joint is lined by synovial membrane, it will react like any other to trauma or to inflammatory conditions. It may be that rest facilitates a reduction in inflammation and oedema, and where there is torsion general relaxation and gentle non-weight-bearing movements in the bed may allow the joint to return naturally to its normal position.

Don Tigny (1985) suggests the use of TNS in conjunction with corrective and preventative therapy. As always with TNS, it is important for the patient to understand that this temporarily masks the pain rather than curing its cause.

Sciatica

When a pregnant woman complains of sciatica, her obstetrician will probably tell her that it is the baby sitting on a nerve. Except near term this seems a little unlikely, and would in any case respond to changes in maternal positioning. Sciatica may accompany backache and sacroiliac joint dysfunction; it will rarely occur alone. The L4 and L5 component of the sciatic nerve runs immediately in front of the sacroiliac joint and so would become involved in any dysfunction or inflammatory reaction at this site. An increased lumbar lordosis would also change the lie of these roots, possibly with traction in lying and standing. Increased loading may result in the spinal foramina being reduced in size with consequent root compression. As already suggested disc lesions are not unknown; and is it impossible for abdominal adhesions, e.g. following infection or surgery, to be another causative factor?

Treatment

Bed rest or, at the very least, reduced activity for one or two weeks has been shown to be the best treatment for acute sciatica (Bell and Rothman, 1984).

Osteitis pubis, diastasis (separation) of symphysis pubis

The width of the symphysis pubis has been shown to increase in pregnancy from about 4 mm to 9 mm (Abramson, 1934); occasionally the joint separates completely. Women complain of transient and sometimes incapacitating pain in and around the joint and radiating down the medial aspect of the thighs. The possible connection with laxer sacroiliac joints has already been discussed. Movements such as turning over in bed and hip abduction cause pain, and walking may be impossible except with a walking aid.

Treatment

Where the condition is acute, bed rest with the legs adducted and flexed is the only solution. The old-fashioned remedy of binding the hips with a long roller-towel may give some relief. Where pain is less severe a strong trochanteric belt worn around the hips, a Tubigrip 'roll-on' or a maternity pantie-girdle can help a woman to continue with her essential daily tasks. A walking frame, sticks or crutches should be supplied where necessary. Ice packs over the painful area two or three times per day may ease the pain.

Coccydynia

Previous injury to the coccyx predisposes to this problem in pregnancy, but otherwise this condition is rare antenatally unless caused by a fall.

Treatment

The most help is gained from a rubber ring to relieve pressure in sitting, but gentle mobilizations – grasping the coccyx using a gloved index finger in the anus and the thumb posteriorly – ice packs, heat, ultrasound and TNS are all worthy of consideration.

Thoracic spine pain

A few pregnant women complain of pain over the thoracic spine. As already discussed (see p. 145), Fraser (1976) claimed a distinctive right–left pattern of spinal pain associated with sacroiliac joint dysfunction. Other possible causes include the effect of the increased thoracic kyphosis (Bullock et al., 1987), the flaring of the ribs towards term causing strain at the costovertebral or costotransverse joints, and the increasing weight of the breasts.

Treatment

If sacroiliac joint dysfunction is confirmed then reduction should be attempted; mobilizations may ease costovertebral or costotransverse joints. Posture correction and a well-fitting brassière should also be considered.

Postural backache

Frequently the backache complained of during pregnancy will be just that – a 'tired ache' in the lower back – often at the end of the day or after particularly heavy effort. There are many comfortable positions to relieve this sort of discomfort (Fig. 5.3, see p. 150); they can be demonstrated and used during antenatal classes, and will give relief at work and at home too. A mid-day rest may be prophylactic.

Osteoporosis of pregnancy

Osteoporosis of pregnancy is a rare event, but it can be important clinically and the obstetric physiotherapist must be aware of its possibility when considering back and hip problems in pregnant women. Back pain, together with vertebral collapse and consequent loss of height, are the most frequent features, although hip fractures have also been reported. It has been suggested (Smith et al., 1985) that there may be a transient failure of the usual changes in calciotrophic hormones which prepare the maternal skeleton for the stress of

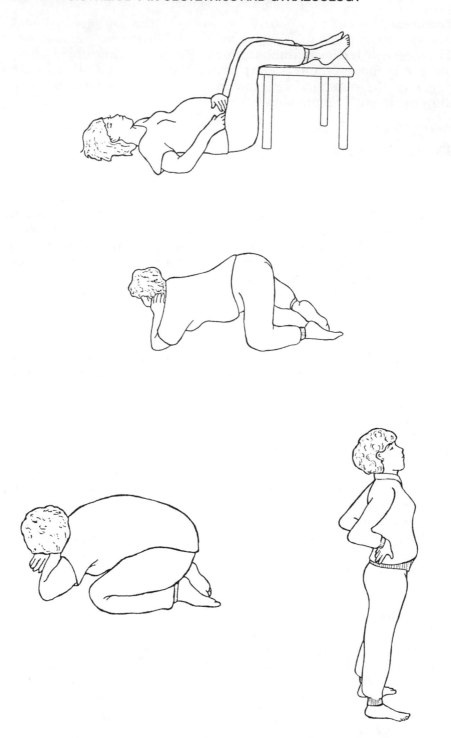

Figure 5.3 Women may find these positions helpful when dealing with tired, aching backs.

childbirth. Most women find that their back pain improves spontaneously a few months following delivery, and that the condition does not necessarily recur in subsequent pregnancies.

NERVE COMPRESSION SYNDROMES

During the third trimester of pregnancy fluid retention can lead to oedema which, as well as being visible in the ankles, feet, hands and face of the pregnant woman, can lead to reduced joint mobility and a variety of nerve compression syndromes.

Carpal tunnel syndrome

Carpal tunnel syndrome, the most common of the nerve compression syndromes, is clinically recognized as impairment of sensory and sometimes motor nerve function in the hand, caused by compression of the median nerve as it passes through the narrow carpal tunnel under the flexor retinaculum at the wrist. Ekman-Ordeberg et al. (1987) reported that 2.5% of a population of pregnant women had symptoms of carpal tunnel syndrome, although other authors show much higher incidence of up to 50% (Melvin et al., 1969; Gould and Wissinger, 1978; Voitk et al., 1983). It appears to be associated with the generalized oedema suffered by some women in the final trimester of pregnancy, although a purely localized oedema can also cause the symptoms.

The median nerve supplies the thenar muscles and the first and second lumbrical muscles, and gives a sensory supply to the thumb, index and middle fingers. A frequent complaint from a woman presenting with this condition is paraesthesia and pain, which is commonly experienced at night – it may wake her. It can be at its worst first thing in the morning, and sufferers may have difficulty holding objects and performing fine movements. Phalen's test (paraesthesia in the three radial fingers provoked by maximal palmar flexion of the wrist for at least one minute), and diminished sensory function in the hand to touch, are two objective diagnostic signs for this condition.

The ulnar nerve, although it passes in front of the flexor retinaculum, may also suffer compression at the wrist or at the elbow. This could lead to numbness and tingling in the fourth and fifth fingers, and sometimes to weakness of the interossei muscles as well as those of the hypothenar eminence.

Treatment

Ekman-Ordeberg et al. (1987) showed that by wearing a wrist splint at night 46 out of 56 women became symptom-free. These splints, which prevent full wrist flexion, could also be worn during the day if necessary.

Physiotherapeutic measures, ice packs (a small bag of frozen peas wrapped in a wet handkerchief could be used at home), resting with the hands in elevation, and wrist and hand exercises may give relief. Some clinicians have found ultrasound to be helpful. While the syndrome usually resolves spontaneously following delivery, decompression surgery may rarely be necessary.

Brachial plexus pain

Some women complain of pain and paraesthesia in the shoulder and arm. Fluid retention and postural changes are thought to cause this, but a familial factor has been noted which could be associated with some anomaly such as a cervical rib.

Treatment

Shoulder girdle exercises and elevation of the arm may prove helpful.

Meralgia paraesthetica

Generalized fluid retention can result in compression of the lateral femoral cutaneous nerve of the thigh as it passes under the inguinal ligament. Symptoms of meralgia paraesthetica – burning paraesthesia over the anterolateral aspect of the thigh, together with mild sensory loss to light touch and pin-prick – can vary from mild to severe. This condition may occur as early as 25 weeks' gestation.

Treatment

TNS has been successfully used to alleviate symptoms. Fisher and Hanna (1987) placed electrodes along the course of the nerve. They described this technique as being highly successful, non-invasive, non-neurolytic and carrying no fetal risk.

Posterior tibial nerve compression

Ankle oedema can compress the posterior tibial nerve as it passes behind the medial malleolus. This will lead to paraesthesia of the sole of the foot and the plantar aspect of the toes.

Treatment

Resting with the legs in elevation plus foot and ankle exercises, and ice packs may be used to relieve discomfort.

CIRCULATORY DISORDERS

Varicose veins in the legs

The hormonally induced hypotonia of the walls of the veins (see p. 33) and raised intra-abdominal pressure together with the presence of incompetent valves, leads to varicosities which are unsightly and often uncomfortable too.

Treatment

Attention to leg circulation is important. Women should be aware that standing or sitting for long periods, with the legs dependent or the knees crossed, is unhelpful. Frequent and vigorous ankle dorsiflexion and plantar flexion – for at least 30 seconds at a time – can promote more efficient venous return. Sitting or lying with the feet raised is also useful. Raising the foot of the bed on bricks is often suggested.

Support tights or stockings may be prescribed and should be put on in bed *before* the woman gets up in the morning. Elastic support stockings are firmer than tights, but are difficult to keep up. If the woman is prepared to wear a maternity pantie-girdle (she will probably have to buy suspenders separately and stitch them into place), she will have good support along the whole length of her legs. However, tights and stockings do tend to slip down and gather into tight ridges just below the knee and around the ankle. Women must understand that this unevenness of pressure could contribute to superficial thrombophlebitis. Tights or stockings will therefore need to be rolled down to the ankles and then gradually eased up the leg again several times a day. Ideally this should be done on a bed or the floor to reduce the effects of gravity on the veins.

Vulval varicose veins

Fortunately this incredibly painful and restricting condition is not common.

Treatment

Rest with the foot of the bed raised, a sanitary pad in a pantie-girdle for support, and frequent pelvic floor contractions may give relief.

Haemorrhoids

Together with the venal hypotonia there is a relative relaxation of the intestinal smooth muscle, resulting in slowing of faecal material through the gut, consequent increased fluid absorption and harder stools, often leading to constipation. Straining to move the bowels can cause ballooning of the veins in and around the anus; these are called haemorrhoids or piles, and are a frequently unmentioned source of discomfort.

Treatment

Once again this is not strictly a problem for the obstetric physiotherapist, but if it is mentioned during an antenatal class, attention to diet – plenty of fibre and fluid – can be reiterated. Pelvic floor contractions will improve perineal and anal circulation, and a small ice pack will relieve pain. In severe cases a foam-rubber ring may increase comfort.

Cramp

Many women suffer from cramp during pregnancy, this often occurs at night. The most common site is the calf, although this painful problem can also occur in the feet and thighs. Different theories as to the cause have been suggested – calcium deficiency, ischaemia and nerve root pressure among them. Towards term increased fluid retention together with reduced activity, particularly in the evenings, may be an additional factor. Calf cramp is almost always triggered by the woman stretching in bed and plantar flexing her feet.

Treatment

A method of preventing calf muscle spasm is to stretch with dorsiflexed feet. Knee extension and dorsiflexion will also release calf cramp if it should occur; deep kneading massage plus vigorous foot exercises will prevent the bruise-like pain which often follows an attack. A pre-bedtime walk, a warm bath and foot exercises may be prophylactic.

Thrombosis and thromboembolism

Thrombosis is not common in pregnancy, but is significant because of the possibility of thromboembolism. The raised level of fibrinogen together with a slowing of venous blood flow, particularly in the legs as pregnancy progresses, predisposes to this condition. Pulmonary embolism, rare but potentially fatal, may be the result.

Treatment

Patients must wear full-length antiembolic stockings, and anticoagulant treatment (e.g. heparin) will be given in severe cases. Physiotherapy consists of an antithrombotic regimen, including foot and leg exercises and deep breathing.

OTHER PROBLEMS

Costal margin pain (rib ache) and intercostal neuralgia

In the final trimester women often complain of pain along the anterior margin of the lower ribs, sometimes accompanied by unilateral thoracic back pain. As the growing uterus rises in the abdomen it forces the ribcage out sideways with consequent stretching of the softened costal interarticular tissues. The 'flaring' can increase the diameter of the chest by as much as 10–15 cm. 'Intercostal neuralgia' is a term sometimes used to describe the intermittent pain, usually unilateral, which can radiate around the chest and may be referred to the lateral abdominal wall.

Treatment

'Rib lifting' techniques are helpful in dealing with these discomforts. Raising both arms over the head with the hands clasped, or side flexion (with arm raised) *away* from the pain may give relief. Sitting astride a chair 'backwards' is often more comfortable than using it conventionally (Fig. 6.2d). A hot-water bottle or an ice pack may also be soothing.

Chondromalacia patellae

Because of the increased ligamentous laxity, slightly wider pelvis and femoral torsion, chondromalacia of the patella can occasionally be a problem. The woman will complain of aching at the front of her knee which is exacerbated by prolonged sitting or by knee flexion–extension activities. Although symptoms may disappear after the baby is born, it is possible that the increase of knee flexion necessary to squat or kneel when picking up toddlers can lead to a recurrence of this troublesome condition months later.

Treatment

Ice packs two or three times per day, plus a strengthening routine for the quadriceps muscles can be helpful.

Restless leg syndrome

The restless leg syndrome is an unpleasant creeping sensation deep in the lower legs causing an irresistible desire to move the leg in order to relieve the sensation; a leg may even involuntarily twitch or jump. The aetiology is uncertain but it is strongly associated with pregnancy. Of 500 women interviewed at an antenatal clinic, 97 (19%) were diagnosed as having this syndrome (Goodman et al., 1988), so it is important for the obstetric physiotherapist to be aware of it. The symptoms seem to be associated with fatigue, and also anxiety or stress. Bed rest or a period of reduced activity, such as giving up work, often give some relief, and the vast majority of women will be symptom-free soon after the birth of their baby. Reassurance and understanding, coupled with advice to rest more, will help to alleviate their worries.

Uterine ligament pain

The 'remodelling' undergone by the skeletal ligaments and collagenous connective tissue also is thought to affect the uterine suspensory ligaments, but they must also be under considerable stretch from the rapidly growing uterus. The sudden, sharp stabs of lower abdominal pain or the constant dull ache, often unilateral, in the iliac fossa are not only distressing but can make the woman wonder if she is in labour. It is often helpful to explain that the uterus is 'tethered' to the pelvis like a tent or a hot-air balloon, and that the worrying 'cramps' are not significant and are not damaging the baby. Warmth or cold may help, as does massaging or stroking the skin over the site of the pain.

Pain from abdominal adhesions

Obstetric physiotherapists, working in centres where various abdominal investigations and surgery for infertility are carried out, may be presented with subsequent abdominal or pelvic pain in pregnant women. Doctors often attribute this to tension on, or subsequent stretching of, postoperative intra-abdominal adhesions. Perhaps also the anxieties brought about by problems in conceiving, lead to a lowering of the pain threshold when the long-awaited pregnancy is finally achieved. Frequently these women will need extra emotional and physical support. Repeated explanation and reassurance with suggestions for the symptomatic treatment of these troublesome pains is necessary, e.g. warmth, abdominal support and TNS.

It should be remembered, though, that abdominal adhesions may occur in the absence of surgery – for example following pelvic inflammatory disease.

Fibroids

These benign tumours (see p. 296) tend to hypertrophy during pregnancy, when they can give rise to pain as a result of red degeneration. Sometimes they are actually visible and palpable through the abdominal wall; women will need reassurance that nothing untoward is occurring. TNS can be used to relieve pain. Following the birth of the baby, and as part of the process of involution, a decrease in size can be expected.

Fatigue

The tiredness so often experienced in the first trimester (p. 102) is usually less noticeable in the middle trimester, but becomes increasingly severe towards term as weight increases and the body is more cumbersome.

Women, their partners and their employers must be prepared to accept the possible need for a reduction in the expectant woman's total daily activity. At the very least, a daily lunch-time rest is essential, horizontal if possible! Weekends should be used wisely; the temptation to complete at any cost tasks such as redecoration, before the birth of the baby, should be resisted.

Insomnia and nightmares

Very many women experience sleep problems as their pregnancies progress. Some find it difficult to get to sleep at night, they are uncomfortable and cannot find a satisfactory sleeping position; others initially fall asleep easily but are unable to drop off again after one of their many night-time visits to the toilet. The enormous psychosocial changes of pregnancy and impending labour and parenthood naturally give rise to anxieties, fears and worries, conscious or unconscious; and vivid and sometimes frightening dreams are also common, especially in the last trimester.

Because most young women are used to an uninterrupted night's sleep of 7–9 hours, many become tense and feel that they will not be able to deal with the coming day. It can help them cope with the problem if they regard it as a 'dress rehearsal' for the broken nights of new motherhood. As well as making every effort to create a sharing atmosphere at each antenatal class so that women feel able to talk about their experiences (it is very helpful for them to realize they are not alone in their predicament), the obstetric physiotherapist can give invaluable advice about the use of pillows, bean bags and alternative sleeping positions. Sometimes the simplest suggestion – such as supporting the abdomen and top leg with pillows in side lying – can mean the difference between sleep or anxious wakefulness. Relaxation has a very important place in the solution of insomnia too. Suggesting to women that instead of tossing and turning in desperation, they get out of bed, eat something light and have a warm drink, and then go back and practise a relaxation technique in a comfortable, well-supported position, can often solve the insomnia problem without resort to sleeping pills.

Pruritus

Distressing skin irritation sometimes presents during the third trimester. The aetiology is uncertain. If simple advice such as discontinuing the use of perfumed soaps, talcs and bath oils, taking cold baths, applying calamine and wearing light cotton clothes is not successful, the mother should be encouraged to consult her doctor.

Heartburn

Although not strictly a problem for the obstetric physiotherapist, this unpleasant condition – a direct consequence of the 'relaxing' effect of pregnancy hormones on the smooth muscle of the cardiac sphincter at the base of the oesophagus – is often mentioned in antenatal classes. The reflux of acid stomach juices into the oesophagus actually burns its mucosa, and this problem is increased by upward pressure of the growing uterus.

Treatment

Apart from suggesting that women consult their general practitioner to have suitable antacids prescribed (free during pregnancy in the UK), it may be helpful to advise them to eat 'little and often'. Raising the head of the bed on two bricks and using extra pillows can give night-time relief.

Morning sickness

Nausea and vomiting often affect women during the first trimester of pregnancy, although it is certainly not restricted to the morning. The raised level of human chorionic gonadotrophin (HCG) (see p. 36) at this stage has been suggested as the cause, and it is often more severe in multiple pregnancies. Fry (1986) has described the use of acupressure to the front of the wrist to relieve postoperative vomiting. The patient's wrist is held so that pressure is evenly applied by the flexor surface of the index, middle and ring fingers of the therapist to the distal 5 cm of the forearm. The thumb gives counterpressure underneath. The force applied should be similar to that of a firm handshake. Fry (1988) also suggests that this technique could be used during pregnancy where sickness is a problem. The acupuncture point that is stimulated is P6. Pressure is applied for 30 seconds at a time. The non-invasive nature of this technique could be attractive to pregnant women, who could apply thier own pressure. A rounded button stitched to a 2 cm wide elastic bracelet and worn so that the button presses on the acupuncture point may also give relief.

Urinary frequency

During the first trimester, when the still anteverted growing uterus presses against the bladder, and again in the final trimester when bladder compression between the abdominal wall and the much enlarged uterus prevents normal volumes of urine being comfortably contained, frequency of micturition is a common and often annoying problem. Nocturia in the first trimester is often a sign of pregnancy to many women who are unused to having to empty their bladder at night. Additionally, the increased volume of urine produced during pregnancy is partly responsible for frequency.

Stress incontinence

This troublesome and embarrassing symptom can present during pregnancy, particularly in the third trimester. It is a condition that should be discussed regularly in antenatal classes – very few people have the courage to volunteer that they are experiencing bladder leakage, and it can be very helpful for them to realize that they are not alone. For most women it will be a transitory problem, but they should be aware antenatally that if stress incontinence continues after the birth of their baby it can be treated. Midwives and doctors may need reminding that it is a pregnancy ailment that possibly can be relieved.

Treatment

Women may be able to control leakage by bracing the pelvic floor before coughing, sneezing or lifting (see p. 369). If they are not already exercising their pelvic floor muscles regularly – it is never too late to start! If there is uncertainty as to whether they are contracting the pelvic floor correctly, the suggestion that they try to stop their flow of urine in mid-stream may be useful. Where the problem appears to be severe, or the woman claims to be unable to feel a pelvic floor contraction, it is advisable to investigate further. Inspection of the perineum will help ascertain if the woman is actually able to use her pelvic floor muscles. In view of the fact that vaginal examinations should be avoided where possible in pregnancy the obstetric physiotherapist should ask the professional who may perform the procedure to check if the woman is able to contract her pelvic floor. A note should be made for a follow-up appointment to be offered postnatally should the stress incontinence persist.

References

Abramson D., Roberts S.M., Wilson P.D. (1934). Relaxation of the pelvic joints in pregnancy. *Surgical Gynaecology and Obstetrics*, **58**, 595.

Bell G.R., Rothman R.H. (1984). The conservative treatment of sciatica. *Spine*, **9**, 1., 54–6.

Berg G., Hammar M., Möller-Nielsen J. et al. (1988). Low back pain during pregnancy. *Obst. Gynec.*, **71**, 71–75.

Bullock J., Jull G.H., Bullock M.I. (1987). The relationship of low back pain to postural changes during pregnancy. *Austr. J. Physiother.*, **33**, 10–17.

Calguneri C., Bird H., Wright V. (1982). Changes in joint laxity occurring during pregnancy. *Ann. Rheum. Dis.*, **41**, 126–8.

Cats A. (1986). Inflammatory disease and the spine. *International Back Pain Society Seminar*, London.

Consumers Association (1986). Back pain. *'Which' Magazine*, February.

Coxhead C.E., Inshipp H., Mead T.W. et al. (1981). Multicentre trial of physiotherapy in the management of sciatica symptoms. *Lancet*, i, 1065.

Don Tigny R.L. (1985). Function and pathomechanics of the sacroiliac joint. *Phys. Ther.*, **65**, 35–44.

Ekman-Ordeberg G., Salgeback S., Ordeberg G. (1987). Carpal tunnel syndrome in pregnancy. *Acta Obstet. Gynecol. Scand.*, **66**, 233–5.

Fast A. et al. (1987). Low back pain in pregnancy. *Spine*, **12**, 368–71.

Fisher A.P., Hanna M. (1987). Transcutaneous electrical nerve stimulation in meralgia paraesthetica of pregnancy. *Brit. J. Obstet. Gynaec.*, **94**, 603–5.

Fraser D. (1976). Postpartum backache; a preventable condition? *Canadian Family Physician*, **22**, 1434–6.

Fry E.N.S. (1986). Acupressure and postoperatve vomiting. *Anaesthesia*, **41**, 661–2.

Fry E.N.S. (1988). Acupressure and morning sickness. *J. Roy. Soc. Med.*, **81**, 44.

Golightly R. (1982). Pelvic arthropathy in pregnancy and the puerperium. *Physiotherapy*, **68**, 216–20.

Goodman J.D.S., Brodie C., Ayida G.A. (1988). Restless leg syndrome in pregnancy. *Br. Med. J.*, **297**, 1101–2.

Gould J.S., Wissinger H.A. (1978). Carpal tunnel syndrome in pregnancy. *Southern Med. J.*, **71**, 144–9.

Grieve G.P. (1981). *Common Vertebral Joint Problems*, p. 398. Edinburgh: Churchill Livingstone.

Haldeman S., Meyer B.J. (1977). Why one cause of back pain? In *Approaches to the Validation of Manipulation Therapy* (Buerger A.A., Tobis J.S., eds.) Ch. 10. Springfield: Thomas.

Hall D.C., Kaufmann D.A. (1987). Effects of aerobic and strength conditioning on pregnancy outcomes. *Am. J. Obstet. Gynecol.*, **157**, 1199–1203.

Lewit K., Knobloch V., Fakterora Z. (1970). Vertebral disorders and obstetric pain. *Manuelle Medizin*, **4**, 70.

Mannheimer J.S. (1985). TENS – uses and effectiveness. In *Pain, International Perspectives in Physical Therapy*, (Hoskins M.T., ed.) p. 77. Edinburgh: Churchill Livingstone.

Mantle M.J. (1988). Backache in pregnancy. In *Obstetrics and Gynaecology International Perspectives in Physical Therapy* (McKenna J., ed.) Ch. 5. Edinburgh: Churchill Livingstone.

Mantle M.J., Greenwood R.M., Currey H.L.F. (1977). Backache in pregnancy. *Rheum. Rehab.*, **16**, 95–110.

Mantle M.J., Holmes J., Currey H.L.F. (1981). Backache in pregnancy. II: Prophylactic influence of backache classes. *Rheum. Rehab.*, **20**, 227–32.

Melvin J.L., Brunett C.N., Johnsson E.W. (1969). Median nerve conduction in pregnancy. *Arch. Phys. Med.*, **50**, 75–80.

Nwuga V.E.B. (1982). Pregnancy and back pain among upper-class Nigerian women. *Aust. J. Physiother.*, **28**, (4), 8–11.

Scholey M., Hair M. (1989). Back pain in physiotherapists involved in back care education. *Ergonomics*, **32**, 179–90.

Sims-Williams H., Jayson M.V., Young S.M.S. et al. (1978). Controlled trial of mobilisation and manipulation for patients with low back pain in general practice. *Br. Med. J.*, **2**, 1338.

Smith R., Winearls C.G., Stevenson J.C. et al. (1985). Osteoporosis of pregnancy. *Lancet*, **i**, 1178–80.

Voitk A.J., Mueller J.C., Farlinger D.E., Johnston R.U. (1983). Carpal tunnel syndrome in pregnancy. *Can. Med. J.*, **128**, 277–282.

Further Reading

Chamberlain G., ed. (1984). *Pregnant Women at Work*. London: Royal Society of Medicine/Macmillan.

Cherry N. (1987). Physical demands of work and health complaints among women working late in pregnancy. *Ergonomics* **30(4)**, 689–701.

Grieve E. (1980). The biomechanical characterisation of sacroiliac joint motion. MSc Thesis, University of Strathclyde.

Grieve G.P. (1976). The sacroiliac joint. *Physiotherapy*, **62**, 384–400.

Mullinax K.M., Dale E. (1986). Some considerations of exercise during pregnancy. *Clin. Sports Med.*, **5**, 559.

Potter N.A., Rothstein J.M. (1985). Intertester reliability for selected clinical tests of the sacroiliac joint. *Phys. Ther.*, **65**, 1671–1675.

Wilder E., ed. (1988). *Obstetric and Gynecologic Physical Therapy*. Edinburgh: Churchill Livingstone.

CHAPTER 6

Preparation for Labour

Before beginning a course of 'preparation for labour' classes, obstetric physiotherapists must always remember that women have different hopes, fears and aims for their labour. Some will want to handle this immense physical and emotional experience on their own, with as little intervention as possible. Others will plan to make use of whatever technology is available to help them speedily and painlessly through the event. It is essential that physiotherapists do not impose their own opinions on the client. They may well feel that the 'right' way to cope with labour is for a woman to use her own resources without resort to the 'big guns' of analgesia, and that breast-feeding is the only way to feed a baby. However, there will probably be women attending the classes who would like to 'book' their epidural anaesthetic in advance, and for whom the mere thought of breast-feeding is repulsive. Although it is wrong to generalize, surveys have shown that middle-class women are more likely to demand a natural childbirth, while working-class mothers-to-be are not so concerned with this; they tend to see childbirth as a means to an end and want it to be as comfortable, painless and safe as possible (McIntosh, 1989; Nielson, 1983).

Fashions come and go in obstetrics, as they do in everything else; antenatal teachers must not only be aware of developments and changes in obstetric and midwifery practice, but should also follow trends and views that will concern pregnant women and their partners. Subjects such as 'water birth' may only interest the dedicated few initially; but if it is shown that this method of birth can be used safely by low-risk women, then it is likely to be adopted by maternity units who feel that choice in childbirth is the right of all their clients. Thirty to forty years ago husbands were not allowed in most labour wards; then they were allowed to remain with their wives if they were found to be 'suitable' on interview, but only for the first stage of labour. Today they are welcomed as part of the team, and the emotional and physical support they give is acknowledged by carers as well as by labouring women. What started as a demand from articulate middle-class women in the late 1950s and early 1960s, when women were often left unattended for many hours in the first stage of labour, has evolved into accepted practice.

The use of procedures such as routine episiotomy and the use of forceps as opposed to vacuum extraction have also been challenged, and discussion often follows in the media. Women will want to talk about such matters in class, and antenatal teachers must be aware of current controversies and the scientific basis behind both sides of each argument.

Many women, and possibly their carers too, regard labour as the 'grand finale' of pregnancy; an ordeal which must be gone through before 'life goes back to normal'. It is perhaps better regarded as a continuation of pregnancy, the 'overture' to parenthood and a totally new lifestyle. Labour is undoubtedly a physical and emotional marathon, and, whereas in some cultures it may be accepted on a more natural physiological level, in developed countries its importance has assumed gigantic proportions – an event that must be prepared and even 'trained' for. While formal antenatal classes are not advocated by some authorities (Michel Odent felt they were unnecessary when he was at Pithiviers), there is no doubt that a woman feels more in control, confident and able to cope if she has 'something' she can do or use during her labour contractions. There is a natural anxiety in all women about their ability to withstand the crises of labour and birth. While childbirth preparation will not alter the primary causes of labour pain, it can modify women's perception and interpretation of these signals, increase their confidence in themselves and their carers, and give them 'tools' to use which will help them deal with whatever eventualities labour brings. This 'tool-kit' of coping skills, non-invasive and without deleterious side-effects, can make the difference between confidence and fear, satisfaction and disappointment. This is important, because since childbirth has become safer for mother and baby and simple survival is no longer the main aim, attention has turned towards making it a psychologically rewarding experience too.

The drawback to this aspect of antenatal education is that sometimes women and their partners, in spite of every effort on the part of their antenatal teachers to present the realities of labour without minimizing the intensity of the experience, will set themselves goals which, in some cases, prove unrealistic and unattainable. It now seems that it is not enough for the mother to survive and give birth to an undamaged baby; some women will be looking for the ultimate psychosexual and orgasmic experience; others hope for labour without pain relief and with an intact perineum. While some may recall their experience of giving birth as a high spot in their lives – a pinnacle of achievement – there are many who do not have their hoped-for pattern of labour. These latter women can be desperately disappointed, feel like failures, and have the early days, weeks or even months with their new babies blighted by their inability to handle labour as they had planned. With the right preparation and support it is possible for a woman to be satisfied with a 'high-tech', actively managed birth with every possible intervention, even when she may have been hoping for a natural labour which started spontaneously, and progressed via endurable contractions to a normal delivery with an intact perineum.

It is important for antenatal educators to impress upon their clients the tremendous variability of labour, and to prepare them for the way in which it will be managed in the unit they have chosen to use for the birth. It is downright harmful to present a picture of contractions which will merely be 'uncomfortable', a labour ward where 'anything goes' and where intervention is reserved for the very few, when the teacher knows that labour ward protocol in the place where the woman will be delivering is rigid and governed by strict criteria, for example as to the time allowed for cervical dilatation and for the management of the second and third stages of labour. Nor can it be a good preparation for birth to present the controversies that surround so many obstetric procedures these days, to condemn the very methods with which the women will have to deal and send them in to 'do battle' at what will be an emotionally and physically vulnerable time. It is far better for the teacher to help mothers plan their hoped-for labours, encourage them to put their wishes in writing on the birth plan most hospitals now use, and suggest that they discuss and make requests *in advance* with senior personnel. Where a teacher feels strongly about the inadvisability of some labour ward procedure, it is the *teacher's* duty to discuss it with midwives and doctors, making sure that this concern is backed by research and hard facts, rather then by feeling or intuition.

In addition to a clear, factual explanation of the physiology of labour and the way women are cared for at this time, the coping skills that should be presented as a preparation for labour ought to include relaxation, imagery, breathing awareness, positioning, massage and other strategies such as a warm bath or music.

RELAXATION

It is interesting to trace the philosophies underlying the use of relaxation for labour in modern obstetrics, because the original concept that the mother should 'lie back and breathe' has today largely been replaced by a more positive attitude and active approach towards coping with the pain and stresses of labour.

Grantly Dick-Read, one of the pioneers in this field, advocated the use of relaxation as a means of breaking the vicious cycle of pain–fear–tension (Dick-Read, 1942) and began teaching it as early as 1933. Randall (1953) has a chapter in her book *Fearless Childbirth* called 'Relaxation makes you fit and fearless'. She suggested that there were two reasons for teaching relaxation to use in labour:

1. To prevent the mother becoming unduly tired, thereby causing 'nervous fatigue'.
2. To help her control her thoughts and feelings or emotions.

Heardman (1951) said that in order to displace disturbing and worrying thoughts some positive idea must be given to the mind. Rhythm is a mental release, and the natural breathing rhythm is incorporated in her scheme of progressive relaxation. These three authors used the 'tense–relax' relaxation technique.

Since 1963 the Mitchell method of physiological relaxation has been widely used by obstetric physiotherapists. In the latest edition of her admirable book (Mitchell, 1987) she suggests that a woman should use pre-labour Braxton Hicks contractions for practising relaxation during a muscular wave of activity over which she has no control. She feels that relaxation should be used during the first stage of labour as a method of conserving the mother's energy for the 'hardest work she will ever do'. In the second stage, relaxation fits well into the cycle of maximum activity during contractions followed by maximum rest in between, which appears to be nature's intention for an efficient, quick and safe emptying of the uterus. The beauty of her method is that by performing the movements necessary to put trigger areas in positions of ease and comfort, the mother can produce relaxation in the space of a few seconds.

Hassid (1978) draws attention to the fact that during labour the body is required to perform hard physical work for long periods of time under stress, and that the intensity of the pain experienced by women will be partly affected by cultural variables, previous pain experience, anxiety and fatigue. A system of controlled relaxation based on psychoprophylaxis is described. To learn this, the woman lies supine, fixes her eyes on a spot to enhance concentration, and tenses and relaxes legs, arms and face while inhaling and then exhaling. Her 'labour coach' works with her – 'tapping' working areas, feeling muscles for 'quality' of tension and then stroking and moving the relaxed limb. This progresses to tensing one limb or the 'key' areas (jaw and perineum) while relaxing everywhere else. The labour coach constantly assesses the woman's tension and relaxation so that in labour she is able to release tension in response to gentle stroking.

Noble (1980) says that relaxation is more than rest or stillness; it involves recognizing and releasing excess tension – whatever the cause. The passive relaxation practised in pregnancy should be replaced by an alert but 'non-striving' state of relaxation in labour. She describes a sequence of 'dissociation' – selective relaxation which develops the body's ability to maintain a state of general release when one part of it (the uterus) is working hard. In 1983 Noble wrote that 'relaxation is the key to awareness and energy' (Noble, 1983). 'Unblocking' the muscular system and breathing freely can be a blissful release when tension has developed. She points to the fact that women who have found ways to release tension in labour experience contractions that are very different to those felt by women without this 'safety valve' – the contractions are almost pleasurable.

Williams and Booth (1985) feel that the kind of relaxation where women are left to doze while the teacher goes away to make a cup of tea is inappropriate as a preparation for the use of relaxation in labour.

One of their suggestions for experiencing relaxation during discomfort is for a partner to squeeze the inside of a woman's thigh, increasing the pressure until it becomes unpleasant, while she tries to minimize the sensation by deliberately relaxing towards the pressure – concentrating on deep, slow breathing. Kitzinger (1987) discusses the concept of 'touch relaxation', where a woman relaxes towards the touch of her partner. While this may be useful for some people, it should be remembered that many women cannot bear to be touched during labour contractions; another possible disadvantage is that a woman's partner may not be able to be with her during labour, which could reduce her confidence and the ease with which she is able to cope with her birth experience, should she have planned for her partner's active involvement.

Whichever method of achieving relaxation the obstetric physiotherapist decides to teach, it must be with a full understanding of the way in which it reduces tension, gives ease and comfort, and enables women to deal with the stress and pain of labour. The piecemeal amalgamation of parts or aspects of different methods of teaching relaxation, most particularly without full understanding and consideration, is to be deprecated, for conflicting effects may actually be produced. For example Jacobson (1938) activates both antagonists and agonists maximally, while Mitchell (1987) activates only antagonists moderately. However, it is important to realize that simply 'relaxing' during contractions will not usually be enough to enable women to cope with their intensity. To an awareness of relaxation in the 'trigger areas' (face, shoulders, hands) must be added other self-help techniques (movement, breathing, massage etc.). While relaxation is initially taught in well-supported positions (lying, side lying, sitting), women must also practise relaxing in postures that are possibly not so comfortable. There is little use in being able to relax perfectly while lying on your side but be unable to release tension in prone kneeling, if during labour prone kneeling is the one position that relieves your backache!

Relaxation practice must never be hurried. Although a dark, quiet room is not necessary (it may even be a disadvantage because labour wards are certainly rarely dark *or* quiet!), class participants must be given time and freedom to explore the uniquely personal state that relaxation can bring. It is inadvisable for the obstetric physiotherapist to move around the room, lifting arms and legs to 'test' relaxation; this is distracting and stressful, and should be unnecessary. With experience, it is easy to recognize relaxation; the position of the body, the rate of respiration, eyes open or closed, whether a person fidgets or not, and the overall look of comfort are all clues which point to the success or failure of the method being used. Women must be encouraged to change position if they are uncomfortable; they should be covered if they are cold; the antenatal teacher must be swift to provide extra pillows for support (one wedge and one pillow per participant are *not* sufficient), and above all she must encourage and praise. After all, it is often difficult to relax in the safety and comfort of your own bed – how much harder to become deeply relaxed on the floor of a parentcraft room!

Relaxation once a week for the length of the antenatal course is unlikely to produce a level of awareness in all women that will enable them to cope with a stress such as labour. Women should be urged to bring the art into their daily lives. They must become aware of stress and tension when they queue in the bank or post office, sit in traffic jams, peel potatoes (hunched shoulders often accompany the simplest chores), deal with difficult toddlers, give blood in the antenatal clinic and experience abdominal or vaginal examinations. They should be encouraged to use their relaxation response to cope with irritating, worrying or painful events; in this way they will become more confident of their ability to use the technique during labour. Formal relaxation sessions, in bed when they cannot sleep, or on a chair or couch in the middle of the day, are also important. It is useful to discuss with each group, week by week, *when* they practised and what problems they were able to ease by utilizing the relaxation skills they are gradually accumulating. Finally, although relaxation will be a valuable tool during the comparatively few hours of labour, antenatal teachers must never lose the opportunity to impress upon class participants that the ability to control the body's response to stress is a skill that will last for a lifetime.

When a relaxation session draws to a close it is important that people 'come back' slowly. They should take a deep breath in, stretch, and stretch again (feet pulled up to prevent calf cramp), and then stay where they are until they feel ready to slowly sit and then stand up. Participants should also be given the opportunity to discuss their opinion of the session – was it comfortable, easy, nice? Did they enjoy the experience? Was it uncomfortable or difficult? In this way the obstetric physiotherapist will learn from the clients which techniques work and are helpful, and which do not succeed in giving a successful experience of deep relaxation.

IMAGERY

A person's thoughts and emotions can produce powerful effects on their physiology, and imagery is a way of harnessing these thoughts to complement physical relaxation. The suggestion should be made, while people are relaxing, that they imagine they are somewhere pleasant, perhaps a place they know – their garden, a park or the beach. It is warm and sunny, birds are singing, people are talking in the distance but are not intruding; they can smell cut grass or beautifully perfumed flowers; maybe birds are flying overhead. Alternatively, they hear the waves gently rolling on to the sand, and then the sound of the water being sucked back again. The smell of the seashore and perhaps the sun lotion they have smoothed on their body is in the air. Children are playing and laughing but not disturbing their rest; and all the time – whichever place they choose to escape to – the sun is warming their body, making them feel heavy and very comfortable. Their special place is safe, and they can go back there whenever they like. Each person should 'paint' her own environment – the grass or sand, the rug she is lying on, the colour of the sky, the trees and flowers or rocks and dunes – all contribute to her personal scenario. Such vivid, personal thoughts can greatly assist the process of relaxation.

BREATHING

Breathing is normally involuntary; it continues, at different rates and depths depending on what we are doing, from the moment of birth until the moment of death. It can, however, also be a voluntary activity – consciously controlled and manipulated. Noble (1981) draws attention to the many physiological adjustments that occur in the respiratory and cardiovascular systems during pregnancy. Alveolar ventilation, tidal volume, cardiac output and blood volume are all increased. The whole system is perfectly designed so that maternal and fetal blood gases are adequately exchanged. It is difficult, she says, to understand the justification for altering something as fundamental as normal breathing, especially during the increased metabolic demands that occur in labour. And yet, over the years, this is precisely what some authorities have recommended: 'controlled' respiration, with both the rate and depth consciously altered. In some cases breathing techniques are even dictated by a labour coach. Historically, different authors have suggested different ways of using breathing during labour (Table 6.1, see pp. 170–174).

Stradling (1984) states that the average person has a respiratory rate of approximately 15 breaths per minute with a tidal volume of 333 ml. This gives a total volume of around 5 litres per minute (15 × 333 ml). However, 133 ml per breath do not reach the alveoli, being wasted in filling up the airways. Alveolar ventilation is therefore 3 litres per minute (15 × 200 ml). He presented figures (Table 6.2, see p. 175) which show that even when the overall ventilation is kept constant at 5 litres per minute, slow and deep breathing gives much better alveolar ventilation – and therefore oxygen absorption and carbon dioxide release – than fast, shallow respiration.

During heavy exercise alveolar ventilation may increase ten- to twenty-fold to supply the additional oxygen needed and excrete the excess carbon dioxide produced (Vander, 1980). Stradling (1984) states that during labour there is a considerable increase in the oxygen requirements of the body and its carbon dioxide production. More alveolar ventilation is necessary and this is often doubled or quadru-

Table 6.1 Recommendations for breathing during labour

Author	First stage	Transitional stage	Second stage
Dick-Read (1942)	Natural free respiration which increases in rate and depth as labour progresses; 24–28 full breaths per minute. Abdominal and upper thoracic respiration	Not specifically mentioned, but breathing will probably be at its fastest and deepest	Women were 'trained' to hold their breath to push; 2–3 full deep breaths were taken after each expulsive effort. Rapid shallow panting for delivery
Heardman (1951)	Abdominal breathing *very* slow. The mother attempts to take one breath in and out in 30 seconds, progressing to 40–50 seconds	Costal and sternal breathing with an open mouth, drawing deep breaths. This may sound 'noisy'	Holding a lungful of air, the mother bears down until she can hold her breath no longer; she does this possibly 3 times per contraction. She takes deep breaths when it is over. 'Sternal' panting with open mouth for delivery
Randall (1953)	Although 'deep' breathing (a slow breath in through the nose and out through the mouth with an 'Ah-h' sigh), 'deeper' breathing (prolonged expiration followed by a deep breath in), and 'easy long breathing' (a slow, gentle, deep breath in and out through the nose, without allowing the abdomen to move and with the breath held for 3 counts) are all mentioned as aids to relaxation – the way a woman 'should' breathe during labour is not actually described anywhere in the book		

Table 6.1 Recommendations for breathing during labour (continued)

Author	First stage	Transitional stage	Second stage
Karmel (1959) (Lamaze)	Slow, deep, costal breathing (in through the nose, out through the mouth). This changes to lightly accelerated and superficial breathing or panting (through nose or mouth). Almost silent, no abdominal movement	Panting with a forced blow 'out' every 20 seconds to resist premature pushing urges	A breath in and then out; then a deep breath, in through the nose, which is held for 20–30 seconds. Two pushes for contractions of 70 seconds
Kitzinger (1962)	Slow breathing 'all down the back' is used to aid relaxation and to gain control between contractions. 'Contraction-led' breathing, ranging from slow full chest, via quicker, shallow chest, to 'mouth-centred' (very shallow and rapid) breathing	Mouth-centred 'hummingbird wing' breathing, punctuated every so often by a crisp blow 'out'	Breathe in, blow out; then take a deep breath in through the mouth, fixing ribs and diaphragm; hold the breath and squeeze baby gently and evenly down, releasing pelvic floor muscles

Table 6.1 Recommendations for breathing during labour (continued)

Author	First stage	Transitional stage	Second stage
Wright (1964) Describes the practice of psychoprophylaxis and the 'levels' of breathing and 'disassociation' drill favoured by this regimen	Conscious, controlled breathing in four levels: *Level A* – deep breath in through the nose, blow out through the mouth. Notice how diaphragm goes down. *Level B* – breathe in and out through the mouth, expanding lower ribs; less deep than level A – emphasize breath out. *Level C* – 'breast-bone' breathing in and out through the mouth; mentally say 'out' with each outward breath. *Level D* – stop concentrating on breathing – let it happen automatically. Sing a song in the head and tap the rhythm with the fingers The breathing accelerates gradually from level A to level C and there is formal practice with the number of breaths at each level being suggested by the teacher. Level D is used for 20–50 seconds in the middle of the strongest contractions	A controlled response to contractions where there may be an urge to push: 1 breath in level B 3–4 breaths in level C 5–8 breaths in level D Then silently count '1, 2, 1, 2' as air is allowed into the chest, followed by blowing it out through pursed lips. This is accompanied by a 'sit up' and 'slump' movement if the mother is sitting, and by a movement of her upper arm like a rudder if she is in side lying	Two breaths in level A while getting into the pushing position (sacrum flat and horizontal, 3–4 pillows behind upper body, legs lifted and held with the feet off the bed, supported by the mother's hands under her knees). The third breath in is held for 10 counts, the chin goes on to the chest, ribs and shoulders pushed down, and the abdominal muscles and pelvic floor pushed forwards. This 'blocks' the air in the chest. This is repeated so that there is a 'block-and-push' cycle. Panting breaths in deep level C for the actual birth

Table 6.1 Recommendations for breathing during labour (*continued*)

Author	First stage	Transitional stage	Second stage
Hassid (1978)	'Rhythmic chest breathing' – 7–8 breaths per minute progressing to a faster rhythm of 12–16 breaths per minute. Breathe in through the nose – count '1'; passive exhalation through the mouth – count '2, 3'	Shallow breathing – 1 breath per 2 seconds, increasing to 1 per second and then decreasing the rate. 'Puff-blow' – shallow breathing punctuated every few seconds by a short, staccato blow out	Breathe in and out, breathe in and out, breathe in, hold and push. Relax perineum. Breathe out, relax
Noble (1980)	Continue with normal breathing as long as possible – concentration on outward breath enhances relaxation. Allow breathing to become lighter and faster ('panting'). Breathing rate and depth inversely related: slow= deep, faster=shallow	Combination of blowing and panting: 6 pants and blow, or 3, 2 or 1 pants with a blow, known as 'hoo-hah' or 'choo-choo' breathing	'Spontaneous' pushing with the air audibly exhaled. One or more pushes per contraction, depending on the urge. Pant for delivery – relax pelvic floor throughout
Balaskas (1983)	Deep 'belly' breathing, concentrating on exhalation. When contractions become intense, groaning, moaning, humming or singing may help	Keep up deep breathing, still concentrating on breath out; if breathing naturally becomes shallower, allow this to happen. Some women will need to make a noise and others to be very quiet	Give in to the natural urges of the body. Do not hold the breath to push; release the pelvic floor and allow whatever cry or scream, which will happen instinctively, to emerge

Table 6.1 Recommendations for breathing during labour (*continued*)

Author	First stage	Transitional stage	Second stage
Williams and Booth (1985)	'Easy breathing' – a little slower and deeper than usual (12 breaths per minute). 'Lighter breathing' – the upper chest rises and falls 'like a pigeon ruffling its breast feathers' (24–28 breaths per minute)	Breathing to prevent pushing: 'fairly deep' breathing to move the diaphragm up and down, together with a sharp blow out through relaxed lips	One or two deep breaths in and out, then hold the breath making the diaphragm 'piston' go down. Repeat when breath runs out, after a gulp of air. Slow 'St Bernard dog' panting for crowning

In a chapter entitled 'Some new ideas' the following is suggested:

	Ignore contractions in the beginning; when they become distressing give a long, easy breath out through the mouth and then breathe through the nose at any rate or depth the body chooses	SOS technique – sigh out slowly through the mouth, breathing in through the mouth. 'Tune in' to the demands each contraction makes on the body	Strong breath holding is discouraged – short pushes are made – and the woman can 'hiss' gently out to prevent 'throat pushing'

Table 6.2 Comparison of breathing rates (Stradling, 1984)

	Slow & Deep	Normal	Fast & Shallow
Respiratory rate (per minute)	10	15	20
Tidal volume (ml)	500	333	250
Total ventilation (litres)	5	5	5
Alveolar ventilation (litres)	3.7	3.0	2.3

pled. It must follow, therefore, that slow, deep breathing will be more beneficial to mother and fetus during labour, and that techniques that stipulate a rapid increase in respiratory rate and a reduction in depth interfere with the natural physiology of breathing and the gaseous exchange. Buxton (1965) showed that where 'levels' of breathing were taught antenatally (psychoprophylaxis, Lamaze, Wright), marked hyperventilation accompanied their use.

Hyperventilation and blood gases

Breathing is primarily controlled by carbon dioxide levels via the brain stem. Rises in carbon dioxide levels are not tolerated and are followed by hyperventilation to wash out the excess and restore normal levels. Hypocapnia (a low level of carbon dioxide) is tolerated, however, and results from voluntary or involuntary hyperventilation. Rises in oxygen levels are tolerated, but not falls. Carbon dioxide is acid; low levels will cause respiratory alkalosis (raised pH) leading to a decrease in calcium ionization, which can affect nerve conductivity (Table 6.3).

Table 6.3 Effects of hyperventilation

Signs and symptoms	Cause
Dizziness, 'wooziness', eventual unconsciousness	Cerebral hypoxia due to constriction of cerebral vessels and reduced blood pressure
Numbness and tingling in the lips and extremities; paraesthesia and muscle spasm	Changes in ionized calcium caused by alkalosis which affects nerve conduction
Pallor, sweating, feelings of panic and anxiety	Possibly due to cerebral anoxia

Theoretically, maternal hyperventilation could affect the fetus:

1. Low maternal carbon dioxide levels lead to reduced uterine blood flow (caused by lowered blood pressure and uterine vasoconstriction).

2. Haemoglobin 'hangs on' to oxygen when the blood is alkalotic; this reduces the amount of oxygen available to the fetus in the placenta.

However, it has not been shown that hyperventilation, which probably occurs physiologically in all labouring women, actually affects the normal fetus which is not compromised. What might possibly affect the fetus is the maternal apnoea (sometimes prolonged) that follows periods of hyperventilation. As the carbon dioxide level falls the oxygen level rises; neither of these states stimulate the brain to continue respiration. Until the carbon dioxide level rises again, the message 'breathe' will not be given – it is this apnoeic episode that could add to distress in the compromised fetus. It is advisable, therefore, for women to be encouraged to continue breathing gently when a contraction finishes; talking will also result in their taking in breaths. Symptoms of hyperventilation can be relieved and the condition reversed if the mother breathes into her cupped hands or a paper bag, thus replacing carbon dioxide.

Breathing for labour

When asked, many women state that their reason for attending antenatal classes is to be 'taught the breathing' to use during labour contractions. It can now be seen that teaching rigid patterns of respiration has the potential not only of reducing the oxygen supply to mother and fetus, but by actually causing hyperventilation and low carbon dioxide levels, of giving rise to distressing maternal side-effects, i.e. panic, anxiety, 'wooziness', paraesthesia. This in turn will further affect the rate and depth of respiration, intensifying the symptoms.

A useful introduction to breathing awareness can be made when relaxation is taught. With the class sitting or lying comfortably, ask the women how many times they think they breathe out in one minute. Replies can vary between 4 and 64 breaths per minute! Next, ask them to count each outward breath made during a timed minute. Of course everyone will be different because there is not a completely uniform respiratory rate. The observed number of expirations will range from 10 to 25 or so (a useful indicator of people who may be hyperventilating in day-to-day life). Hasten to reassure them that they are all normal – everyone is different! Now ask them to notice what happens when they breathe at rest – cool air can be felt entering the nostrils, warm air coming out. Suggest that they focus on their own individual pattern of breathing: a breath in – momentary tidal pause – a breath out – and then a rest between breaths. Now ask them to feel where movement takes place as they breathe; resting their fingers lightly on their 'babies', can they feel a rise and fall of the abdomen? Explain how slow, 'low', or 'deep', calm 'abdominal' breathing has a soothing, tension-releasing effect at times of stress. O'Brien (1988) suggests that we 'breathe out tension, breathe in peace'. Tell the class to move their hands to the lower rib cage and ask what happens here as they breathe. Mention that our bodies receive more oxygen when our breathing is slow and deep rather than fast and shallow, and this will be better for their babies in labour. Now build this slow, calm, easy breathing into relaxation practice; explain how expiration can increase the depth of relaxation and relieve tension. When people are under stress, as well as adopting the 'tension' posture to a greater or lesser extent, they will tighten or pull in their abdominal muscles: can they feel the ease and release gained from allowing the abdominal wall to swell and fall back instead? Ask them to practise calm, easy breathing when they relax at home and also to use it in stressful situations. Be wary of introduciing too much scientific jargon. Explanations must always be geared to the level of understanding of each class.

Coping with contractions

When discussing labour contractions it is most important to emphasize their positive nature. Yes, they will probably be painful – but it is a life-giving pain. Although the mother knows for certain that a contraction is going to come and will build up to a peak, she should also concentrate on the fact that each contraction, having done its work, will then decline and die away, allowing her to rest and 'recharge her batteries'. She must deal with each 'rush of energy' (Gaskin, 1977) as it comes – there is only one contraction to cope with at a time; those that have passed and those yet to come are irrelevant to the task in hand.

Although the obstetric physiotherapist will have described the physiology and mechanics of labour, it is helpful to describe the use of imagery as well, so that women and their partners can better cope with their experience. Perhaps compare labour to the sea: usually calm and flat, with just the odd 'ripple' or 'wavelet' of Braxton Hicks contractions. As labour progresses, the sea gradually gets rougher: waves last longer, are higher and more demanding and they come closer together. The woman's aim is to let it happen, to ride the 'waves' produced by her working uterus; her breathing and relaxation, helped by positions of comfort and perhaps massage too, are surfboards or rowing boats taking her up, over the top, and down the other side. Each wave takes her nearer the shore and the birth of her baby.

Alternatively, the image of a range of hills can be used: low and easy to climb at first, becoming steeper and more rugged, and, eventually, overwhelmingly difficult. Each contraction becomes a 'mountain' (some low and short, others high and long-lasting); each mountain starts with a walk up grassy slopes (mention the buttercups, daisies, sheep and cows), and becomes steeper as the paths turn into stones. Then come the sheer rock faces and, finally, the ice, snow, glaciers and avalanches. Just as they feel they cannot go any higher, the mountain goes down the other side and they descend, via the rocks and stony paths, until they reach the green meadows at the bottom. Obviously not all the contractions will reach the 'glaciers' every time – class practice must include all sizes of waves or mountains!

Some teachers compare the course of labour to taking a walk up a mountain. The latent phase of the first stage allows the mother to walk through undulating meadows; the established active phase means she has to make her way up steeper paths and rocks (the end of the first stage, or transition as it is sometimes called, can seem like an insurmountable face of rock); her baby will be born at the summit of the mountain.

It is helpful to draw diagrams of contractions, perhaps on a black-board, to show the likely progress of labour see Appendix 1. It is also useful to 'draw' each contraction in the air with a hand as the class is talked through it. It is an aid to relaxation if every first-stage contraction begins with a breath out and the word 'relax'; every contraction should be consciously welcomed, each one brings the woman nearer to the birth of her baby. Women should notice their 'trigger areas' of tension (jaw, shoulders, hands) and release these as they breathe slowly and comfortably up and over each contraction's peak. Some people find it helpful to say, in their head or out loud, 'relax', 'let go' or 'out' with expiration, linking it with the release of tension and relaxation. Every contraction should end with at least one deep breath in and then out – 'Hooray, I've done it, that's one less!'

Deep, slow, calm breathing – pausing between expiration and inspiration – may be all that some women use in the first stage. Most, however, will be unable to maintain this and a modification will be needed. Untrained women may either hold their breath or uncontrollably hyperventilate when contractions progressively become stronger and more painful. Bearing in mind that by using slow, deep breathing the mothers will have alveolar ventilation of about 3.7 litres per minute, they may find it helpful to take breaths that are very slightly lighter and a little faster (3.0 litres per minute alveolar respiration). After all, the respiratory response to exercise and effort is for breathing to become faster. In the class this can be introduced as gentle 'feather' or 'candle' breathing. They could imagine that an ostrich feather or a candle is in front of their faces, and that they are very gently breathing in and out (this will probably be more comfortable through the mouth) so that the feather or candle flame would barely move on the outward breath. Each contraction will still start with the outward, relaxing, welcoming breath and continue with slow, deep, calm breathing; the lighter breaths will only be used at the contraction's summit. There should still be a momentary 'pause' between the outward and inward breath and respiration should be as slow and deep as is comfortable.

The end of the first stage (or transition) is a very special time for the labouring woman. The contractions are probably unremitting in strength and ferocity; the pain may well be intense. The woman may feel desperation, hopelessness, exhaustion and perhaps irritation, aggravated, perhaps, by annoying symptoms such as limb shaking and nausea or belching. She will become withdrawn and find it difficult to articulate her needs. Occasionally she may feel the urge to bear down before full cervical dilatation is achieved. For a great many women this is the worst and most difficult time of all. Nothing seems to work, they are convinced labour will never end; their body cannot 'do it'; they want an epidural, forceps or a caesarean section! When discussing this time in the antenatal class two points should be made:

1. These are all good, positive signs that the second stage of labour is not far away.
2. Before accepting or requesting an injection of pethidine or an epidural anaesthetic, women should ask for a vaginal assessment, unless one has recently been carried out. The cervix may well be very nearly fully dilated and both these procedures could delay progress of the imminent second stage by impairing the woman's ability to cooperate.

It is at this point in labour that hyperventilation, with its unpleasant side-effects, will be most noticeable, so thought must be given when suggesting 'coping' techniques not to worsen the respiratory situation. Various strategies have been recommended:

1. SOS – 'sigh out softly' – gentle expiratory sighs, released at the peak of contractions.
2. Sighing the breath out while saying 'hoo-hoo-hah' gently and slowly. Breathing in and out continues; only the 'hah' is a long expiration.
3. Saying 'I won't push'; breathing in and out for the first two words, and giving a long sigh out for the word 'push'. This should also be gentle, and as slow as possible.
4. 'Puff, puff, blow'; this should be a gentle panting interspersed with a sharp blow out, and is useful to overcome premature pushing urges.

Some women find gently tapping the rhythm of their chosen breathing pattern an added distraction and therefore helpful. Others find that when all else fails, singing or reciting a well-known song or poem sees them over the crisis.

Because respiration during labour, particularly at this stage, will spontaneously become faster and more 'laboured', it is essential that women are warned about this possibility. It is also important whenever any of these techniques are practised that the rate is kept as slow and gentle as possible. Women should be reminded that it may be necessary to breathe into their cupped hands or a paper bag to counteract hyperventilation symptoms.

Many women worry about making a noise during labour. They should be encouraged to use their voices to express the difficulty they are having; the groans, moans and sighs will be those of effort, not necessarily pain. The suggestion has been made (Balaskas, 1983) that making sounds stimulates the production of endorphins and alters the level of consciousness. Simkin (1988) asks antenatal teachers to consider the use of 'role play' during classes. It is helpful for women and their partners to see and hear the very things they are fearing: panic, tension, crying out in pain. Working with a colleague, the teacher can show – using her body and voice – how it may be for them in labour. Her partner will demonstrate how calm, competent support can help the labouring woman deal with the extremely painful contractions of late first stage and the accompanying nausea, trembling, panic and irritation. This technique requires experience, a real familiarity with labour, and great confidence on the part of the teacher!

Simulating contractions

While it is impossible to enable women to experience 'dress rehearsal' labour contractions in advance, there are techniques that will allow them to gain an impression of what it will be like to relax through, and cope with, muscle work over which they have no voluntary control. Some of these methods for simulating contractions involve the use of discomfort or pain, while others rely on pressure to create a 'contraction'.

1. Working in pairs, a partner places his or her hands over the bottom ribs and the top of the abdomen when the instruction 'Here is a contraction, and it is starting *now*' is given. Slowly and gradually pressure is built up so that after 30 seconds maximum 'squeeze' is reached. This is maintained for 10 seconds or so, and then, equally gradually, is released over the next 30 seconds. Women should not experience discomfort – but this way of practising labour contractions does give them a very good idea of what it will be like to relax *around* intense abdominal activity.
2. Escalating 'Chinese burns' (twisting the skin on the wrist), a pinch on the forearm (which starts with a touch and builds up to a nipping, twisting squeeze), pinching the tendo archilles or squeezing the inner aspect of the thigh have all been described as painful methods of giving 'pretend' contractions. Once again, they should last at least one minute.

Following the effort of the transitional phase there is often a lull, a period of rest, when full dilatation is reached. Women used to be urged to begin pushing as soon as this happened. It is more usual today for pushing to be delayed until the fetal head has descended to the pelvic floor and the vertex is seen. The bearing-down urge is not usually experienced until the perineum begins to stretch; premature pushing can be unnecessarily exhausting and uses up the permitted time in labour wards that have a strict protocol in this respect!

Women must be warned about the sensations they may experience in the second stage of labour. The feeling of 'fullness' in the rectum and anus (as if a large grapefruit is waiting to be expelled), the burning stretch of the perineal skin (two fingers in the mouth, pulling the lips out sideways, can mimic this) as it begins to bulge and distend, and the 'opening out' feeling in the sacroiliac, symphysis pubis and sacrococcygeal joints can be frightening if they are not expected. Many women will be relieved that at long last there is something active that *they* can do; they may actually enjoy the wonderful feeling of working with the immensely powerful 'piston' which has developed within their body. The pain of the first stage recedes and all becomes purposeful effort. Others will be frightened of 'joining in'. They may fear that by pushing they will tear the perineum, cause themselves more pain, defaecate, or even harm their baby. For others the embarrassment of exposing this very private part of their body, possibly in that most threatening and vulnerable of postures, the lithotomy position, will be immensely inhibiting. Reassurance and the opportunity to voice their apprehensions antenatally, together with sympathetic and empathetic encouragement and support during labour, will go a long way towards helping women achieve normal delivery. It is difficult for some women to 'tune in' to their internal body sensations and to respond to these by pushing effectively. It must be mentioned during antenatal classes that several contractions may go by before the woman realizes how to push her baby down and out. Each mother should be encouraged to work with her own internal expulsive urge, rather than have to push just because the cervix is fully dilated and the uterus contracting. The desire to bear down usually comes in waves, perhaps three or four 'emptying' urges per contraction, and she may not be able to push well until she actually experiences this. It is essential that she is in a position which is comfortable and feels right to her during this time.

Hopefully the days are gone when a woman was exhorted to 'push, push, keep pushing' (possibly even before the uterus had begun its own spontaneous expulsive efforts). Frequently she became purple in the face, with bulging veins and bloodshot eyes, and felt altogether exhausted with the effort of maintaining unnaturally prolonged pushes which in no way matched what *she* was feeling. Often she was supine, had to heave her body and legs up, gripping behind her knees to stabilize herself, and was in fact pushing her baby 'uphill'. The instructions to push were not linked to her sensations – and the whole performance was most unphysiological! The Valsalva manoeuvre (forced effort with a closed glottis – originally recommended by a seventeenth-century Italian physician for expelling pus from the ear) leads to several undesirable sequelae:

1. Initiallly there is a large rise in blood pressure.
2. The veins in the chest and abdomen are compressed by the increase in intrathoracic and intra-abdominal pressure; blood flow back to the heart is reduced.
3. Cardiac output falls and blood pressure drops.
4. Dizziness results, the Valsalva manoeuvre is released, and cardiac output returns to normal.
5. Blood flow to the placenta is reduced, which can be reflected in fetal heart decelerations.

Noble (1981) suggested that this sequence of events leads to pooling of blood in the pelvis and legs and could predispose a woman to varicosities; the tissues of the rectus sheath, linea alba and the pelvic floor will be unduly strained by artificially prolonged pushing. Caldeyro-Barcia (1979) has associated forced straining with an increased need for episiotomy because there is insufficient time for the perineum to distend slowly and gradually. To avoid these potentially damaging events, the way women push in the second stage of labour is currently being rethought, and it is to be hoped that midwives and doctors will no longer insist on unphysiologically prolonged forced effort.

There are two methods of using breathing to facilitate pushing:

1. The breath can be held while the woman follows her own bodily urge to bear down. Each push should last about five to ten seconds, and each contraction will demand three to four pushes.
2. After an initial breath in, pushing is accompanied by gradual expiration.

Some women will automatically combine these two methods; taking a breath in, beginning the push with a breath out and then holding their breath to complete the effort. Whichever technique best suits the mother, it is important for at least one deep 'pre-push' breath in and out to be taken so that a good supply of oxygen is available to mother and fetus. One or two deep 'parting' breaths should be taken when the contraction is over. Between contractions, the mother should change position as necessary, have her face sponged and take sips of water; and above all she should rest.

Breathing for the delivery of the baby will normally be dictated by the midwife. It will be a combination of short pushes, longer pushes and a gentle sighing and panting – the best combination to enable the midwife to control the birth of the head and then the shoulders. It is advisable to rehearse these events so that women are prepared for the variations that may be necessary. Once again it is essential to discuss with women the fact that their voices will automatically be part of the effort of giving birth. Point to the spontaneous noises weightlifters make before taking up a load. Vocalization is an integreal part of the birthing process – women should expect to hear themselves making noises and *not* feel they must continually apologize for crying out!

If delivery of the placenta is allowed to proceed physiologically, without the use of ergometrine, oxytocin and continuous cord traction, the mother may be asked to push or cough to help its expulsion.

POSITIONS IN LABOUR (see also p. 60)

The 'medicalization' of childbirth saw the gradual immobilization of women, culminating in their restriction to the delivery couch. Further hampered by intavenous drips and monitoring equipment, women have been prevented from following their instinctive internal body 'messages'. The way women moved about and the positions they adopted during the first stage of labour and then for the delivery of their babies have been historically and anthropologically recorded (Attwood, 1976). Many authorities (Smellie, 1974; Vaughan, 1951; Randall, 1953) have drawn attention to the positions women found comfortable and which seemed to facilitate progress. Although the expression 'active birth' is reasonably new – it was originally coined by Janet Balaskas, a yoga teacher and antenatal educator, in the late 1970s – its philosophy is old, and the exercises and postures Balaskas advocates (Balaskas, 1983; Balaskas and Balaskas, 1983) are all included in the early obstetric physiotherapy textbooks (Randall, 1953).

There is now a wide range of research into the benefits or otherwise that can be gained from ambulation in labour, and into the help given by frequent changes of position and the adoption of forward leaning postures (Dunn, 1976; Flynn and Kelly, 1976; Williams and Thom, 1980; Russell, 1982; Calder, 1982; Roberts et al., 1983; Stewart and Calder, 1984; Lupe and Gross, 1986; Pöschl, 1987). Although there is not a consensus of opinion, one fact does repeatedly emerge: the comfort of the mother and her feeling of freedom and well-being are most important. All authorities recommend the encouragement of women who feel that ambulation and the use of different positions enable them to cope better with labour.

Normal uninhibited labour is often a restless time; the mother will walk, squat, sit, stand, kneel and lie down, trying to find comfortable positions by following her own instincts. Passive confinement to the bed is rejected in the concept of 'active birth' – women want to use, and work actively, with their bodies; it is a return to the age-old intuition of womankind since time immemorial.

Because of the anteversion of the uterus during first-stage contractions (see p. 50), many women find that they instinctively need to lean forward on some sort of support; some like to rotate or rock their pelvis (Fig. 6.1). The different postures that women may like to use should be demonstrated and practised during antenatal classes, and

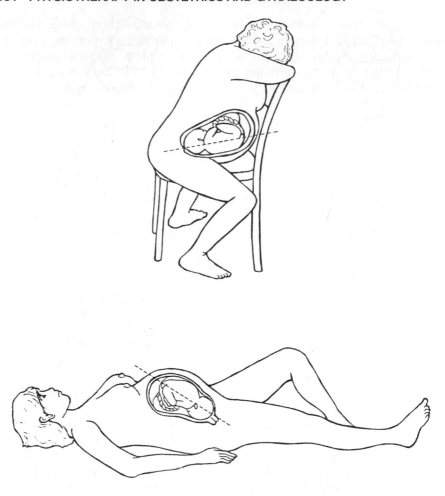

Figure 6.1 During a first-stage contraction the uterus anteverts (see p. 50); the supine position can reduce this movement and many women feel most comfortable leaning forwards, which facilitates anteversion.

their use at home encouraged; women should be able to move easily from one position to another and become used to those which may be uncomfortable or awkward at first (Fig. 6.2). Partners and carers should also be aware of these postures, because during labour it may be up to them to suggest alternatives; some women become so overwhelmed by what they are feeling that they become immobilized and frightened to move in case they make their pain worse. Roberts et al. (1983) showed that it is actually the change from one position to another that stimulates efficient uterine activity. Sometimes the cervix dilates unevenly, so that towards the end of the first stage of labour an anterior lip or rim remains between the presenting part and the pubis, while the rest of the cervix is well drawn up. The woman should be

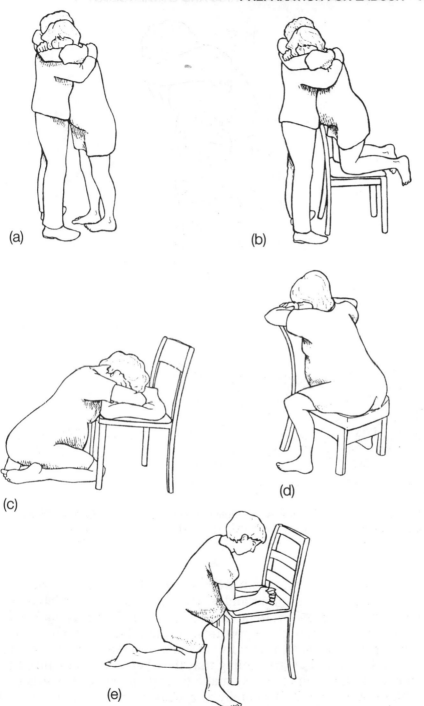

Figure 6.2 a–e Women should be encouraged to change position during the first stage of labour. It is useful to practise a variety of possibilities during antenatal classes. Forward leaning and upright postures are often preferred in early labour.

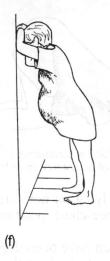

(f)

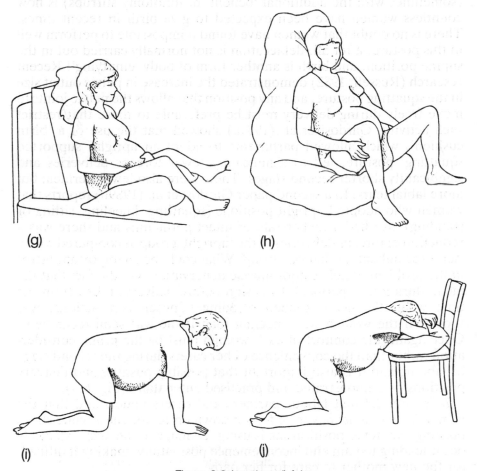

(g)

(h)

(i)

(j)

Figure 6.2 (continued) f–j

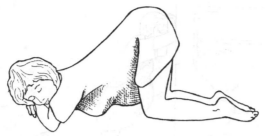

Figure 6.3 The knee-chest position is sometimes helpful in assisting the elimination of an anterior lip of the cervix.

discouraged from pushing; lying on her side with the foot of the bed raised or adopting the knee-chest position can be helpful in this situation (Fig. 6.3).

Throughout history women have been depicted giving birth in many postures, but rarely recumbent. And yet the 'stranded beetle' position (sometimes with the additional 'benefit' of lithotomy stirrups) is how countless women have been expected to give birth in recent times. There is no doubt that women have found it impossible to perform well in this posture; after all, defaecation is not normally carried out in the supine position, and birth is another form of body 'emptying'! Recent research (Russell, 1982) demonstrated the increase in pelvic outlet size in the squatting posture, and any position that allows the pelvic joints to move freely during delivery must be preferable to those that restrict such activity. Gardosi et al. (1989a) showed that the use of a 'birth cushion', which allowed parturients to adopt an upright 'supported squatting' posture, led to significantly fewer forceps deliveries and significantly shorter second stages. There were also fewer perineal but more labial tears. In a second paper Gardosi et al. (1989b) reports that women who adopted upright positions (squatting, kneeling, sitting or standing) also had a higher rate of intact perineums and there was a reduction of forceps deliveries in the 'upright' group as compared with a 'semi-recumbent' or 'lateral' group. What could be an important factor in the problem of pelvic floor muscle denervation was the fact that the mean duration of perineal distension before delivery, taken from the time when the head stopped receding between contractions, was shorter if the woman was kneeling than if she was semi-recumbent. Once again, the comfort of each woman must be the prime consideration rather than the convenience of her carers during the second stage of labour; and it is also important that possible pushing and delivery positions be demonstrated and practised antenatally (Fig. 6.4).

It is essential that labour partners and carers understand that the woman's head must never be forced down on to her chest while she is pushing, whatever position she is using. Damage to the neck can easily occur leading to pain and inconvenience postnatally, making it difficult for the new mother to care for her baby.

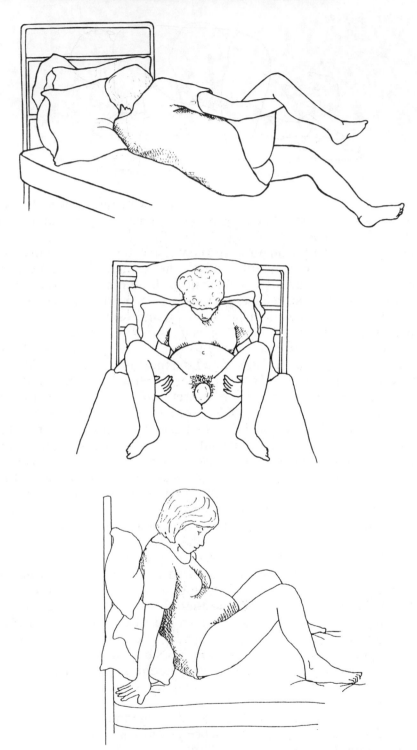

Figure 6.4 Some suggested positions for second stage.

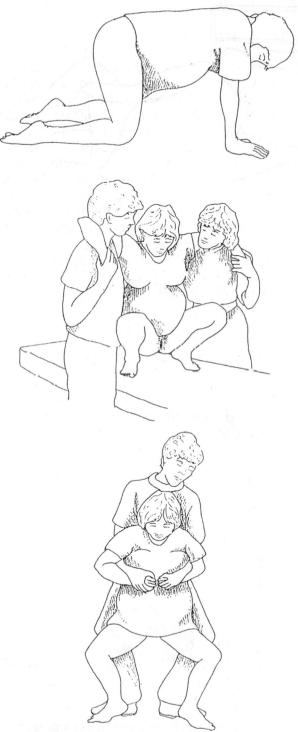

Figure 6.4 (continued)

MASSAGE IN LABOUR

Women who have experienced skilful massage during labour often say afterwards how helpful and pain relieving it was. Although no controlled trials have as yet been conducted to determine the exact neurophysiological mechanisms by which massage moderates pain, it is indisputable that 'rubbing' very often 'makes it better'. Before the advent of the use of anaesthesia during labour iin the mid-nineteenth century, midwives and labour supporters had little else to offer.

It is probable that the soothing sensory input from stroking, effleurage and kneading activates the 'gate closing' mechanism at spinal level (Wells, 1988). It may also be possible by means of tissue manipulation (e.g. deep sacral kneading) to stimulate the release of endogenous opiates. In addition to its pain-relieving potential, massage demonstrates caring and non-verbal support and communication. This is particularly valuable when language barriers exist. It is most important that whoever is giving massage is sensitive to the changing needs of the parturient with regard to site, depth and technique, and uses advantageous well-supported positioning.

The Back

Back pain can be very demoralizing, particularly when it is associated with a prolonged first stage of labour or where the fetus is in the occipito-posterior position. As is shown in Fig. 6.5 back pain is experienced in the lumbosacral region, and it intensifies as labour progresses. Stationary kneading, single-handed or reinforced with one hand over the other, applied slowly and deeply to the painful area is often helpful (Fig. 6.6). Elbows should be bent, and the masseur should use his or her own

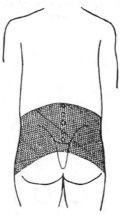

Figure 6.5 Back pain can be experienced in the lumbosacral region in the first stage of labour.

body weight combined with a gentle rotary movement to apply comfortable pressure, without fatigue, for a long period. Partners and midwives must be warned how easy it is to increase pain by over-enthusiastic and vigorous work. Hands should be relaxed and moulded to the part; uneven pressure, particularly with the heel of the hand, and with straight arms must be avoided, especially where the sacroiliac area is bony; practice is essential both in antenatal classes and at home. Double-handed kneading with loosely clenched fists directly over the sacroiliac joints may be necessary as the pain becomes more severe (Fig. 6.7). Hand-held tennis balls can be a useful alternatiive where hands are small or become fatigued.

Effleurage from the sacrococcygeal area, up and over the iliac crests, will be even more soothing if a little talcum powder is used to overcome the effects of sweating, (Fig. 6.8). Slow, rhythmical longitudinal stroking, from occiput to coccyx, single or double handed, can relieve tension and facilitate relaxation (Fig. 6.9). The strokes may be applied

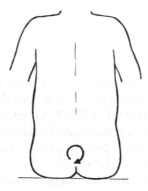

Figure 6.6 Deep kneading, one hand over the other, is given over the painful area.

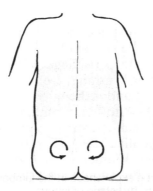

Figure 6.7 Double-handed kneading over the sacroiliac joints can give relief.

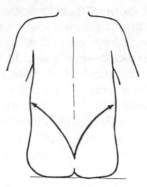

Figure 6.8 Effleurage from the sacrococcygeal area, up and over the iliac crests can be soothing.

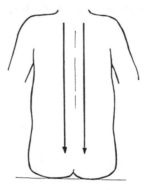

Figure 6.9 Slow, rhythmical longitudinal stroking, from occiput to coccyx, can relieve tension.

with the whole hands or the fingertips, actually over the spine or parallel to it. Pressure can become slightly deeper as the hands descend.

The Abdomen

Pain is most commonly experienced over the lower half of the abdomen, particularly in the suprapubic region (Fig. 6.10). It is often described as nauseating. Deep massage will be totally unacceptable, but light finger-stroking or brushing, from one anterior superior iliac spine to the other, passing under the bulge and over the pain, is often well received (Fig. 6.11). Another technique, best performed by the mother herself, is double-handed stroking ascending either side of the midline and across to the iliac crests (Fig. 6.12); this can be synchronized with easy breathing. Women often spontaneously and instinctively massage themselves; this should most certainly be encouraged and supplemented if it proves helpful.

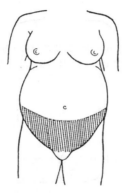

Figure 6.10 Pain is experienced in the lower half of the abdomen in the suprapubic region.

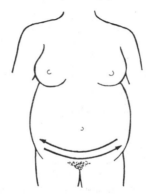

Figure 6.11 Light finger-stroking over the site of abdominal pain, from one side to the other, is often appreciated.

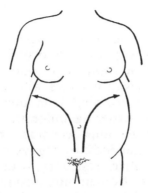

Figure 6.12 Double-handed stroking by the mother herself, synchronized with easy breathing, can relieve abdominal pain.

The Legs

Occasionally labour pain may be perceived in the thighs, and cramp in the calf or foot may also occur; effleurage or kneading can relieve this.

PERINEAL MASSAGE

Some midwives will massage a mother's perineum in the second stage of labour in an effort to encourage stretching of the skin and muscle and thus prevent tearing or episiotomy. Grandmothers in some Eastern cultures also encourage their pregnant daughters or daughters-in-law to practise this simple stretching technique. The suggestion that it is possible to prepare the perineum for birth could be made during an antenatal class while discussing the second stage of labour, and how the mother can best help herself and her midwife to complete the delivery with an intact perineum.

This simple massage technique can be used by the woman herself, leaning back in a well-supported position, or when squatting. Alternatively, some women may prefer their partner to do it for them. A natural oil (olive, wheatgerm, sunflower, etc.) can be used. Both index fingers or thumbs, or the index and middle fingers from one hand, are put about 5 cm into the vagina. A rhythmic 'U' or sling type movement, upwards along the sides of the vagina and with downward pressure, stretches the perineum from side to side. Maintaining a sideways stretch for a few seconds and gradually building up for 30–40 seconds can prepare the woman for the sort of sensation she can expect to feel as her baby's head begins to crown. As elasticity is improved it is suggested that three or four fingers could be used. As an alternative a kneading movement between index finger and thumb could be employed. If the woman contracts her pelvic floor during a perineal massage session she will realize how difficult it will be for her tissues to stretch if she 'holds back' while her baby's head is crowning. This may reinforce the idea of relaxing the pelvic floor during delivery.

Avery and Van Arsdale (1987), two American nurse-midwives, evaluated the effect of perineal massage on 55 women (29 experimental and 26 controls); massage began six weeks before the due date. In the experimental group 52% had an intact perineum or a first-degree laceration; 48% had an episiotomy and/or a second, third or fourth-degree tear. In the control group 24% had an intact perineum or first-degree laceration, and 76% had an episiotomy and/or second, third or fourth-degree tear. When the episiotomy rate was examined, 38% of the experimental group and 65% of the control group had had an episiotomy. Third and fourth-degree tears only occurred when an episiotomy was performed. Some of the women in the trial experienced discomfort and discontinued the massage; they also felt it required a significant time commitment (5–10 minutes daily was suggested).

However, many of the participants noticed a dramatic increase in perineal elasticity in the first two to three weeks of massage, which was maintained but not significantly increased if the massage was continued to term. No comment was made in this trial as to the strength of the pelvic floor muscles postnatally.

OTHER COPING STRATEGIES

Increasingly, maternity units are arranging for baths and showers to be available, because it has been appreciated that some labouring women derive great benefit from them (Lenstrup et al., 1987). Couples should be encouraged to bring tapes of favourite music which is relaxing and distracting. Television and games such as Scrabble or backgammon can be used to help pass the time. Backgammon in particular appeared in one case to have an amusing after-effect: a couple played several games during the first stage of labour before the birth of their fourth child, and for about four months following his birth they were unable to play the game because the rattling of the dice woke the baby who cried and became distressed (Birch and Birch, 1988)! In this case the auditory stimulus was perhaps associated with the unpleasant (to the baby) sensations of labour.

Appendix 2 summarizes a labour sequence.

PAIN RELIEF IN LABOUR

Until the middle of the nineteenth century there were no really effective methods of anaesthesia or analgesia that eased labour pain. With the discovery of ether and chloroform doctors were finally able to relieve the pain of the 'poor, suffering mother'. Many felt, and some still feel, that as Sir James Young Simpson wrote in 1848, 'it is our duty as well as our privilege to use all legitimate means to mitigate and remove the physical sufferings of the mother during parturition' (Moir, 1986).

With the advent of reliable methods of contraception most pregnancies today will have been planned and the vast majority of babies will be wanted. Perhaps it is because of this that a sizeable proportion of women now express the desire to cope with labour 'on my own'. The knowledge that some forms of analgesia adversely affect the fetus and the course of labour will also be a factor. Many feel that labour, in spite of its pain, is the ultimate fulfilment of their femaleness, they are prepared to suffer the pain of parturition, to deal with it as they might the pain of marathon running or mountaineering, in return for an enormous sense of achievement and self-fulfilment. Morgan et al. (1982) showed that a completely painless labour is not always desirable for all mothers, and that analgesia is not the most important determinant of a satisfactory experience of childbirth. Reports of epidural anaesthesia (Crawford, 1972; Billevicz-Driemel and Milne, 1976) noted that some mothers felt 'deprived of the experience of childbirth' by perfect analgesia.

Many mothers regard the support of a sympathetic midwife as the most important factor in relieving their labour pain, and the presence of a *doula* (a lay female companion) during labour has been shown to shorten the interval, and therefore her pain, between the mother's admission and her baby's delivery (Sosa et al., 1980). Melzack et al. (1981) and Charles et al. (1978) showed that antenatal preparation was related to lower levels of pain and higher levels of enjoyment during childbirth. Nevertheless, particularly in primiparous women, some form of analgesia will frequently be requested or be necessary, in addition to each mother's 'tool kit' of self-help techniques: positions of ease, mobility, body awareness and neuromuscular control (relaxation), breathing, massage, distraction techniques, warm baths and showers, music, companionship, imaging. The following analgesic methods are in general use and should be discussed in antenatal classes. Although many women hope that they will manage to cope with labour without resorting to analgesia, it is important that they know what is available to relieve their labour pain and how it can help them, and also something about the side-effects they and their babies may experience.

Pethidine

Pethidine (meperidine in the USA) is a synthetic opioid analgesic derived from morphine, and is the most common narcotic drug used in obstetric analgesia in the UK, although diamorphine is used in some centres. It is generally administered as an intramuscular injection in 100 mg doses, and is one of the drugs midwives may prescribe and give on their own responsibility to a woman in labour, to a maximum of 200 mg. Because the response to any drug is individual, and is related to body mass, 50 mg may be sufficient for some women, while others will need 150 mg. Self-administered controlled doses of intravenous pethidine via a pump have been found acceptable by some mothers. When the drug is administered parenterally it is recognized that there is unrestricted placental transfer from mother to fetus. As with other narcotic analgesics side-effects can and do occur, and these are of particular concern during labour when the fetus must also be considered. However, pethidine is readily available in all maternity units and can help women relax when they become distressed by the intensity of their labour.

Maternal side-effects

Pethidine can cause maternal nausea and sometimes vomiting; an antiemetic is often given simultaneously because of this. Other side-effects include drowsiness, distressing hallucinations and dysphoria, which can interfere with the mother's concentration on her own 'coping' techniques, and affect her cooperation with her attendants. Pethidine is said to reduce the tone of the lower oesophageal sphincter and delay gastric emptying, which could have implications if a general anaesthetic has to be given. It could also give rise to hypotension and respiratory depression. It is not a perfect analgesic by any means; only 20–40% of women experience effective pain relief when given doses by a midwife (Holdcroft and Morgan, 1974; Priest and Rosser, 1991).

Fetal and neonatal side-effects

In common with other drugs, what affects the mother will also affect her baby, and although pethidine can be metabolized in the maternal liver and eventually excreted from the mother's body, this may not be the case for the newborn infant. Because there will be a high concentration of pethidine and its metabolite norpethidine in the mother's blood stream, the drugs will cross the placenta into the baby; in the first two to three hours following an injection up to 70% of the dose plus some norpethidine will have accumulated in the fetus. Even at term the neonate's liver and kidneys are too immature to metabolize and excrete the drug effectively. After three hours, when the level of pethidine has fallen in the mother, the drug again crosses the placenta into the mother where it can be dealt with. Where labour is premature the problems are intensified. The preterm baby, being much smaller, will receive a proportionately larger dose of pethidine, and its more immature organs are even less able to deal with the drug.

Consequently, if the mother receives her dose of pethidine between one and four hours before the birth, it is possible (because pethidine will still be in the baby's blood stream) that prolonged side-effects will be apparent in the neonate in addition to those observed in the fetus before delivery: fetal acidosis, a depressed fetal heart-rate and a slower response to sound have all been reported. Respiratory depression in the neonate can occur following large or repeated doses; this can be reversed by the drug's antagonist naloxone, but as naloxone has a shorter duration of action than pethidine repeated doses may be required. Adverse neurobehavioural effects have been reported which are potentiated in the preterm infant; these include drowsiness (Richards and Bernal, 1972) which can interfere with the early bonding process, and difficulties in establishing breast-feeding (Belsey et al., 1981). Other, more subtle side-effects have been observed, including the baby being less alert, more easily startled, less easily comforted, fretful and slower to respond to faces and sounds. It is easy to dismiss these changes as unimportant, but they could be distressing to new mothers who can lose confidence in themselves unless they have been warned in advance that they may need to persevere and devote more time to establishing breast-feeding and their new relationship.

It is advisable, therefore, for women to have pethidine at the times in their labour that can give them maximum help with least effect on their baby. More than four hours before delivery is said to be reasonably safe for the baby who will then have low levels of pethidine in its blood stream at birth – and although it is difficult to predict exactly when a baby will be born, it is probably advisable for pethidine to be given following vaginal assessment in order to avoid severe neonatal side-effects.

Moir (1986) said that none of the narcotic analgesics provides complete pain relief to all labouring women when given in safe doses, and women must be prepared to feel some labour pain following an injection of pethidine.

Entonox

Various forms of inhalational analgesia have been available to women in labour in the past: 'gas' (nitrous oxide) and air, trichlorethylene (Trilene) and methoxyflurane (Penthrane) among them. They have mainly been superseded in the UK by Entonox, which is a mixture of 50% nitrous oxide with 50% oxygen. It is available in cylinders, but in many delivery suites will be piped in from a central source. Entonox is taken by the mother herself for each contraction, one at a time. It is not, nor should it be, administered by a midwife or labour companion.

Nitrous oxide is a weak anaesthetic but has a good analgesic effect. Ideally women should be instructed in its use antenatally, with a quick revision in early labour. Deep breaths are essential to gain maximum effect, and 20 seconds inhalation or seven breaths are necessary before the mother begins to feel the benefit. It is usually recommended that the woman starts using Entonox before a contraction or immediately it begins; eight to twelve breaths may be all she needs to help her cope with it. Maximum analgesia will be reached after 45–60 seconds, and the effects wear off rapidly. A mask is usually used for the administration of Entonox, but it may also be taken via a plastic mouthpiece – a method many mothers find more acceptable. It is most important for the obstetric physiotherapist to impress upon the mother the need to keep the mask, if used, firmly in contact with her face. A hissing noise will be heard if the apparatus is being used correctly.

Some women complain of nausea as a result of using Entonox, and some will find that analgesia is insufficient or non-existent.

Epidural anaesthesia

Continuous epidural (also known as extradural or peridural) anaesthesia is now widely used in the UK and may be available on demand in obstetric units that have full anaesthetic cover. As well as giving pain relief for labour, epidural anaesthesia may also be used for caesarean section. A full explanation is essential in antenatal classes for women who will have access to this form of pain control. Many 'young wives' tales' abound, and a great many women reject the idea of epidural anaesthesia without fully understanding its method of induction, the way it works, and how they can help themselves in the second stage of labour if they use it.

The benefits of epidural anaesthesia

1. The mother will be fully conscious, her mind unclouded by analgesia; she will be able to welcome her baby with an alert mind.
2. The effects of bupivacaine on the baby are minimal compared to those of pethidine.
3. Epidural anaesthesia may be helpful in cases of pre-eclamptic toxaemia and incoordinate uterine activity.
4. Where a woman is exhausted from a long, painful labour, or is frightened and unable to tolerate her pain, an epidural anaesthetic can transform the experience for her and can reverse maternal and fetal acidosis.
5. For a complicated delivery (i.e. twins, breech, forceps), epidural anaesthesia provides the obstetrician with the conditions needed for control and hence the safety of the baby. The mother has better pain relief than with a local nerve block, and general anaesthesia with its associated complications is avoided.
6. Caesarean section can be carried out under epidural anaesthesia; the mother can be awake, and will escape the unpleasant after-effects of general anaesthesia and its dangers. An important 'plus' is that the father can be present for the birth of his baby.

Technique

An intravenous infusion, usually Hartmann's solution, is always set up beforehand. The mother will either lie on her side, curled up as much as possible, or she may sit with her legs over the edge of the delivery table supported by her labour companion or a midwife. A small amount of local anaesthetic solution is injected into the surrounding skin at L2–L3 or L3–L4 prior to the insertion of a Tuohy needle. Some women may find the technique painful, while others do not seem to experience pain or discomfort. Pain is usually caused by difficulties, such as hitting bone. Relaxation, together with calm quiet breathing, can help mothers cope with what for many is a frightening ordeal. Once the Tuohy needle is inserted the anaesthetist moves it slowly from the resistance of the tough interspinous ligament into the epidural space.

Before a dose of local anaesthetic (commonly bupivacaine, a 0.25% solution is often used) is injected, careful aspiration for blood or cerebrospinal fluid (CSF) is made. The presence of either of these could lead to complications, and the epidural would probably be resited at an adjacent intervertebral space. A fine plastic catheter is threaded through the needle and its tip positioned in the epidural space. The first dose will be given by the anaesthetist (the woman may notice a cold sensation in her back at first), and subsequent top-up doses will probably be given by a midwife. The effect of a good epidural anaesthetic should be to block the sensory nerves and eliminate pain, but leave motor power.

Side-effects and complications of epidural anaesthesia

1. There appears to be an increased rate of forceps delivery with its attendant maternal and fetal trauma. This could be due to three main factors:
   (a) There is normally a physiological increase in maternal oxytocin during the second stage of labour. This neuroendocrine response is said to be due to stimulation of the pelvic stretch receptors by the descending fetus (Ferguson's reflex). However, where epidurals are used Ferguson's reflex is abolished and uterine activity is measurably less, either because this oxytocic surge does not occur or because there is a drop in oxytocic output. Because of this an oxytocin infusion is often necessary to stimulate efficient expulsive contractions.
   (b) The sensory blockade that eliminates labour pain also eliminates pelvic floor sensation, so the woman whose epidural is topped-up will not appreciate the bearing-down reflex.
   (c) Extensive epidural anaesthesia can lead to a relaxation and 'guttering' of the pelvic floor muscles which may interfere with the rotation of the baby's head; additionally the abdominal muscles may be affected.
   The suggestion in antenatal classes that women consciously push in the second stage of labour as if they were trying to open their bowels can be helpful if an epidural has blocked sensation and also led to decreased motor power. It must be remembered, however, that the epidural may have been given *because* a forceps delivery was envisaged – it may not be correct to state dogmatically that forceps deliveries are always a direct result of a woman having had epidural anaesthesia.
2. Alongside the sensory blockade, the sympathetic nerves will also be affected. This leads to vasodilatation of blood vessels in the lower abdomen and the legs (which will be warm to the touch) and a consequent drop in blood pressure. This will be compounded if the mother is supine (although this should never happen), and

could interfere with placental blood flow to the fetus. If this occurs the mother will be turned on her side; she may be given oxygen if there is fetal distress.

3. The mother's legs may feel 'heavy' and she may be unable to move them easily; walking will not be possible.

4. The mother sometimes feels dizzy, and shivering can be a nuisance.

5. Urinary retention may occur if the mother is unable to feel her bladder filling. She should try to micturate every two hours; a catheter will be passed if retention of urine becomes obvious.

6. Unblocked segments and unilateral blocks are common problems and can prove distressing for the woman who was hoping for total pain relief. They can sometimes be relieved by top-up doses in appropriate positions – but women should be warned antenatally that this may happen, also that it takes time to work.

7. The accidental puncture of the dura and consequent release of CSF can give rise to severe postpartum headache. In the past the mother was usually nursed flat for at least 24 hours and the intravenous drip of Hartmann's solution remained in place. In current practice, the drip may remain and the mother is encouraged to drink; she may not be required to remain supine. If the problem is prolonged and severe the anaesthetist may inject a 'blood patch' of the mother's own venous blood into the epidural space at the site of the damage. Women suffering from postepidural headache are usually distressed at their immobility and their inability to care for their baby and respond spontaneously and comfortably to its needs. They will need extra support and assistance, and the reassurance that the condition will resolve and that this initial problem will not interfere with the bonding process between them and their baby.

8. Many women complain of pain and tenderness postpartum at the epidural site, and for some this can be intolerable. The suggestion has been made that a tiny haematoma forms in the epidural space with consequent pressure on sensitive tissues, and women can be reassured if they are reminded that bruising often occurs around ordinary injection sites. The obstetric physiotherapist can help alleviate this problem by offering a 'hot pack' or TNS, and suggesting that the mother rests in prone lying.

9. Total spinal anaesthesia can occur if the dose of local anaesthetic is accidentally injected into the subarachnoid space. This potentially fatal condition (severe hypotension and cessation of spontaneous respiration can occur very quickly) requires instant artificial respiration, the injection of vasopressor drugs and rapid fluid infusion. Rarely, spinal anaesthesia follows a top-up given by a midwife.

10. Neurological complications may persist following epidural anaesthesia. Muscle weakness in a leg or foot, loss of sensation in an area

    of skin and (fortunately extremely rarely) paralysis have been reported.

11. Fusi et al. (1989) have shown that women receiving epidural analgesia during labour are at increased risk of developing pyrexia. It is thought that this may be due to vascular and thermo-regulatory modifications induced by epidural analgesia.

12. Bupivacaine, like other local analgesics, enters the maternal blood stream from the epidural space, crosses the placenta and can be found in measurable (but clinically unimportant) concentrations in the fetal circulation within 10 minutes of epidural injection (Caldwell et al., 1977; Rosenblatt et al., 1981). The neurobehavioural effects are clinically unimportant, unlike those of pethidine.

13. A recent paper has shown an increased incidence of long-term backache following epidural anaesthesia (MacArthur et al., 1990).

Epidural anaesthesia for caesarean section

Because of the risks associated with general anaesthesia in the pregnant woman, especially Mendelson's syndrome and its possible effects (see p. 64), epidural anaesthesia for caesarean section has become increasingly popular. Psychologically, women can have the satisfaction of being conscious and 'there' for the birth of their baby; partners are often present too, so that the new family unit is together from the beginning. When preparing women for an elective caesarean section under epidural anaesthesia it is important to mention that, because of the profound block required to achieve total analgesia, they may experience unpleasant side-effects. Hypotension can give rise to a feeling of faintness; shivering and vomiting can also be a nuisance, and the mother may feel very cold. Babies born by caesarean section frequently need paediatric assistance to clear mucus and liquor from their lungs. They will not have had the benefit of chest compression in the second stage of labour to achieve this. It is important to warn women that a paediatrician will be present at the operation and may need to help the baby breathe before the parents are able to hold the infant. It is also important to prepare the mother for the fact that although she should feel no pain during the operation, she will be aware of pulling and tugging. One mother described her epidural caesarean section as being similar to having 'the washing-up done in my tummy'! It is also important, where possible, to prepare the father for this type of delivery. Spinal anaesthesia is also used for caesarean section.

Transcutaneous nerve stimulation

One of the most exciting steps forward in the field of pain-relieving modalities available to physiotherapists in the past 20–30 years has been the development of tiny electronic stimulators which can be safely used by patients suffering from acute or chronic pain problems. Transcutaneous nerve stimulation (TNS) involves the transmission of electrical energy through the skin to the nervous system. Its analgesic effects are said to be due to a 'gate-closing' mechanism in the dorsal columns of the spinal cord and the release of endogenous opiates (Mannheimer, 1985; Frampton, 1988; Thompson, 1989). It is also said to interfere with the ability of the brain to recognize pain input patterns (cognitive effect) (Mannheimer and Lampe, 1984). TNS can be an additional tool which the obstetric physiotherapist is able to offer to women in labour. Its non-invasive mode of action and absence of side-effects are very attractive to the woman hoping to cope with labour by relying on her own resources.

The intensity of labour pain experienced varies from woman to woman, and from labour to labour in the same woman. The three P's: power (uterine contractions), pelvis (its shape and size), and passenger (the presentation and size of the baby) will all play a part in the length of labour, and therefore the ability of a mother to manage without invasive analgesia. The level of anxiety experienced during pregnancy is also said to have a bearing on the analgesic needs of a labouring woman (Haddad and Morris, 1982, 1985). TNS may give sufficient additional analgesia (combined with relaxation, breathing, massage, positioning, mobilizing, etc.) to enable a mother to deal with her contractions without drugs. Alternatively it may help her to cope with the early latent phase of the first stage of labour, or with prostaglandin-induced contractions, where an unripe and unfavourable cervix is 'primed' prior to rupture of membranes in induction of labour. This could be an important factor in the outcome of labour. Wuitchik et al. (1989) showed that the levels of pain and distress-related thoughts experienced during the latent phase of labour were predictive of the length of labour and obstetric outcome. Women registering high pain scores and distress-related thoughts during labour's latent phase had longer labours and were more likely to need instrumental delivery. Maternal distress during this time was also related to higher incidences of abnormal fetal heart-rate patterns and the need for neonatal assistance. If women find that TNS gives adequate pain relief during the latent phase of labour this could possibly influence both the length of labour, the mode of delivery and even the condition of the newborn infant. TNS may continue to be used if the mother opts to have additional help in the form of pethidine or Entonox. It may be helpful to retain TNS for post-delivery suturing, and it can also be useful for women experiencing severe after-pains in the early puerperium.

Early reports suggested that electrodes should be positioned on the mother's back, paravertebrally, over the dermatomes T10–L1, the innervation of the uterus and cervix. These were used during the first stage of labour. For the second stage, additional electrodes over the dermatomes S2–S4, the inneravation of the birth canal and pelvic floor,

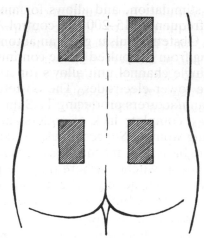

Figure 6.13 TNS electrodes can be placed dorsally from T10 to L1 and S2 to S4.

were brought into use. More recent work has been done using all four electrode positions (Fig. 6.13) simultaneously during both first and second stages of labour (Bundsen et al., 1981, 1982; Bundsen and Ericson, 1982; Harrison et al., 1986), and some work suggests the use of abdominal electrodes where suprapubic pain is present (Robson, 1979). Bundsen, in the second of three papers dealing with pain relief in labour by TNS (Bundsen and Ericson, 1982), mentioned the theoretical possibility that high-intensity stimulation with conventional electrodes over the parturient's lower abdomen could, in unfavourable circumstances, induce irregularities in fetal heart function. This did not occur during their trials. Women may find that four dorsal electrodes together with abdominal massage give sufficient relief during contractions. Bundsen also mentioned TNS interference on the cardiotocograph tracing of the fetal heart. Although this can happen if a scalp clip is in use, when the heart is being monitored electrically, it does not seem to happen if external monitoring is being used, i.e. the heart rate is being monitored ultrasonically. The interference may disappear if the intensity of stimulation is decreased. This problem could probably be solved if the manufacturers of both monitoring equipment and TNS units cooperated in the development of a filter.

TNS units

Several manufacturers are now producing TNS units specifically for use in labour; most of these are existing stimulators with simple modifications. The Obstetric Pulsar (Spembly Medical) is a versatile dual-channel unit which has a finger-controlled (light pressure and release) patient demand switch. It can deliver pulsed low-frequency or continuous high-frequency stimulation, and allows for amplitude (0–48 mA into 1kΩ load) and frequency (15–200 Hz) control. The pulse width is fixed at 200 μs. The Obstetric Pulsar gives an automatic 10% boost in intensity on switching from the pulsed to the continuous mode. A dual as opposed to the single channel unit allows for stronger intensity of stimulation from the lower electrodes. The obstetric physiotherapist should beware of manufacturers producing TNS units intended for use in labour who show a complete lack of understanding of the special needs of the labouring woman. Suggested electrode placement can be without any scientific basis; the machines are restricted in what they offer; and patient control switches, where they exist, require constant pressure throughout a contraction. The amplitude of stimulation available from some of these units is insufficient to cope with the intensity of labour pain.

Electrodes, leads and electrotransmission gel

A variety of electrodes are available: self-adhesive and disposable (rather expensive, particularly if a mother decides after twenty minutes that TNS is not for her!); self-adhesive and reusuable and the conventional carbon-impregnated rubber electrodes, which are probably the most suitable from the point of view of cost. The size best suited for obstetric use is 110 mm × 40 mm. Leads can be bifurcated into two or four, so that if six electrodes were to be used a dual-channel unit could accommodate them.

Various manufacturers produce electrotransmission gels for use with TNS stimulators, all of whom claim that their product is hypoallergenic. These gels seem to work equally well, and from the user's point of view it is probably better to buy the largest size available. Obstetric TNS is unlikely to be used for long enough to produce an allergic reaction to the gel, but where a mother knows that she is very sensitive to creams and gels or to rubber, Karaya gum pads can be used instead. KY Jelly is an unsuitable medium because it is not electrotransmissive. Some form of strapping will be necessary even with self-adhesive electrodes; something like Mefix (Molynlyke) which is flexible and light is probably better than a non-flexible strapping; a heavy adhesive plaster is uncomfortable and unsuitable.

Technique

1. Test the battery.
2. Attach electrodes to the leads, plug into the unit and test the machine. Disconnect the leads.
3. Spread gel over the electrode surfaces so that they are completely covered – no dry spots should be apparent.
4. Cut suitably sized strapping.

5. Place electrodes on the mother's back and secure with strapping.
6. Plug the leads into the machine and allow the mother to switch on the current and adjust it to her own needs. The pulsed mode should be used between contractions, with a switch to the continuous mode during a contraction.
7. When TNS is no longer needed removal should be as follows: switch off the machine; disconnect the leads; carefully lift the electrodes (do not pull on the leads to do this); separate the leads from the electrodes; wash and dry the electrodes.

Poor results

1. There may be too little gel, or it may have dried out. After four to six hours' use the electrodes should be removed, the skin washed and dried, more gel applied, and the electrodes repositioned.
2. There may be too much gel, the electrodes may have slipped and come in contact with each other.
3. The electrodes may have become detached.
4. The battery may be running out.
5. Accommodation – the mother may have become used to the intensity of stimulation, and it needs to be increased.
6. The mother's labour pain may be of such a degree that it cannot be controlled by TNS.

Introduction of TNS to pregnant women

Ideally TNS should be discussed and experienced as a possible analgesic for labour during antenatal classes. It can be described as a pain-relieving stimulator, and women who may not like the idea of 'electricity' being attached to their body will be reassured to see the size of the battery powering the unit! Physiotherapists tend to test current output of modalities such as faradism or TNS by holding electrodes between their fingers. This is *not* suitable for mothers or for midwifery and medical colleagues. Mitchell (1987) mentions the acute sensitivity of the fingers and thumb, so that people unaccustomed to and nervous of electricity may perceive TNS as unpleasant and painful. The level of sensory innervation of the back gives a totally different sensation to those experiencing TNS for the first time. Those who are interested in using TNS during labour should try the electrodes on their back either during the antenatal class or during a special TNS instruction class preferably for both partners. Where it is possible for women to borrow a TNS unit to use in early labour at home, the obstetric physiotherapist should prepare a simple list of instructions as to preparation and placement of electrodes and the use of the machine in labour. It is important for the correct electrode position to be marked on each woman's back. It is essential to keep a record of women borrowing TNS units and a signed receipt should be obtained. They should be told specifically to return it to a particular person and *not* to leave it on the labour ward if it does not belong there! Many women are happiest at home in early labour which is when TNS should be applied for the best results. If it is not possible to lend out units women will only be able to begin using TNS once they are admitted to hospital, when the contractions may already be severe and demanding.

Women should understand that TNS will not give them total pain relief – labour pain will still be felt – but for many it can give the extra assistance necessary to deal with this intense experience. In 1984 Clifford Woolf wrote in the *Textbook of Pain*: 'The ability of the clinician to reduce pain in a patient by exploiting the patient's own inbuilt neurophysiological control mechanisms must surely rank as one of the greatest achievements of contemporary medical science' (Woolf, 1984). Melzack and Wall (1982) described the concept of multiple influences on the transmission cells (T cells) in the central nervous system. Many variables, both psychological and physical, will affect the level of pain felt. They also mention the multiple convergent theory of pain relief, whereby two or three therapies, which alone give only slight analgesia, may give significant pain relief when combined. TNS should be regarded as an adjunct to other coping strategies, not as the sole source of pain relief in labour. The obstetric physiotherapist should be constantly alert to advances in this fascinating field, and should look into the effects of varying pulse widths and current frequencies, as well as possible alterations in electrode placement.

Midwives and TNS

In June 1986 the UK Central Council accepted the recommendation of its Midwifery Committee that midwives should not, on their own responsibility, use TNS for the relief of pain in labour. However, they are allowed to use TNS under supervision provided that they have been instructed in its use in accordance with Rule 41(1) and (3) of the Nurses Midwives and Health Visitors (Midwives Amendment) Rule 1986. In many centres this is taken to mean that within a 'blanket' referral from the consultants in charge of the obstetric unit, and with proper tuition and constant updating from obstetric physiotherapists, midwives are able to use TNS in labour for those mothers who wish to use it as a form of analgesia.

Acupuncture

This ancient method of relieving pain is sometimes used in labour. Doctors, midwives and physiotherapists are all showing new interest in this field. Jackson (1988) describes general techniques and modern explanations for the pain-modulating effects of acupuncture, but although he suggests that it may be used for childbirth pain he does not describe how this may be done. Skelton (1988) gives a comprehensive description of acupuncture techniques that have been successfully used in the treatment of labour pain, and suggests that this modality may be beneficially used.

Hypnosis

Anaesthetists, obstetricians and general practitioners have all described the use of hypnosis for the relief of labour pain, and also for the relief of tension and the promotion of relaxation in pregnancy. Women are usually treated individually, which is time-consuming for the practitioner. Attempts at group treatment have been made in antenatal classes. It certainly works for some women; one of the authors of this book saw her own father (a general practitioner) perform a forceps delivery on one of his patients who had been trained to put herself into a hypnotic trance for each labour contraction and for the delivery. Freeman et al. (1986), in a randomized trial of hypnosis in labour, showed a trend for labour to be more satisfying for women who used hypnosis, although analgesic requirements were similar in hypnosis and control groups. Women who were good or moderate hypnotic subjects reported that hypnosis had been instrumental in reducing anxiety and helping them cope with labour.

THE THIRD STAGE OF LABOUR (see also p. 67)

The third stage of labour has been called the most dangerous (Sleep, 1989) because of the risk of haemorrhage. It can be managed actively or passively, and it is important to prepare women antenatally for what is likely to happen and what may be expected of them. Couples are usually so overwhelmed by joy and excitement, and the wonder of actually seeing and touching their new baby, that this phase often passes by in a blur.

If the third stage is actively managed, a method in widespread use because it is said to reduce blood loss (Prendiville et al., 1988), the mother will receive an injection of syntocinon and ergometrine as the anterior shoulder is delivered. She will be asked to lie back so that the midwife can palpate the uterine fundus, and the placenta will be delivered by continuous cord traction once it has separated from the wall of the uterus, which is achieved by strong uterine contractions.

Where passive physiological management is used to deliver the placenta, the mother will probably have to adopt an upright posture so that gravity and intra-abdominal pressure can play their part in helping the process. Once the midwife feels the strong uterine contraction that results in placental separation and its descent into the lower uterine segment, the mother will be asked to bear down in order to help push the placenta out. If the baby sucks at the breast, oxytocin is produced which stimulates contractions and a 'clamp down' on the uterine blood vessels, thus aiding the physiological process. This is important because oxytocic drugs are not normally used when the third stage is passively managed. It is helpful for women to know that they may notice a gush of blood from the vagina as their baby suckles, a sign that the uterus is contracting well.

While the mother is made comfortable and has her perineum and vagina inspected for damage, the father can cuddle their new baby. This is often the time when parents want to talk about their experiences with the staff who cared for them in labour.

BIRTH PLANS

The birth plans which many hospitals now suggest their clients should prepare evolved from a reaction to the managerial approach of some obstetricians and midwives. The professionals thought that they 'knew best' when it came to childbirth. Women who felt that their needs and wishes would not be met by their carers wrote down their requests for the management of their labours and the care of their new baby. Because these early birth plans were sometimes written in an aggressive and demanding manner they were often met by hostility. But, as is often the case, the establishment began to realize that it was on the losing side in this confrontation, and hospitals began to produce their own formal printed plans for women to complete. This, of course, does make it seem as if women are being consulted and given choices, but in many cases hospitals' ready-printed birth plans do nothing of the sort. They are often just a series of statements requiring a yes/no answer or a tick in the relevant box, and the kind of questions women are asked only deal with trivial, superficial matters. Further, these birth plans are frequently handed out in antenatal clinics, without explanation, before women have started their course of antenatal classes – as early as 26–28 weeks. They will not yet have discovered what options are available to them.

Kitzinger (1987) has written wisely of the special importance of birth plans where women do not know in advance who will be caring for them in labour, and also how they can help midwives and doctors understand what matters to each mother. She also mentions the anxiety some professionals feel when they are confronted by a birth plan that has been compiled by a well-informed woman. Articulate women and their partners tend to read widely and also attend the sort of antenatal class that questions interventionist obstetric practices. Some have very pronounced views on labour and how they hope their own experience will be managed.

An example of a birth plan is given below.

Birth plan

Deborah and Anthony Smith

We have attended a course of antenatal classes and would like to experience as natural a birth as possible based on breathing and relaxation techniques which we have practised.

We would like the following points to be taken into consideration, and look forward to having a good relationship throughout with midwives and doctors. We acknowledge the medical expertise of staff and accept that unforeseen complications may necessitate alternative action to our wishes.

1. Please discuss everything with us first.
2. Anthony would like to be present at all times.
3. Please do not perform amniotomy – we would like labour to be as natural as possible.
4. Please use a fetoscope to monitor the baby.
5. Please offer a drink before a glucose drip.
6. Please check the dilatation of the cervix before any intervention.
7. We would prefer a small tear to a routine episiotomy.
8. Deborah hopes to be able to change position and move around frequently, so would prefer not to be electronically monitored.
9. We would like to listen to music and relax with the help of breathing techniques, and would welcome any advice from medical staff to achieve this end.

Pain relief. We intend to bring a TNS machine with us, and have been taught how to use it by an obstetric physiotherapist. We hope to use Entonox if necessary. Diamorphine should be given only if requested by us, and in the smallest doses possible.

Please deliver the baby onto the mother's abdomen. We would prefer the lights to be dimmed and minimum noise at the birth. Deborah would like to help lift the baby out, if possible.

Third stage. Please do not inject Syntometrine unless postpartum haemorrhage is suspected. If this is the case, please clamp the cord. We would prefer the cord not to be clamped until it has stopped pulsating. We would prefer the placenta to be delivered in an upright position, by pushing.

Please allow the baby to stay with the mother for demand feeding at all times. No glucose or water should be given.

Time should be devoted, during preparation for labour courses, to the consideration of birth plans and how they can be used to communicate to the caring staff not only each woman's feelings about her labour, but how she hopes necessary interventions such as caesarean section would be managed (e.g. epidural versus general anaesthesia), and also how she would like her baby to be handled after the birth. A birth plan is a good place to express the mother's feeding intentions and her attitude towards complements such as artificial baby milk and dextrose.

If birth plans are discussed by a class, women who find it difficult to voice their feelings, needs and preferences can be helped to express their wishes by the encouragement of their fellows and the teacher. However, women and their partners must understand that, as obstetricians and midwives are responsible for the consequences of *their* decisions, so too are they.

A useful booklet, *Your Baby – Your Choice* has been produced by the Maternity Alliance to help women prepare their birth plans.

VARIATIONS IN LABOUR

It is important for possible variations in the pattern of labour to be discussed during antenatal classes – not necessarily in great detail – as a preparation for mothers who may not experience 'textbook' births. The antenatal teacher must keep abreast of changes in labour ward protocol and be able to give accurate, up-to-date information on the management of breech and multiple births, for example, and also give guidance on the handling of such eventualities as occipito-posterior presentation. The following possibilities should be mentioned.

First stage

The powers

Hypotonic contractions. Weak, infrequent hypotonic contractions with slow progress may necessitate oxytocin infusion.

Hypertonic contractions. Very powerful, frequent hypertonic contractions can lead to precipitate labour and delivery, and possible fetal distress. The mother should try to remain calm and relaxed, and will probably need to use lighter, quicker breathing.

Induction of labour. If the cervix is unripe, prostaglandin in one form or another will be administered. This may be followed by artificial rupture of the membranes (ARM) and intravenous oxytocin. Mothers must be warned that prostaglandins can give rise to unpleasant, 'colicky' contractions (TNS may be helpful), and that induced or accelerated contractions will be stronger, possibly more painful, and with shorter resting intervals than those of normal labour. In addition the woman may be immobilized by drips and monitoring equipment. She will need extra support and may require additional analgesia.

The passages

Cephalopelvic disproportion. The pelvis is too small for the fetus. Squatting may help overcome this in the second stage (see p. 71).

Cervical dystocia. Failure of the cervix to dilate (see p. 68).

Placenta praevia. This can obstruct descent (see p. 41).

The Passenger

Occipito-posterior presentations. These account for approximately 30% of labours (see p. 70). An aching, 'boring' backache will be apparent; it may persist between contractions. The first stage of labour can be long-drawn-out, with irregular contractions. The mother will be more comfortable in positions that take the weight of her uterus away from her back, e.g. prone kneeling; between contractions, pelvic rocking and circling may help alter pressure within the pelvis. Deep back massage or pressure, heat or ice packs and resting in a warm bath may relieve discomfort. The fetus may rotate or be delivered face to pubes. An epidural anaesthetic may be necessary.

Breech birth. Labour may be no different to a vertex presentation, but is likely to be actively managed with epidural anaesthetic in most hospitals. Pelvimetry and an ultrasound scan at 38 weeks will attempt to identify women whose babiies will need delivery by elective caesarean section (see p. 69).

Malpositions or malpresentation. These may be associated with an obstruction, such as disproportion or placenta praevia.

Second stage (see p. 74)

Episiotomy. The possibility of this enlarging cut being used must be pointed out.

Forceps delivery (or ventouse extraction). Most forceps deliveries today will be 'lift-out' procedures. Women should be shown the lithotomy position in antenatal classes. It sometimes helps to describe the use of forceps as a shoe-horn, helping a baby out of a tight fit!

Caesarean section. Women must be prepared for this eventuality; the reasons for both elective and emergency operations should be described. It is most important that women know how they may feel postoperatively, and how they can best help themselves in the immediate postpartum period.

Third stage (see p. 72)

Lacerations and tears. These must be mentioned; also the role of pelvic floor exercises in the relief of postpartum discomfort.

Retained placenta. Although this is uncommon, women should be aware of its possible occurrence. A regional block or short general anaesthetic may be necessary to remove the placenta.

THE PUERPERIUM

It is important that some time is devoted antenatally to the problems women may encounter postnatally. Even where there has been a spontaneous vaginal delivery with an intact perineum, perineal pain or loss of sensation and pelvic floor muscle power may occur. These problems will be exacerbated after perineal tearing or an episiotomy; and if forceps have been used or a vulval or vaginal haematoma has developed, pain can be intense. It is thoroughly unfair to women if they are not warned that these problems often arise; self-help measures must be discussed in advance of the event. Pelvic floor exercises, the use of a bidet and warm baths; alternative feeding positions; the use of foam rings or pillows; resting flat in prone lying – all these techniques can be instituted by the woman herself before an obstetric physiotherapist arrives on the scene.

The possibility of the 'maternity blues' developing and the early signs of postnatal depression must be mentioned in view of the very large proportion of women who experience them. The emotional reactions and sense of anxiety felt by many mothers following childbirth should also be pointed out (mixed antenatal classes of primigravid and multigravid women will give the physiotherapist a better insight into this aspect of postnatal change), and the tremendous fatigue which often follows the initial period of elation should likewise be discussed by each group.

Women and their partners should be encouraged to look ahead to the early weeks at home with their new baby, and to the tremendous disruption in their lifestyle that follows every birth. The advent of a first baby dramatically alters the one-to-one relationship that exists between a couple; and the introduction of a new baby into an existing family can be traumatic for siblings too. Probably no amount of antenatal discussion can prepare parents-to-be for the realities of the disorganization which often follows birth – but maybe forewarned is slightly forearmed!

Sources of postnatal help should be pointed out antenatally; the family doctor, the community midwife, health visitors and voluntary organizations (National Childbirth Trust, La Leche League, Association of Breastfeeding Mothers and organizations devoted to specific problems) should all be included.

All must not be gloom; the joy and fulfilment which also accompany birth will reward parents for the hard grind and physical chores new babies bring. As the months pass the 'light at the end of the tunnel' draws closer, and for most families the transition to the new family state will be reasonably painless. It is important to discuss the practicalities of going home with a new baby. Will the father be able to spend some time at home? If a female relative is coming to stay, will she understand that *her* job is to look after the home and the new mother, and the new mother's job is to look after the baby? Postnatal exercises shoud be discussed; why they are important, when they should be done and the arrangements for teaching them postnatally must all be mentioned. Where women will only be in hospital for a very short period following the birth, the early exercises must be taught antenatally and 'reminder' leaflets given in advance.

LOSS OF A BABY

Childbirth is usually a happy event for all concerned, and the vast majority of parents will be blessed with a normal, healthy baby who survives into childhood. Although most pregnant women and their partners automatically expect this to happen, tragedies can and do occur. Little can be done to prepare a couple for coping with their baby's illness or death, yet the possibility of such a trauma occurring should be mentioned, and discussed if necessary, in antenatal classes.

Miscarriage

Miscarriage is the spontaneous termination of a recognized pregnancy before 28 weeks. While most miscarriages will take place before obstetric physiotherapists meet their clients, some of the women coming to 'early bird' classes may suffer a miscarriage and others, admitted to gynaecological or antenatal wards because of miscarriage, may be known to them. The emotional consequences of miscarriage can be great, and it is important that parents are allowed to mourn the loss. Sympathetic support is essential, both in hospital and once the woman returns home. Remarks such as 'Never mind, you can always have another baby', or 'You've got a lovely family already' can be wounding and do nothing whatsoever to help ease the pain (see p. 131 for supportive aftercare organizations).

Premature delivery and ill babies

Premature babies are those born after the 24th week and before the 36th week of pregnancy. With intensive care, many tiny early infants now survive, although not all will grow into undamaged children. Some special care baby units today allow antenatal classes to visit, and women who are hospitalized because of the risk of preterm birth are often introduced to the staff and the kind of care their babies may require.

Where removal of a pre-term or ill baby to intensive care is unexpected, the emotional trauma to the parents can be overwhelming, and in the past was often underestimated. The sight of frail wisps of humanity struggling for life, surrounded by monitors and machines, is almost too much for some parents to bear; many women find it impossible to visit their tiny baby unless accompanied and supported by their partner. The mother's physical contact with her baby is reduced or almost non-existent, and instead of a plump, pink bundle nestling in her arms, she will not only have an empty belly but empty arms too. She may well feel a failure because her body was not able to grow a full-term baby; she may also be frightened to bond with a baby who might not survive.

Women need immense empathetic support as this time and often turn to their obstetric physiotherapist, whom they may already know from antenatal classes, for reassurance. Almost certainly, the last thing they will have a mind for will be themselves. Many will have had an elective caesarean section to prevent damage to very undersized or ill babies, and they will have to cope with their own physical discomfort as well as their emotional distress and anxiety. Carers must look out for the welfare of the distracted mother.

Stillbirth

If a member of an antenatal group has experienced a stillbirth it is comparatively easy to raise the subject. Whether this is the case or not, it is a topic that must be introduced at some stage in the course, and it is probably better to do so at the beginning rather than at the end.

Occasionally a baby dies *in utero* (IUD) and the mother will have to cope with the knowledge that her baby, although still within her body, is dead; and sometimes a baby will die during the course of labour. A stillborn baby is one born after 28 weeks, gestation. This catastrophic experience is something no parent believes will happen to them, and one which carers often find very difficult to cope with themselves. Women are often discharged from hospital very quickly and, while many will want to be in the security of their own environment again, this is sometimes done to spare the staff the pain of the parents' grief. Stillborn babies used to be whisked away and were often buried in anonymous graves; parents were not given the time or encouragement to allow the normal grieving process to take its natural course. Bourne and Lewis (1983) described some of the long-term problems that may follow the inability to grieve properly. These include mothering difficulties with subsequent babies, marital problems, severe disturbances at anniversaries, puerperal psychosis in the next pregnancy and fracturing of the doctor–patient relationship. Today a much more humane, therapeutic approach is recommended. Parents are encouraged to look at and hold their baby, and photographs are often taken to provide a memento of the person who only existed inside the mother's body. It is indeed difficult to bring this subject up in antenatal classes; some women have a superstitious inability to think of such things, but it must be mentioned. An obstetric physiotherapist who is in contact with bereaved parents postnatally must not be ashamed of sharing their grief with them.

Cot death

There can be very little that is worse than the discovery that the baby who was apparently healthy a short while ago is cold and dead in its cot or pram. There are many causes of cot death or sudden infant death syndrome (SIDS). This unthinkable eventuality does happen, and while the obstetric physiotherapist may not be in contact with women when it does, the subject often arises in antenatal classes if a woman has experienced this, or a stillbirth, previously.

Professionals undoubtedly have difficulty coping with the distress experienced by parents whose babies are ill and more particularly with the despair of those whose babies are stillborn, handicapped or have died. Junior staff may not have received guidance in dealing with the anguish such tragic events can cause, and may well avoid bereaved and suffering parents. Thoughtless remarks which are meant to be consoling can add to the pain, but isolation and avoidance can be equally hurtful. Parents often appreciate the opportunity to talk about their lost baby and the events leading to the death; and although this can be upsetting for carers, the knowledge that it helps those who are distressed makes the discomfort easier to bear.

Courses are often arranged for professionals on how best to help parents cope with miscarriage, stillbirth and neonatal and cot death, and obstetric physiotherapists would be well advised to attend these.

References

Attwood R.J. (1976). Parturitional posture and related birth behaviour. *Acta Obstet. Gynecol. Scand.*, suppl., **57**, 5–25.

Avery M.D., Van Arsdale L. (1987). Perineal massage: effect on the incidence of episiotomy and laceration in a nulliparous population. *J. Nurse-Midwifery*, **32**, 181–4.

Balaskas J. (1983). *Active Birth*. London: Unwin Paperbacks.

Balaskas J., Balaskas A. (1983). *New Life*. London: Sidgwick & Jackson.

Belsey E.M., Rosenblatt D.B., Liebermann B.A. et al. (1981). The influence of maternal analgesia on neonatal behaviour: I. Pethidine. *Brit. J. Obstet. Gynaec.*, **88**, 398–406.

Billevicz-Driemel A.M., Milne M.D. (1976). Long term assessment of extradural analgesia for the relief of pain in labour. II Sense of 'deprivation' after extradural analgesia in labour: relevant or not? *Br. J. Anaesth.*, **48**, 139–144.

Birch M., Birch A.D.J. (1988). Fetal 'soap' addiction. *Lancet*, **ii**, 40.

Bourne S., Lewis E. (1983). Letter. *Br. Med. J.*, **286**, 145.

Bundsen P., Petersen L.E., Selstam U. (1981). Pain relief in labour by transcutaneous electrical nerve stimulation – A prospective matched study. *Acta Obstet. Gynecol. Scand.*, **60**, 459–68.

Bundsen P., Ericson K. (1982). Pain relief in labour by transcutaneous electrical nerve stimulation – safety aspects. *Acta Obstet. Gynecol. Scand.*, **61**, 1–5.

Bundsen P., Ericson K., Petersen L.E., Thringer K. (1982). Pain relief in labour by transcutaneous electrical nerve stimulation – testing of a modified stimulation technique and evaluation of the neurological and biochemical condition of the newborn infant. *Acta Obstet. Gynecol. Scand.*, **61**, 129–136.

Buxton R. StJ. (1965) Breathing in labour: the influence of psychoprophylaxis. *Nursing Mirror*, viii–ix.

Calder A.A. (1982). Posture during labour and delivery. *Maternal and Child Health*, **7**, 475–85.

Caldeyro-Barcia R. (1979). Physiological and psychological bases for the modern and humanised management of normal labour. In *Recent Progress in Perinatal Medicine and Prevention of Congenital Anomaly*, pp. 77–96. Tokyo: Ministry of Health and Welfare.

Caldwell J., Moffatt J.R., Smith R.L. et al. (1977). Determination of bupivacaine in human fetal and neonatal blood samples by quantitative single ion monitoring. *Biomed. Mass Spectrom.*, **4**, 322–5.

Charles A.G., Norr K.L., Block C.R. et al. (1978). Obstetric and psychological effects of psychoprophylactic preparation for childbirth. *Am. J. Obstet. Gynecol.*, **131**, 44–52.

Crawford J.S. (1972). Lumbar epidural block in labour: a clinical analysis. *Br. J. Anaesth.*, **44**, 66–74.

Dick-Read G.D. (1942). *Childbirth Without Fear*. Oxford: Heinemann.

Dunn P.M. (1976). Obstetric delivery today: for better or for worse? *Lancet*, **i**, 790–3.

Flynn A., Kelly J. (1976). Continuous fetal monitoring in the ambulant patient in labour. *Br. Med. J.*, **2**, 842–3.

Frampton V. (1988). Transcutaneous electrical nerve stimulation and chronic pain. In *Pain: Management and Control in Physiotherapy* (Wells P.E., Frampton V., Bowsher D., eds.) Oxford: Heinemann.

Freeman R.M., Macaulay A.J., Eve L., Chamberlain G.V.P. (1986). Randomised trial of self-hypnosis for analgesia in labour. *Br. Med. J.*, **292**, 657–8.

Fusi L., Steer P.J., Maresh M.J.A., Beard R.W. (1989). Maternal pyrexia associated with the use of epidural analgesia in labour. *Lancet*, **i**, 1250–2.

Gardosi J., Hutson N., B-Lynch C. (1989a). Randomised controlled trial of squatting in the second stage of labour. *Lancet*, **ii**, 74–77.

Gardosi J., Sylvester S., B-Lynch C. (1989b). Alternative positions in the second stage of labour: a randomised controlled trial. *Brit. J. Obstet. Gynaec.*, **96**, 1290–1296.

Gaskin I.M. (1977). *Spiritual Midwifery*. Tennessee: Tennessee Bible Books.

Haddad P.F., Morris N.F. (1982). The relationship of maternal anxiety to events in labour. *J. Obstet. Gynaecol.*, **3**, 94–7.

Haddad P.F., Morris N.F. (1985). Anxiety in pregnancy and its relation to use of oxytocin and analgesia in labour. *J. Obstet. Gynaecol.*, **6**, 77–81.

Harrison R.F., Woods T., Shore M. et al. (1986). Pain relief in labour using transcutaneous electrical nerve stimulation (TENS). A TENS/TENS placebo controlled study in two parity groups. *Brit. J. Obstet. Gynaec.*, **93**, 739–46.

Hassid P. (1978). *Textbook for Childbirth Educators*. New York: Harper & Row.

Heardman H. (1951). *Physiotherapy in Obstetrics and Gynaecology*. Edinburgh: E.&S. Livingstone.

Holdcroft A., Morgan M. (1974). An assessment of the analgesic effect in labour of pethidine and Entonox. *J. Obst. Gynaecol. Br. Commonwealth*, **81**, 603–7.

Jackson D.A. (1988). Acupuncture. In *Pain: Management and Control in Physiotherapy* (Wells P.E., Frampton V., Bowsher D., eds.). Oxford: Heinemann.

Jacobson E. (1938). *Progressive Relaxation*. Chicago: University of Chicago Press.

Karmel M. (1959). *Babies Without Tears*. London: Secker & Warburg.

Kitzinger S. (1962). *The Experience of Childbirth*. Harmondsworth: Penguin.

Kitzinger S. (1987). *Freedom and Choice in Childbirth*. London: Viking.

Lenstrup C., Schantz A., Berger A. et al. (1987). Warm tub during delivery. *Acta Obstet. Gynecol. Scand.*, **66**, 709–12.

Lupe P.J., Gross T.L. (1986). Maternal upright posture and mobility in labour – a review. *Obst. Gynec.*, **67**, 727–34.

MacArthur C., Lewis M., Knox E. G., et al. (1990). Epidural anaesthesia and long-term back ache after childbirth *Br. Med. J.*, **301**, 9–12.

McIntosh J. (1989). Models of childbirth and social class: a study of 80 working-class primigravidae. In *Midwives, Research and Childbirth 1* (Robinson S., Thomson A.M., eds.). London: Chapman & Hall.

Mannheimer J.S. (1985). TENS: uses and effectiveness in pain. In *International Perspectives in Physical Therapy 1* (Michel T.H., ed.). Edinburgh: Churchill Livingstone.

Melzack R., Taenzer P., Feldman P., Kinch R.A. (1981). Labour is still painful after prepared childbirth training. *Canadian Medical Association Journal*, **125**, 357–63.

Melzack R., Wall P.D. (1982). *The Challenge of Pain*. Harmondsworth: Penguin.

Mitchell L. (1987). *Simple Relaxation*. London: John Murray.

Moir D.D. (1986). *Pain Relief in Labour – a Handbook for Midwives*. Edinburgh: Churchill Livingstone.

Morgan B.M., Bulpitt C.J., Clifton P., Lewis P.J. (1982). Analgesia and satisfaction in childbirth (the Queen Charlotte's 1000 mother survey). *Lancet*, **ii**, 808–10.

Nelson M.K. (1983). Working class women, middle class women and models of childbirth. *Social Problems*. **30**, 284–97.

Noble E. (1980). *Essential Exercises for the Childbearing Year*. London: John Murray.

Noble E. (1981) Controversies in maternal effort during labour and delivery, *J. Nurse-Midwifery*, **26**, 13–22.

Noble E. (1983). *Childbirth with Insight*. Boston: Houghton Mifflin.

O'Brien P. (1988). *Birth and Our Bodies*. London: Pandora.

Pöschl U. (1987). The vertical birthing position of the Trobrianders, Papua New Guinea. *Aust. NZ J. Obst. Gynaecol.*, **27**, 120–5.

Prendiville W.T., Harding J.E., Elbourne D., Stirrat G. (1988). The Bristol third stage trial: 'active' versus 'physiological' management of the third stage. *Br. Med. J.*, **297**, 1295–1300.

Priest J., Rosser J. (1991). Pethidine – a shot in the dark. MIDIRS. *Midwifery Digest*, **1**, **4**, 373–5.

Randall M. (1953). *Fearless Childbirth*. London: Churchill.

Richards M.P., Bernal J.F. (1972) An observational study of mother-infant interaction. In *Ethological Studies of Child Behaviour*, (Jones ed.) Cambridge: Cambridge University Press.

Roberts J.E., Mendez-Bauer C., Wodell D.A. (1983). The effects of maternal position on uterine contractility and efficiency. *Birth*, **10**, 243–9.

Robson J.E. (1979). Transcutaneous nerve stimulation for pain relief in Labour. *Anaesthesia*, **34**, 357–60.

Rosenblatt D.B., Belsey E.M., Liebermann B.A. et al. (1981). The influence of maternal analgesia on neonatal behaviour. II. Epidural bupivacaine. *Brit. J. Obstet. Gynaec.*, **88**, 407–13.

Russell J.G.B. (1982). The rationale of primitive delivery positions. *Brit. J. Obstet. Gynaec.*, **89**, 712–5.

Simkin P. (1988). Role play of labor: a unique and valuable childbirth education technique. *Int. J. Childbirth Education*, **3**, 14–15.

Skelton I. (1988). Two non-pharmacological forms of pain relief in labour. 1 Acupuncture. In *Obstetrics and Gynaecology*. (McKenna J., ed.) International Perspectives in Physical Therapy 3. Edinburgh: Churchill Livingstone.

Sleep J. (1989). Physiology and management of the second stage of labour. In *Myles' Textbook for Midwives* (Bennett V.R., Brown L.K., eds.). Edinburgh: Churchill Livingstone.

Smellie W. (1974). *A Treatise on the Theory and Practice of Midwifery*. A facsimile printing of the 1752 edition. London: Ballière Tindall.

Sosa R., Kennell J., Klaus M. et al. (1980). The effect of a supportive companion on perinatal problems, length of labour, and mother-infant interaction. *New Eng. J. Med.*, **303**, 597–600.

Stewart P., Calder A.A. (1984). Posture in labour: patients' choice and its effect on performance. *Brit. J. Obstet. Gynaec.*, **91**, 1091–5.

Stradling J. (1984). Respiratory physiology during labour. *Midwife, Health Visitor and Community Nurse*, **20**, 38–42.

Thompson J.W. (1989). Pharmacology of Transcutaneous Electrical Nerve Stimulation (TENS). *Journal of the Intractable Pain Society of Great Britain and Ireland*, **7 (i)**, 33–40.

Vander L.S. (1980). *Human Physiology*, 3rd edn. New York: McGraw-Hill.

Vaughan K. (1951). *Exercise Before Childbirth*. London: Faber.

Wells P.E. (1988). Manipulative procedures. In *Pain: Management and Control in Physiotherapy* (Wells P.E., Frampton V., Bowsher D., eds.). Oxford: Heinemann.

Williams M., Booth D. (1985). *Antenatal Education*. Edinburgh: Churchill Livingstone.

Williams R.M., Thom M.H. (1980). A study of the benefits and acceptability of ambulation in spontaneous labour. *Brit. J. Obstet. Gynaec.*, **87**, 122–6.

Woolf C. (1984). Transcutaneous and implanted nerve stimulation. In *Textbook of Pain* (Wall P.D., Melzack R., eds.). Edinburgh: Churchill Livingstone.

Wright E. (1964). *The New Childbirth*. London: Tandem.

Wuitchik M., Bakal D., Lipshitz J. (1989). The clinical significance of pain and cognitive activity in latent labour. *Obst. Gynec.*, **73**, 35–42.

Further Reading

Balaskas J. (1989). *New Active Birth*. London: Unwin Hyman.

Bennett V.R., Brown L.K., eds. (1989). *Myles' Textbook for Midwives*. Edinburgh: Churchill Livingstone.

Flint C. (1986). *Sensitive Midwifery*. Oxford: Heinemann.

Inch S. (1982). *Birthrights*. London: Hutchinson.

Kitzinger S. (1987). *Freedom and Choice in Childbirth*. London: Viking.

Mannheimer J.S., Lampe G.N. (1984). *Transcutaneous Electrical Nerve Stimulation*. Philadelphia: F. A. Davis.

Maternity Alliance. (1990). Your baby your choice: A guide to planning your labour. London: Persil in association with the Maternity Alliance.

Mitchell L. (1987). *Simple Relaxation*. London: John Murray.

Wall P.D., Melzack R., eds. (1989). *Textbook of Pain*. Edinburgh: Churchill Livingstone.

Useful addresses

International Centre for Active Birth
55 Dartmouth Road
London NW3 1SL

Maternity Alliance.
15 Brittania Street
London WC1X 9JP

Miscarriage Association
PO Box 24
Ossett
West Yorkshire
WF4 4TP

National Childbirth Trust
Alexandra House
Oldham Terrace
Acton, London W3 6NH

Twins and Multiple Births Association (TAMBA)
41 Fortuna Way
Grimsby
South Humberside
DW37 9SJ

CHAPTER 7

The Postnatal Period

Immediately after the birth of her baby the new mother's body begins its period of recovery and its return to normal. However, the normality following the birth of a first baby will not be identical to the prepregnant state but will be a new normality, that of a mature female body that has experienced pregnancy and birth. Before a woman becomes pregnant she may or may not be happy with her shape, but it is the one that she is used to seeing. During pregnancy she will have noticed her body gradually change and grow. At the end of nine months she sees a ripely swollen abdomen, enlarged breasts, possibly oedema of the face, hands and legs, deposits of fat on her upper arms, hips, buttocks and thighs, and even stretch marks. Although in the first few postpartum hours she may be thrilled with the softness and relative flatness of her abdomen, once she is mobile and sees herself in a mirror she will be confronted with a third body; an empty, sagging and still enlarged abdomen, maybe with crêpey wrinkled skin. As she moves, talks and laughs she will become aware of an almost complete lack of abdominal muscle control. She may have experienced an episiotomy or a tear which may be made more painful by bruising and oedema; she may have difficulty in initiating micturition, or the converse may be true – an inability to control her bladder when the desire to void becomes apparent; she may also experience leakage when the intra-abdominal pressure is raised by coughing, sneezing or laughing. Her immediate postpartum emotional state can vary between euphoric exhilaration with an inability to sleep, and disillusioned disappointment (especially if medical intervention proved necessary or the baby was the 'wrong' sex), accompanied by total exhaustion.

For many newly delivered women this will be their first experience of hospitalization. Unfamiliar surroundings, overwhelming responsibilities, and intense fatigue may result in a lowered pain threshold. The obstetric phsiotherapist should be aware of this and complaints of 'aches and pains' should be taken seriously and properly assessed. Minor discomforts, which would almost certainly not normally bother the woman, respond well to physical treatment delivered with empathy and understanding.

POSTPARTUM PHYSICAL CONDITION

Connective tissue

The body's ligaments and collagenous connective tissue will still be softer and more elastic than prior to pregnancy – it will take four to five months (Calguneri et al., 1982) for full recovery to take place.

Abdominal muscles

The abdominal muscles will have been stretched and are now elongated – a split between the two recti abdominis muscles (known as a diastasis or divarication) will almost certainly be apparent in any woman who was at term prior to labour. This can vary between a small vertical gap 2–3 cm wide and 12–15 cm long, to a space measuring 12–20 cm in width and extending nearly the whole length of the recti muscles (Fig. 7.1). As a result, the entire abdominal 'corset' will be weakened with very little apparent mechanical control. Because of this, in addition to the increased elasticity of its ligaments, the back will be very much more vulnerable to injury resulting from incorrect use. Women with a narrow pelvis, those who carried large babies or who had a multiple birth, and multiparae are most at risk of developing a gross diastasis. Women whose pregnancies necessitated prolonged inactivity or those who habitually take very little exercise will almost certainly find that their abdominal muscles are extremely weak.

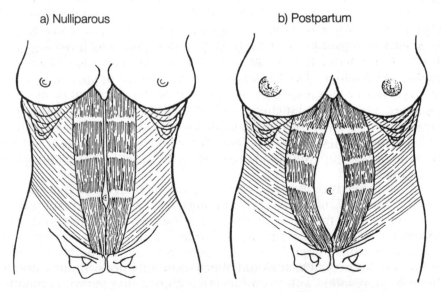

Figure 7.1 Diastasis recti abdominis.

Pelvic floor

The pelvic floor will almost certainly be weaker than it was prior to the pregnancy. In addition to the stretching and trauma sustained during delivery, its muscles and connective tissue will, by the end of the nine months, have been partly responsible for continuously supporting as much as 6 kg of extra pelvic and abdominal weight (i.e. baby, uterus, placenta and liquor). The perineum itself will have been considerably stretched. It may have been cut (episiotomy) or torn, and then sutured, and extensive bruising and oedema is sometimes seen. An additional cause of acute discomfort can be the presence of haemorrhoids. The obstetric physiotherapist should be aware that neurological damage may also be sustained during the birthing process, resulting in temporary (days or weeks), longer-lasting (months) or permanent loss of sensation and muscle weakness (Snooks et al.,1984; Allen et al., 1990).

Legs

Many women will complain of heavy, aching legs – and even if swollen feet and ankles were not a problem before the baby was born, they can become so in the immediate postpartum period. One or both legs may be affected. This could be due to prolonged pushing or pelvic congestion; even the temperature of the postnatal ward can play a part!

Back

Back pain may not have been troublesome during pregnancy but it frequently develops following the birth. For many women the passage of the fetus through the pelvis and the resultant stretching and movement of the lax joints is a causative factor. It can also be present following an epidural anaesthetic (MacArthur et al., 1990), or the lithotomy position for delivery or perineal repair (especially if the legs were not placed and removed from the stirrups simultaneously). Poor, unsupported feeding positions and bad nappy-changing postures, in addition to tension and fatigue, can all give rise to this troublesome condition.

Breasts

The breasts may become engorged when lactation begins on the third or fourth postnatal day. They may feel hot, full and very painful; the pain can extend into the axilla where a 'tail' of breast tissue lies.

Mood

A state of primary maternal preoccupation (Winnicot, 1987) has been described; the mother's attention is fixed on her baby and she is often hypersensitive to every nuance of its behaviour. Her initial elation can change after a few days to a flattening of her mood. She may well be more concerned with her baby than she is for herself.

ROUTINE POSTNATAL CARE

Length of hospital stay

Historically there was a lying-in period of three weeks, during which the new mother largely remained in bed, resting. Over the years this has progressively been reduced, until today most women expect – and are expected – to return to normal activity within a very few days, often regardless of the number of children for whom they have to care. Along with the reduction in the postnatal resting period has come a much earlier discharge from hospital where most births now take place, partly in order to optimize NHS bed usage, and partly because some mothers wish to return home as soon as possible after the birth. The length of postnatal hospital stay is becoming progressively shorter, and varies between six hours following a normal delivery, and seven to ten days, where there have been complications or a caesarean section. Most units will discharge women between two and five days following delivery.

Midwifery

There is a mandatory requirement for a midwife to attend the mother for the first ten postpartum days; if necessary, this can be extended to 28 days. The midwife will be concerned with the mother's well-being, the establishment of lactation and the condition of the baby. She will daily monitor temperature, pulse, respiration and blood pressure. She will also inspect the mother's breasts, abdomen and perineum. A check on the level of blood haemoglobin is made 24 hours after delivery; and this is repeated later so that anaemia can be treated and prevented.

Medical care

If there are no complications the mother may only see a doctor once before she leaves hospital. Following the intensive medical care during the antenatal period and labour, many women feel bereft of their doctor's care and interest; comments about this are often made during their hospital stay, and reassurance may be necessary.

Postnatal establishment of breast-feeding

For some women, putting their new baby to their breast, very soon after birth, is an instinctive reaction; and some babies, once they are presented with their mother's breast, will instinctively latch on to it to enjoy their first feed. But for many breast-feeding will have to be a 'learned art', and these mothers and babies will need the sympathetic and expert help of their midwife to establish successful breast-feeding. Motivation, confidence and support can help women overcome initial difficulties such as a sleepy baby, sore nipples and engorgement, so that they are able to continue happily feeding one, two or occasionally even three babies for many months (Appelbaum, 1970).

Salariya et al. (1978) have shown that where babies were put to the breast within 10 minutes of delivery instead of 4–6 hours after birth, and were then fed 2-hourly until the mother's milk came in, that lactation was induced at least 24 hours earlier than when babies were fed 4-hourly, and that the duration of breast-feeding was significantly extended. De Chateau and Wiberg (1977) also found that putting the baby to the breast early, within one hour of birth, considerably extended the period for which lactation continued when compared with babies whose first experience of suckling was delayed several hours. The implications for these findings are clear – women should be encouraged antenatally to begin breast-feeding as soon as possible.

Position of mother and baby

A mother may choose to sit up in bed or sit in a chair, or she may feel most comfortable and relaxed lying on first one side and then the other. When sitting, her back should always be well supported, and the baby raised to her breast by means of a pillow on her lap. A footstool is essential for total comfort if a chair is being used. When the mother is lying on her side, her head should be properly supported with pillows pulled well in to her neck. Whatever the mother's position, the baby must lie on its side facing the breast, *not* on its back with its head turned to the mother. Although it may be advantageous initially for the mother to lean forward so that the baby can be properly positioned on the breast, she should be encouraged to relax back on adequate support as soon as the baby is feeding well.

Many women, perhaps having been overexposed to bottle-feeding, may attempt to 'bottle-feed' their baby at the breast, and will offer just the nipple, instead of coaxing the baby to take not only the nipple but also a sizeable portion of areola into its mouth as well. The nipple should be drawn into the baby's mouth against the hard palate, and the tongue should be underneath. To be properly 'fixed' on the breast the baby's mouth needs to be well open, with the chin resting on the breast and the lower lip curling down. The mother should not need to support her breast unless it is very heavy, in which case she can slip her hand underneath. The habit of using the fingers to press the breast away from the baby's nose is to be discouraged, as it could cause a blockage in the ducts leading to the nipple (RCM 1991). Colostrum, and later milk, is drawn out by a wave of pressure from the baby's tongue on the lactiferous sinuses, and by a gentle, compressive milking action of the baby's lower jaw. This stimulates the 'let-down' or milk ejection reflex (oxytocin from the posterior pituitary causes the myoepithelial cells surrounding the alveoli to contract, thus releasing the milk). The response is highly individual: for some mothers it may give rise to sharp, needle-like pains in the breast; others may only feel a mild tingling sensation; and a proportion will feel nothing at all. This increase in oxytocin can also cause the characteristic 'afterpains' experienced by so many women during the early days of breast-feeding, as the uterus contracts in response to the varied level of the hormone (p. 79). Deep breathing and conscious relaxation can help the mother cope with these discomforts.

The obstetric physiotherapist must be alert to the pain problems of women who have experienced difficult surgical deliveries, because pain can often prevent the mother being relaxed and comfortable. It is vital that special help, e.g. support, positioning, TNS, ice, pulsed electromagnetic energy (PEME), foam-rubber rings, etc., is given; the establishment of breast-feeding may depend on it.

Length and timing of feeds

Earlier this century very rigid feeding schedules were imposed on mothers and babies; four-hourly feeding was recommended, the length of feeds was restricted, and frequently the night feed was forbidden. Apart from the stress and misery these strict routines caused, they were probably the single most important cause of the failure to establish breast-feeding. Today 'demand feeding' is accepted practice, although the earlier attitudes may still exist here and there. Feeding on demand implies feeding when the baby asks for a feed (but not necessarily every time he cries) and not restricting the length or the frequency of the feeds (see p. 80). Nevertheless the mother's needs must be considered too, so that if, for instance, her breasts are full and uncomfortable, her baby should be roused and offered a feed. Feeding more often will usually increase milk supply if this is insufficient, and it has also been shown that unrestricted feeding is likely to increase the time (in weeks) for which a mother breast-feeds her baby (Slaven and Harvey, 1981).

Table 7.1 Breast-feeding problems

Problem	Possible causes	Solution
Engorgement	Oedema due to temporarily increased blood supply, tends to occur when colostrum begins to be replaced by milk. Possible initial overproduction of milk	Improve position of the baby on the breast; do not restrict length of feed; express milk if the breast is still uncomfortable; good breast support; warm bathing before a feed. Ultrasound
Sore cracked nipples	Poor position, baby not grasping breast properly; possibly soggy breast pads or sensitivity to creams and sprays, infection	Reposition the baby (Inch, 1987, RCM, 1991). Nipple shields are said to be ineffective. Expose nipples to the air and sunlight, rest the breasts if there is no improvement
Blocked ducts – tender, hot, red lump	Engorgement, pressure on a duct from tight bra, baby held too tightly against breast	Check baby's position and mother's bra, feed baby lying down from an exposed breast. Gentle massage towards nipple, warm compresses. Ultrasound
Mastitis – inflamed segments of the breast, pyrexia	Initially may be non-infective, but if unresolved it is usually a staphylococcal infection or blocked duct	If resistant to antibiotics, use hot poultices, ultrasound
Conflicting advice	Lack of knowledge and communication, adherence to outdated concepts	The establishment of an agreed code of practice within the maternity unit and its enforcement

Common problems

Common breast-feeding problems are summarized in Table 7.1.

The early days of breast-feeding can be the 'make or break' period for very many women trying to establish lactation. Good, consistent support from knowledgeable staff can help the mother over the early problems. In today's climate of staff shortages, the amount of time midwives are able to spend with women is sometimes severely restricted. Nevertheless, if *correct* advice is given from the start, even a short time will suffice. Although obstetric physiotherapists are most certainly *not* the professionals in charge of this activity, they will be constantly dealing with women in the early puerperium (and often later on at postnatal community classes), who will understandably often ask them questions. The obstetric physiotherapist should read widely in order to keep abreast of the best available information for a full understanding of the physiological control of lactation, practical ways of helping, and how best to respond to these mothers. Mothers must never be interrupted during a feed for any form of treatment; the establishment of breast-feeding must take priority over all other routines – although a reminder that they can use feeding times to gently exercise the abdominal wall and pelvic floor muscles once things are going well will not come amiss.

It has been suggested (Romito, 1988) that even well-established breast-feeding can bring dificulties not experienced by bottle-feeding women; breast-fed babies feed more often during the night and can be more colicky, which can increase fatigue at an already tiring time. Even if women are not able to arrange a long daily rest, the obstetric physiotherapist can help by discussing the use of relaxation postnatally during antenatal classes, and by reminding women of its positive role when they are seen in the puerperium prior to their discharge from hospital. Most women are aware that they may experience a decline in sexual interest during the early postnatal months; Alder and Bancroft (1983, 1988) have shown that breast-feeders resume sexual intercourse later than bottle-feeders. For the vast majority of women breast-feeding is not an instinctive activity, but rather an art which mother and baby have to learn together. For those who succeed it can be an experience of closeness and nurturing which will remain with the woman for the rest of her life – it is the logical continuation of conception, pregnancy and birth. One mother has said: 'It's so enjoyable to be able to feed your baby with your own milk. She is ours, we made her, we were capable of such a thing, and then in addition you can feed her. And in that moment you feel as if you're a small universe in your own right' (Romito, 1988).

THE POSTNATAL CHECK

It is traditional for a woman to be examined and assessed by a member of the obstetric team six weeks postpartum. However, there is no good physiological reason for this timing apart from the fact that the uterus should have returned to its prepregnancy size by then, lochia should have ceased and any wounds healed. The good obstetrician or general practitioner should also be interested in the mother's emotional state and how she and her family are adapting to, and coping with, the stress a new baby can bring, as well as her physical recovery. Many women will be grateful for and will benefit from a further check, perhaps when their baby is three months old – many new mothers feel abandoned following the six-week examination, particularly if their antenatal care was hospital-based. Women are extremely vulnerable postnatally; they have experienced a tremendous life change, and, particularly for

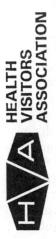

Your post natal check list

Name ....

Name of Health Visitor ....

This list has been produced to help you get the best care for yourself after the birth of your baby. We suggest that you take it with you when you see your Doctor who will be happy to discuss any of these points with you or anything else that concerns you or your partner. Alternatively you might wish to use it for jotting down important items as a memory jogger.

Your health and well being are important. Having a baby is a big change in your life and it may take time to adjust.

Emotions

How are you feeling? ....

How have your other children reacted to your new baby? ....

Rest

Are you getting enough rest?   yes ☐ no ☐

Eating

Are you managing to eat proper meals?   yes ☐ no ☐

Feeding

Are you happy with the method of feeding you have chosen for your baby?   yes ☐ no ☐

Your body

Are your breasts comfortable?   yes ☐ no ☐

Have you got backache?   yes ☐ no ☐

Have you had any further bleeding?   yes ☐ no ☐

If you have had an episiotomy you can expect tenderness and swelling from your stitches for about three weeks. Are you still experiencing pain?   yes ☐ no ☐

Everybody regains their figure at a different rate. Don't expect miracles. It takes nine months for your body to change and it can take nine months to get back to your former shape. Appropriate exercise can help.

Are you constipated?   yes ☐ no ☐

It can take some weeks for the bowel and bladder muscles to return to normal. You can help this process by remembering to practise your post natal exercises every time you go to the toilet.

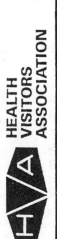

HEALTH VISITORS ASSOCIATION

Your post natal checklist continued

You and your partner

Have you made any arrangements for your post natal check and family planning appointment?   yes ☐ no ☐

Some couples make love before their post natal check. If you have, was it comfortable?   yes ☐ no ☐

Help

Have you got anyone nearby you can rely on for help?   yes ☐ no ☐

Are you able to get out easily?   yes ☐ no ☐

Would you like to be in touch with other mothers?   yes ☐ no ☐

What your post natal examination should include

1. Blood Pressure check
2. Breasts examined
3. Check that the womb has returned to normal size
4. Stitches, if any, checked
5. Discussion about your plans for contraception.

The postnatal examination is an opportunity for you to discuss anything that concerns you, associated with your recent pregnancy. If you are not able to obtain all the information that you require from your Doctor, it is suggested you should talk to your Health Visitor.

Figure 7.2 Postnatal check list (reproduced by permission of the Health Visitors'

primiparae, nothing will ever be quite the same for them again. The obstetric physiotherapist who will be meeting mothers at a 'mother and baby' group is in an ideal position to remind them of the importance and purpose of the postpartum examination – to make sure that their bodies have recovered from the experience of childbirth. Where this is not the case, the subject should be introduced either in antenatal classes or before the woman leaves hospital after giving birth.

Regrettably some postnatal six-week checks are cursory, to say the least, and it is well for women to know exactly what this *should* entail. Ideally the mother's blood pressure will be taken; her breasts and perineum examined, urine sample checked, and abdominal and vaginal examination carried out to ascertain uterine involution and the state of the cervix. The strength of the abdominal and pelvic floor muscles should be tested (and suggestions for improving this made if necessary) and a smear taken. Most doctors take this opportunity to discuss contraception and any health problems the woman may be experiencing (MacArthur, 1991).

Because of the demands of life with a new baby many mothers neglect themselves and put their needs after those of their families. The Health Visitors Association, together with the Association of Chartered Physiotherapists in Obstetrics and Gynaecology, the Royal College of Midwives and other interested groups, drew up a useful postnatal check list to draw women's attention to the importance of caring for themselves, to remind them of the purpose of a postnatal medical examination and the sort of questions they should ask their doctors (see Fig.7.2).

Contraception

Although obstetric physiotherapists are not responsible for giving full contraceptive information and advice, this is a subject which many women want to discuss in the friendly atmosphere of the ante-natal or postnatal class. In 1921 when Marie Stopes set up the first birth-control clinic, the estimated number of women practising contraception was around 10%. Today this is the percentage of women who do not practise contraception and who are therefore at risk of pregnancy. Nevertheless, misunderstandings and 'young wives' tales' about this vitally important subject abound; physiotherapists working with women of reproductive age therefore need up-to-date information about the methods that may be used to prevent conception (Table 7.2); obstetric physiotherapists need to be particularly conversant with methods that can be used by breast-feeding women.

Table 7.2 Methods of contraception

Method	How it works	Advantages and disadvantages
Combined oral contraceptive pill (COC) – oestrogen and progestogen	Inhibits ovulation (oestrogen) and produces endometrial changes and a hostile cervical mucus (progestogen)	Easy and convenient to use, gives a regular monthly cycle; often reduces bleeding, dysmenorrhoea and PMT. Not suitable for women over 45 or for smokers over 35; contraindicated where there is a history of circulatory or liver diseases. Should not be used by breast-feeding women
Progestogen-only pill (POP), minipill	Works primarily by causing a hostile cervical mucus and an atrophic endometrium. Also interferes with the ovulation process	Its efficacy is age-related (increases as fertility decreases), therefore best suited to women over 35. Suitable for diabetics and women with sickle-cell disease. Recommended during breast-feeding; does not inhibit lactation or affect the baby. Can cause irregular bleeding patterns
Injectable progestogens (e.g. Depo-Provera)	High-dose progestogen inhibits ovulation in addition to endometrial and cervical mucus effects. Given every 12 weeks	Eliminates user error; reduces incidence of pelvic inflammatory disease; very suitable for sufferers from sickle-cell disease. Delays return of fertility; causes weight gain and maybe acne; can increase depression where this is a problem. The side-effects have to be tolerated for 3 months since once it is administered the hormone cannot be removed
Intrauterine contraception	Plastic copper-bearing devices inserted by a doctor. Acts as a foreign body, possibly preventing implantation. Alters uterine and tubal fluids; this may impair the viability of gametes and impede fertilization	Effective immediately after fitting; does not interfere with love-making; gives protection as long as it remains *in situ* and only need changing infrequently (2–5 years). Not suitable for nulliparous women because of the risk of pelvic infection; there is a small risk of pregnancy; the device can be expelled by uterine contractions. Periods may be heavier initially and the woman may also experience discomfort in the first few months

Table 7.2 Methods of contraception (*continued*)

Method	How it works	Advantages and disadvantages
Barrier methods	Diaphragm or cap plus spermicide; spermicide-impregnated sponge; condoms	Barrier methods work by preventing the sperm reaching the ovum. They are non-invasive with no side-effects or interference with menstruation. Can interfere with the spontaneity of love-making
Natural methods	Aim to predict ovulation so that the most fertile period can be avoided. Mucus or Billings method requires several months of instruction for the woman to learn to recognize cervical mucus changes prior to ovulation (see p. 22). Symptothermal method combines knowledge that there is a rise in basal body temperature following ovulation, with the mucus method and the recognition of physiological signs of ovulation	No side-effects; acceptable to many women who want to control their own fertility; couples share the responsibility for family planning. Does require dedication, and expert and long-term instruction. Unreliable where there are irregular menstrual cycles, following recent pregnancy, during lactation or at the menopause. The menstrual cycle can be affected by travel, environmental changes, illness, dieting and by the use of drugs that result in amenorrhoea
Sterilization	Vasectomy prevents the passage of sperm into the male urethra; female sterilization closes or divides the fallopian tubes and prevents the ovum reaching the uterus	Both these methods must be regarded as a 'once and for all' procedure for couples who have completed their families; reversal may not be possible

POSTNATAL PHYSIOTHERAPY

Because of the current trend towards a briefer hospital stay, obstetric physiotherapists must continually address how best to deliver an effective postnatal service. Much innovative thinking is urgently required, because there will have to be substantial changes in the provision of immediate postnatal care and rehabilitation in hospital and its continuation in the community. At present, even where a maternity unit purports to have an obstetric physiotherapy service, many women simply receive a greeting and an exercise leaflet, and some even leave without any contact having been made at all.

Assessment

Ideally, at a mutually convenient time within the first 24 hours, the obstetric physiotherapist should assess each new mother to determine her priority needs. Immediate advice and initial exercise instruction is best given individually, and specific therapies, where necessary, should be commenced as soon as possible. However, after this it is more cost-efficient, more effective and much more pleasurable for the women to participate in postnatal classes. Most new mothers enjoy being in a group and benefit from the opportunity to exchange experiences, moan and laugh, discuss problems and work through ways of solving them together. There is a wealth of information and advice, over and above simple exercise instruction, which is particularly important for those women who did not attend antenatal classes.

The postnatal class can be taken in the parentcraft room, if it is nearby, or the ward day-room. Most women are happy to participate, but only if their babies can come too. This should definitely be encouraged because it enables valuable teaching to be presented regarding the new activities, especially baby feeding and nappy changing, which if carried out incorrectly can lead to neck and back ache. Where women are cared for in single rooms and no common room exists, obstetric physiotherapists will be very restricted in what they can offer at this special time.

Diastasis Recti Abdominis

If the diastasis is less than two fingers in width (see p. 223), abdominal exercises may progress rapidly. If the gap is greater, rotation and side flexion exercises should be delayed until the size of the gap has been reduced. Such movements may increase the gapping because of shearing forces (Noble, 1980). Static and gentle dynamic inner-range exercise may be performed with crossed hands (see p. 251).

Pelvic floor

Ideally the obstetric physiotherapist should inspect the perineum of every postnatal mother to ascertain if she is able to contract the muscles of the pelvic floor. This inspection is essential following forceps delivery, ventouse extraction, episiotomy, second- and third-degree tears, and for any woman complaining of intense perineal pain or those who say they cannot feel their muscles working. The aim is to identify women who are initially unable to contract the pelvic floor musculature, so that they can be followed up if necessary. It has been suggested that some women lose cortical control of their pelvic floor muscles following intense postpartum perineal pain (Shepherd, 1980). Neuropraxia and even denervation has also been reported (Snooks et al., 1984; Allen et al., 1990).

Initial postnatal exercises

Breathing

Deep breathing is beneficial for its circulatory and relaxing effects.

Leg exercises

Foot, ankle and leg exercise will help to improve circulation.

Pelvic floor exercises

Pelvic floor exercises are valuable for their strengthening and pain-relieving properties. They will also speed healing by reducing oedema and encouraging good circulation. These exercises can be started in the delivery room; most women should be able to begin once they have reached the postnatal ward. Pelvic floor tightening can be done quickly ('Hold, relax, hold, relax') or slowly ('Pull your pelvic floor in and up, hold – two – three – four (or more) and let go'). This exercise should be done little and often. Ideally the mother should try to contract her pelvic floor 200 times a day – not as impossible as it sounds if she does 20 pelvic floor 'lifts' (in groups of 4 at a time) during every feed. The mother with an acutely painful perineum or who has stitches may be very apprehensive at the thought of exercising her damaged muscles. She must be coaxed to attempt this because even three or four muscle contractions will begin to give relief by virtue of the pumping action on the local circulation. If a woman complains that she is unable to appreciate a pelvic floor contraction while she is lying or sitting, she will probably find that standing with legs slightly apart makes all the difference.

Two essential pieces of early advice which can give these women relief and confidence are:

1 The pelvic floor muscles must be contracted (counter-braced) every time the mother coughs, sneezes or laughs.
2 The sutures should be supported with a sanitary towel or a pad of soft toilet paper when defaecation is attempted and until the perineal pain subsides.

For some women the memory of the postpartum perineal pain they experienced, often lasting several weeks, is worse than their memory of labour pain; it has been called the 'fourth stage of labour'!

Abdominal muscle exercises

The primary aims are to shorten stretched muscle fibres, close any diastasis and strengthen weakened muscles. The first step in abdominal muscle re-education should be the initiation of a simple contraction; for example, drawing in the anterior abdominal wall in crook lying. It is most efficient when it is combined with expiration. However, many women cannot do this easily. The physiotherapist may find it helpful to suggest that women 'Breathe in; breathe out, draw the tummy in – and then relax'. A common fault is attempting to combine abdominal wall retraction with inspiration and breath holding. This has the effect of raising the rib cage with its abdominal wall attachments, thereby taking up the slack, possibly without any muscle contraction. For some women it will be much easier to initiate an abdominal muscle contraction in side lying. Because the abdomen protrudes and sags sideways the muscle fibres are in their outer to middle range – their pre-delivery state – and this seems to make it easier to activate a contraction. A similar situation exists in sitting – women can both see and feel their abdominal movement.

Pelvic tilting

Pelvic tilting can also be taught in crook or side lying; again, it can be done slowly, holding the abdominal wall in while the mother counts to four, or it can be done quickly (tilt, relax, tilt, relax). This second technique is often very helpful for the woman who has afterpains or backache. The obstetric physiotherapist must be vigilant because it is possible to tilt the pelvis in crook lying without contracting the abdominal muscles. Rhythmical gluteal contractions will help ease the pain from haemorrhoids or bruising.

The early postnatal class

All too often postnatal exercises are only taught to women who are lying down; this may well be one of the reasons why many of them fail to continue exercising once they return home. If a woman does not realize that it is possible to strengthen her abdominal and pelvic floor muscles while she is standing or sitting, early exercises will not be done simply because she may never have time to lie down!

Postnatal exercises

Sitting. The early hospital class can begin with the women sitting comfortably and well supported on chairs which have been placed in a circle; pillows should be used where necessary for sore perineums and to support backs. Women must realize that one of their first postnatal exercises is *how they sit when feeding their babies.* Once everyone is settled, attention should be drawn to the main areas of muscle weakness (abdomen and pelvic floor) and the problems that can follow misuse of their backs. Multiparae are often important sources of advice, and their previous experiences can be very useful. The obstetric physiotherapist will find it helpful to have some simple, large diagrams that illustrate the pelvic floor and possible episiotomy sites, as well as the abdominal muscles and the diastasis recti abdominis. The Birth Atlas can be used to demonstrate the extent to which their muscles have had to stretch; women are fascinated by the changes experienced by their bodies during pregnancy and labour, and this realization is often the trigger that stimulates them to continue exercising in order to repair the weaknesses caused by childbirth.

Back care advice for feeding, nappy changing, baby bathing, lifting and carrying should all be discussed. Correct heights for cots and pram or buggy handles should be mentioned (Fig. 7.3). Crying babies can be usefully used to explain the value of slings and how they should be worn, with the baby high on the mother's chest (Fig.7.4, see p. 238). The woman should know that simple abdominal retraction and pelvic floor work can be done while feeding (once they feel confident that both their babies and themselves are doing this correctly!). Other easy exercises which may be done in sitting are side-flexion and rotation (with the abdominal muscles well drawn in), elbow and head circling, and foot exercises.

Standing. Similar movements can be carried out while standing; 'hip-hitching' and gentle trunk forward flexion for its relaxing effect are also useful exercises for the woman who just can't find the time or energy during the first few weeks to exercise lying down. While they are standing the women's attention should be drawn to their posture, which in many cases will still reflect its adaptation to pregnancy or to any postpartum pain they are experiencing. The dramatic difference between the measurement of the abdominal girth when a woman sags compared to that when 'standing tall' (5–12 cm) is wonderfully motivating! Women spend a large part of their day standing – if all they

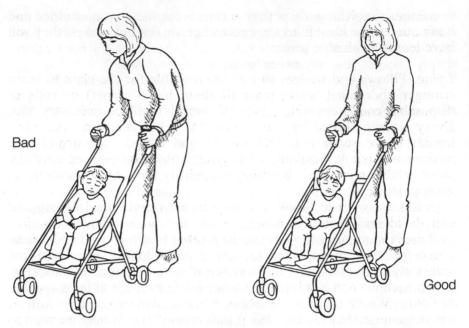

Figure 7.3 Pram and buggy handles should be the correct height to avoid back problems.

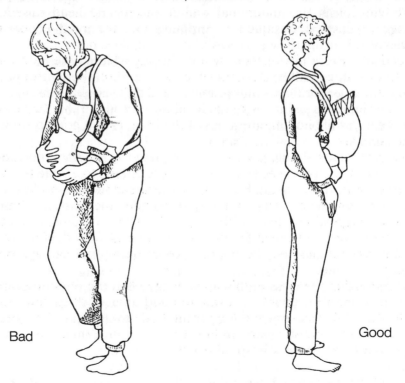

Figure 7.4 The value of carrying slings should be discussed postnatally.

remember from this early postnatal class is the fact that post office and bank queues are ideal places to practise pelvic floor exercises, they will have learnt a valuable lesson!

Lying. Pillows and wedges should be available for the class to learn stronger abdominal work; mats (if there is no carpet) or rolls of disposable couch covering paper (if there is) will be necessary too. Every woman should be shown how to feel if her recti abdominis muscles have separated, and should understand that strong side flexions and trunk rotations, while lying, should be omitted until the anterior abdominal wall is strong enough to allow these movements without shearing.

In this class pelvic tilting can progress to include head raising and then head and shoulders raising. Prior to any postnatal abdominal exercise it is important to remind the mother to draw in the abdominal wall *before* the movement commences. If the abdomen bulges or ridges anteriorly it indicates extreme weakness of the recti abdominis muscles, and in such women head-raising should be delayed for at least another 24 hours. Where there is a diastasis of more than two finger-widths it has been suggested (Noble, 1980) that crossed hands may be used to approximate and support the diverging recti muscles, although in fat women it may be difficult to find them! Alternate single leg sliding from crook lying, with the abdominal wall retracted and head raised, is another excellent technique for strengthening the recti abdominis muscles if it is properly supervised and ridging does not occur.

Practically every new mother will be having at least one bath each day, so the concept of exercising while bathing should be introduced. Pelvic tilting, pelvic floor contractions, head and shoulder raising and alternate single leg sliding, with the head raised and the chin tucked on to the chest, while holding the sides of the bath, are all good postnatal 'aqua exercises'.

This early class should always be completed by a short relaxation session. Women need to be shown how to use pillows to enable them to lie prone comfortably again. Following a caesarean section mothers can enjoy lying on their backs with a wedge under their knees. Simple relaxation suggestions linked with deep, calm, slow breathing will often result in one or two women falling asleep – this usefully demonstrates their intense fatigue and the importance of occasional catnaps once they return home.

By organizing the class in this manner the obstetric physiotherapist can give women invaluable information and advice which can really lead to their full recovery and long-term 'body awareness'; how much more useful and realistic than teaching three or four formal exercises to women lying flat on their hospital beds!

Feeding

The new mother may be feeding her baby eight or more times each day; unless she is shown (preferably antenatally) how best to sit, what should be a happy, relaxed time can turn into an uncomfortable chore. The obstetric physiotherapist will see women daily feeding their babies while sitting slumped, legs dangling over the side of their bed; or sitting bolt upright or slumping, unsupported by the chair back, because their bottom is only halfway on to the chair seat (Fig.7.5). Even women sitting in bed can have unsupported backs, or be lying much too flat. Baby feeding times should give each mother the opportunity to rest and restore her energy – she should welcome each feed and not dread it because of the resulting backache.

When using a chair, the mother should sit right to the rear of the seat; her waist must be supported with a cushion, another should be on her lap to raise the baby and prevent her stooping; finally, for complete comfort, she should have a footstool available (Figs. 7.5, 7.6). This applies to women who bottle-feed as well as those breast-feeding. Modifications for breast-feeding can include side-lying (Fig.7.7) – the ultimate in relaxation!

Where women complain of a painful perineum or haemorrhoids it is essential to find means of relieving this discomfort. A foam-rubber ring, or two folded pillows with a space between them, can prevent pressure; cross-legged sitting in bed with the back well supported is a further alternative.

Thoracic backache postnatally is almost always due to poor, unsupported feeding positions and fatigue; an obstetric physiotherapist who can prevent or alleviate this exhausting problem will long be remembered by the grateful mothers.

Nappy changing

Nappy changing is another activity that can lead to incapacitating pain. Nappies are often changed more than a dozen times a day; if this is carried out on a low surface, so that the mother is bending over her baby, or sitting on the edge of a bed, stooping and twisting, back pain will result. Many hospitals today insist that nappy changing is carried out in the baby's cot; if this is low or if the mother is tall, once again the mother's back will give her problems. Nappies can very satisfactorily be changed on the mother's lap if she sits on a low chair or has a footstool; in this way her back will be upright and supported. Alternatively the baby can be changed on a surface that is approximately waist height, thus preventing the woman stooping (Fig.7.8). Many young mothers like to change their babies on the floor; yet kneeling on both knees will give rise to a painful, stooping posture; half-kneeling can be the solution (Fig. 7.9).

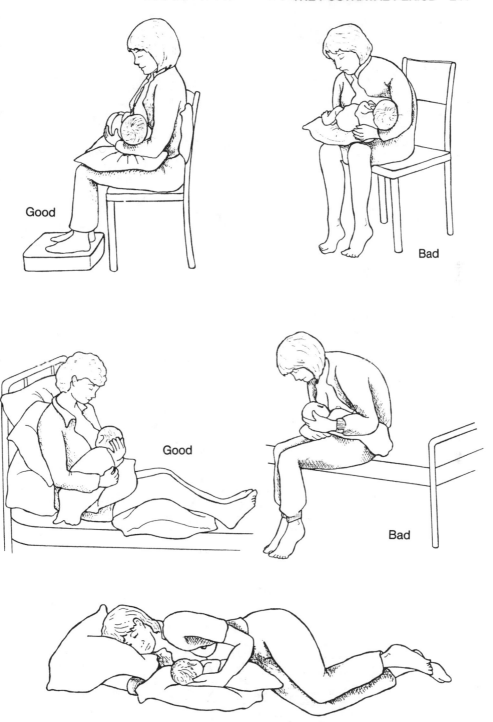

Figure 7.5–6–7 Because women will spend a great deal of time feeding their babies, they must know how to be really comfortable.

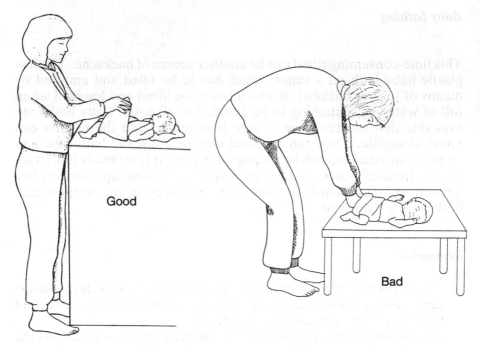

Figure 7.8 Nappy-changing positions.

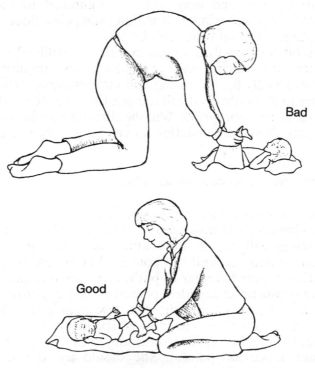

Figure 7.8–9 Changing a nappy at floor level.

Baby bathing

This time-consuming ritual can be another source of backache. The low plastic baby bath on a stand, which has to be filled and emptied by means of jugs or buckets, or which has to be lifted and lowered when full of water, is something to be avoided at all costs. Baby baths are available that can rest over a large bath-tub so that the mother can kneel alongside. They can be filled directly from the bath taps and emptied into the bath-tub by pulling out a plug. It is probably less strain on the mother's back if she uses a special washing-up bowl on her kitchen draining board, or else baths her baby in the well-cleaned bathroom hand basin!

Remember

1. It is important that the obstetric physiotherapist motivates, encourages, and is enthusiastic! Many women will not want to exercise, and may have to be persuaded to participate.
2. Do not burden new mothers with too many exercises – teach just the essentials plus relaxation, using prone lying if the perineum is sore.
3. Following a traumatic delivery the woman will probably be lying comparatively still and may well be frightened to move. It is important for her to begin leg, breathing and pelvic floor exercises – leave anything else until she feels better.
4. Although birth is usually a joyous experience, stillbirths, abnormal or ill babies and neonatal deaths do occur. These are difficult for all staff but especially for the young and inexperienced. The obstetric physiotherapist should establish the priorities and teach the mother exercises that are appropriate. She should not be afraid of empathizing with parents in their anxieties or even joining them in their grief.

Postnatal exercises for continuation at home

To improve circulation during the first few weeks the new mother should try to have a daily walk with her baby in a sling or a pram: the change of scene will benefit her emotionally as well. Pelvic floor exercises can be done around the house. They should be keyed into other activities; it may help her to put notices up to remind her – the toilet and wardrobe doors are ideal places! If the gap between the recti muscles is closing satisfactorily she can now include side flexion and rotation exercises as well as 'curl-downs' (curling down halfway from crook sitting, holding briefly, and returning to the upright position), if her perineum is not too painful. She should try to rest and relax regularly on her bed or in a chair.

Postnatal exercise classes in the community

Individual assessment before a new mother joins an ongoing class is important because the condition of the recti abdominis and pelvic floor muscles will vary from woman to woman. Perineal pain, stress incontinence and backache are the most common conditions that may still be giving problems. Ideally the hospital obstetric physiotherapists should refer, where necessary, to their colleagues in the community. Often women will be most concerned with the parts of their body that are visible, i.e. abdomen, hips and thighs. As well as improvement to their 'outside' figures, long-term benefit will result if women can be persuaded to become aware of their 'inside' figures (pelvic floor and vagina) too! The classes should include exercises together with the babies. Examples of suitable exercises can be found in *The Postnatal Exercise Book* by Polden and Whiteford (1992).

The formal part of the session should end with relaxation; women can lie on their sides, backs or fronts. Sitting at a table resting their heads on their hands is useful as a suggestion for a quick 'rest and relax' during busy times of the day. The social aspect of this type of class is invaluable – mother-to-mother support can make all the difference between being able to cope during the early months or not; cold drinks, tea or coffee should be available (no one should baulk at 10–20p if finance is a problem), and time allowed to feed babies, change nappies and chat before returning home.

The obstetric physiotherapist would do well to introduce the following topics into the conversation.

Fatigue

Fatigue (see p. 260) can be overwhelming in the early days, especially if the new baby is demanding and there are other small children. Women should be encouraged to try to fit in adequate rest and sleep during the day – perhaps when the children are sleeping. Where this is impossible, perhaps the mother could occasionally go to bed immediately after supper early in the evening. When the baby wakes for the next feed her partner could bring the infant to be fed in bed, after which he can change the baby while the mother continues sleeping. Another way to catch up on her sleep debt is for her to arrange that all the children are taken out on Saturday or Sunday afternoon while she sleeps for two or three hours. It is important for the woman to recognize her fatigue and not feel guilty about it, so that she can attempt to relieve it; frequent visitors, unless they are prepared to do the chores, should be discouraged!

Women who are used to being 'in charge' of their lives (perhaps professionals and executives) often find the first few weeks of life with a new baby (particularly if it is their first) totally shattering. There will be an emotional as well as a physical aspect to their fatigue, and it is important for stress-coping devices to be discussed by the group.

Housework

It is very difficult for houseproud women, especially if they have previously combined this with a full-time job, to accept that vacuuming, dusting and paint washing does *not* have to be done daily. It is easy to become obsessive about housework. If they can keep the home tidy the dirt won't be so obvious – and once the new baby settles, one morning's hard work will 'clear the decks'!

Postnatal depression and anxiety

Where a group is meeting regularly it is comparatively easy to identify those who are clinically depressed or anxious (see p. 267) but who may not have recognized this themselves. Realizing that they are not alone in their situation; suggestions for more rest, time on their own, daily outings with their baby in adult company, the occasional evening out with their partner (perhaps a friend or relative could babysit) are all self-help therapies. Their general practitioner should be consulted if the situation does not resolve; possible referral to a psychiatrist may be necessary to help the woman become herself again.

Loss of libido

The all-consuming role of new motherhood and the fatigue with which it is accompanied often result in a complete loss of libido. This can be made worse if the woman is still experiencing perineal or vaginal discomfort and is frightened that intercourse will prove painful. A partner who is demanding and lacking in consideration may add to their predicament and sense of guilt – particularly if they had a good sex life before pregnancy. Reassurance that eventually she should regain her interest in sex, suggestions for the use of a lubricant where soreness is a problem, alternative positions if she is fearful that the 'missionary' posture will be too painful, may all help. Self-referral for further help via the general practitioner or family planning clinic may be necessary for some couples. Some women and their partners will worry about what has happened to the vagina and pelvic floor muscles ('too tight' and 'too loose', 'not the same as before') – group discussions and laughter can ease what to some people is an intolerable situation.

Return to sport and exercise

Even the athlete, dancer or dedicated sportswoman will have reduced the intensity and amount of exercise by the end of her pregnancy. After the postnatal period of recovery and gradual restoration of muscle strength, these women will be ready to return to their activity. Where the prepregnancy level of activity considerably decreased prior to delivery, a gradual reintroduction of sport and training schedules is essential. This is particularly important for the non-athletic woman who feels that she should be 'doing something' once her baby has settled down; she should be discouraged from joining a mass aerobics class at the local leisure centre, jogging long distances or cycling many miles if she has not thus exercised for a long time. It is most important that such classes and activities are supervised by properly qualified teachers who understand the limitations of comparatively unfit women.

Swimming, an ideal activity for the fit and for those hoping to become fitter, may be resumed when the lochia have cleared.

Baby massage

In the same way that adults enjoy and feel relaxed by skilful massage, many babies respond with pleasure to simple stroking or kneading techniques. In the East and amongst many ethnic groups in this country, baby massage is practised regularly. In its simplest form, most mothers include a stroking movement when smoothing oil or powder into their baby's skin following a bath or nappy change. A short baby massage session could enjoyably be included in a mother and baby exercise class or postnatal group; and while massage is most successfully performed on the naked body (the room would have to be very warm in this case, and plenty of nappies available), it is perfectly possible to teach this form of massage where the baby is wearing a stretch suit.

Simple effleurage and stroking over the babies' backs, chests, abdomens, arms, legs, hands and feet can be practised by the group together. Mothers are probably most comfortable sitting on the floor with their backs supported by a wall or cupboard. The babies lie across their mothers' laps – if a baby is crying for a feed or has a wet nappy and is uncomfortable, the massage session should be postponed.

At home, mothers should be encouraged to massage their babies when they are not hungry and are likely to enjoy it – although a simple back and abdominal massage can sometimes soothe a distressed baby. Oil or powder can be used sparingly. The most important factor to remember is that the session should be enjoyed by both the baby and the mother (or father), and that it should not become a chore. Experienced physiotherapists can easily adapt conventional massage strokes to their tiny clients; reading about the subject in detail (Aukett,

1988; Balaskas and Gordon, 1987) may give useful insight into this technique, although some of the benefits to the various body organs and systems which are claimed to result from massaging babies may seem rather surprising!

Mother and baby postnatal exercise classes in the community provide an excellent forum for introducing education on preventative health care and can help instil good habits for the entire family. If society will afford this care, problems such as backache, mild prolapse, stress incontinence and osteoporosis in later life may be prevented or alleviated. Educating women as to how they may feel and keep well is an investment for their future. Teaching relaxation and stress-reducing techniques gives women skills for life.

IMMEDIATE POSTNATAL PROBLEMS

Painful perineum

Obvious visible problems can include bruising, oedema, labial tear, haematoma, tight stitches, infection and breakdown of suturing. Haemorrhoids may also be apparent. A vaginal haematoma will not be visible but may be intensely painful.

Before considering the techniques obstetric physiotherapists can use or suggest to women for the relief of perineal pain, it is important to consider the exact purpose of treatment. Because of the high vascularity of the perineal region it is unlikely that physical techniques will accelerate the rate of wound healing. Attempts to show objectively that ultrasound or pulsed electromagnetic energy increase the rate of healing the traumatized perineum have been disappointing (Grant et al., 1989). Initially the physiotherapist's skills are best directed towards the relief of pain, the reduction of oedema and enabling the mother to overcome her discomforts in order to care for her baby.

Treatment

Pelvic floor exercise. One of the most physiologically sound self-help techniques for the relief of perineal pain must be the repeated contraction and relaxation of the voluntary component of the pelvic floor musculature. The resulting pumping action assists venous and lymphatic drainage and the removal of traumatic exudate, thus relieving stiffness. It is also theoretically possible that the muscle activity triggers the 'pain-gating' mechanism and may also stimulate the production of endogenous opiates. Pain tends to be maximal with the first contraction and decreases with repetition as oedema disperses. Certain positions in which to exercise (e.g. stride crook lying, prone lying, stride standing) may be more comfortable than others (e.g. sitting)

Positioning. Women must be helped to experiment in order to find comfortable positions for feeding, relaxation and sleep, using pillows and a foam-rubber ring. Pain relief can occur rapidly if the mother's weight is advantageously redistributed.

Ice. The pain-relieving effect of cold therapy is well documented (Lee and Warren, 1978; Lehmann and deLateur, 1982; Palastanga, 1988; Knight, 1989). Moore and James (1989) compared three topical analgesic agents in the treatment of postepisiotomy pain (Epifoam, *Hamamelis* water and ice). All three agents were equally effective on the first day, although one-third of the women derived no benefit from any agent. Ice, however, gave better pain relief thereafter. It is an analgesic therapy which is readily available in hospital and at home, and is certainly cheapest – a factor which must be taken into consideration in the current economic climate.

The following are suitable techniques for the newly delivered woman who finds that the problem of perineal pain interferes with her efforts to care for her baby, prevents her moving or sitting comfortably, and even intrudes on her sleep.

1. Crushed ice can be wrapped in damp disposable gauze or a disposable washcloth/surgical wipe, and, with the woman reclining, the resulting pad applied lightly to the painful, possibly oedematous area for 5–10 minutes. Alternatively, crushed ice may be put into a plastic bag which may then be wrapped in a damp disposable covering, although some authorities say this is not necessary (Knight, 1989).
2. Massage with an ice cube which is held by means of a tissue and is used by the woman herself, while in bed or over a toilet, can give excellent pain relief.

The benefit of self-treatment is that women know exactly where their pain is situated, and can use the ice whenever this is most severe, and at times convenient to themselves. When using ice in any form, the bed should be protected. Filling latex gloves with water, freezing them, and applying the solid result to the perineum is seldom comfortable, and if the mother uses them for a prolonged period, ischaemia and an ice burn could result. Freezing wet sanitary towels and then applying them tends to be uncomfortable, and they could remain in contact for too long. The most successful techniques seem to be those that use crushed ice in a flexible rather than a rigid form. If an ice machine is not available, a liquidizer or food processor could be used. Ice packs or ice massage should be continued as long as they give the woman some relief. The obstetric physiotherapist must be alert to the possibility of ice burns, particularly because the skin sensation may not be normal.

Warm saline baths and bidets. These are used principally to promote good perineal hygiene. Although not strictly physiotherapeutic, most women experience relief of pain and a relaxed feeling of well-being following the traditional use of a warm saline bath. Women should be actively discouraged from staying in the bath too long, as traumatized skin quickly becomes 'soggy'. Warm saline can also be poured over the perineum from a jug while the woman is sitting on the toilet. This eases the burning sensation some women experience when urinating following the delivery if they have sustained lacerations. The use of a bidet can also be soothing.

Ultrasound. When ultrasound was first used to relieve pain and promote healing in the damaged perineum, it was felt that treatment involving direct contact between the applicator and skin, via a coupling gel, could lead to infection. Treatment was given with the mother seated in a bath (McLaren, 1984); all electrical sockets were outside the bathroom. The inconvenience and impractical nature of this method led to physiotherapists using ultrasound in the manner normally used for recent soft-tissue injuries. Even though the perineal area is far from sterile, it is most important to observe high standards of cleanliness to prevent carry-over of infective organisms. It is currently being suggested that the treatment head is washed with detergent and carefully dried before and after use, and immersed in glutaraldehyde (Cidex or Asep) following every treatment. In view of the current concern about AIDS the physiotherapist must be constantly alert to new directives from the Department of Health and the local Infection Control Officer in matters of hygiene. Where no other specific instructions are given, the authors feel that the minimum precautions taken by an obstetric physiotherapist should include the wearing of good-quality latex gloves, and that the mother should be asked to remove her own sanitary towel and put it into a bag.

Where there is obvious bruising and oedema, treatment should start as soon as possible after delivery and should continue on a daily basis until the woman is pain-free. The treatment is best given in the crook lying position; it is most important to be able to see the perineum and buttock area clearly. Using a cotton-wool swab and warm water, and swabbing from front to back, any lochia is gently washed away. An ultrasound coupling gel is applied and treatment given in the usual way. Normally pulsed ultrasound is used for its analgesic and exudate-removing properties, although it has been shown that the thermal and non-thermal effects of ultrasound are beneficial to all stages of tissue repair (Dyson, 1987). For an initial treatment, a dosage of 3 MHz, 0.5 W/cm^2 and 2 minutes per head-sized area of trauma was used by McIntosh (1988). It is thought unnecessary to increase the dosage if there is improvement in pain and swelling. Where the pain is too intense for direct contact a condom can be successfully used as a water bag – with couplant applied to the patient's skin, the bag and the treatment head. This also makes the application of ultrasound to haemorrhoids much more comfortable.

Pulsed electromagnetic energy. This technique known variously as pulsed shortwave diathermy, pulsed high-frequency energy or pulsed electromagnetic energy (PEME) – is rapidly gaining a reputation for its success in the treatment of recent trauma and is now being used in many maternity units. Both Bewley (1986) and Frank(1984) have described its pain-relieving and therapeutic effects for bruising, large haemorrhoids, extensive suturing, post-caesarean section haematomas and inflamed or infected wounds in the early postnatal period. Its 'no touch' mode of operation must make it particularly suitable in the puerperium. The dosage usually used is mild – its exact parameter must depend on which machine is used. Acute conditions are said to respond well to a pulse width of 40–65 µs pulses with a repetition rate of 10–220 pulses per second (Low, 1988), and it is suggested that treatment should be given at least twice a day, initially for 5 minutes and progressing to 20 minutes at a time. There is a variety of published opinions as to dosage and length of treatment; the obstetric physiotherapist who is able to use this modality for postnatal problems will need to keep an open mind and be alert to newly published trials and their results.

Infrared irradiation. Following skin testing, mild warmth from a non-luminous source with the mother in side or crook lying, with her legs apart and well supported on pillows, can often give pain relief. The surrounding areas are covered to prevent overheating; 50–70 cm is the usual distance from the lamp to the perineum and 20 minutes the length of treatment. The soothing effect may enable the woman, often for the first time, to perform effective pelvic floor contractions. A further benefit is the fact that she has to lie down for the treatment. This enforced rest can result in her feeling refreshed and relaxed.

Diastasis recti abdominis

Diastasis recti abdominis (see p. 223) is a common condition which varies in severity from woman to woman. It will mechanically interfere with the supportive and expulsive function of the abdominal wall unless it is recognized and treated. Noble (1980) and Boissonnault and Kotarinos (1988) both describe the condition, which can appear in pregnancy or be caused by bearing down in the second stage of labour. In some women gross diastasis will actually be visible when they try to sit up or lie down – a wide ridge of bulging tissue becomes apparent when activity involving the use of the recti muscles is undertaken against gravity, particularly from the supine position. The diastasis may simply extend a few centimetres above and below the umbilicus and only be 2–3 cm wide, it may only appear below the umbilicus, or it may involve the major part of the linea alba – extending from just below the xiphisternum to just above the symphysis pubis and can be as much as 20 cm in width. Because the size of the diastasis influences postnatal physiotherapy care it is advisable to examine every newly delivered woman in crook lying; this will only take a moment. The physiotherapist places her fingers, holding her hand widthways, below the level of the umbilicus; the mother is asked to lift her head and reach with her hands towards her knees. The physiotherapist will then be able to feel both the width and length of any recti separation. In severe degrees the 'peaking' of the abdomen will be very noticeable. It is much easier to palpate and diagnose the condition in slender women – thick layers of fat overlying the abdominal wall can make it impossible to estimate the full extent of any problem. Each woman should be shown how to palpate her own abdomen; some may be a little squeamish at first, but most are fascinated by the 'hole' in their middle. It is important to explain that the gap is not dangerous – nothing will fall out! It is also wise to mention that the two recti muscles, even when they are fully rehabilitated, will always lie slightly apart; even when the linea alba was intact the two muscles were separated by 1.5–2 cm. It is reassuring for mothers to know that although their 'unzipped' linea alba will not regenerate, this is not important providing their muscles are strong.

Re-education

It is most important to teach the woman to be constantly aware of her abdomen in all positions. It can be helpful if the obstetric physiotherapist uses the analogy of 'having to get the message through' to the elongated, separated, lax muscles; that the time for 'stretch' is over, and shortening now begins. Abdominal retraction should be repeated frequently; this simple exercise can easily be integrated into all the activities of daily living. Pelvic tilting is an easy dynamic progression which should be taught in crook and side lying, sitting and standing. Careful supervision is required because it is possible to tilt the pelvis without using the abdominal muscles. This exercise can progress to head and shoulder raising in crook lying, always ensuring that the abdominal wall is well retracted first. Initially several pillows can be used to support the head and upper trunk. As abdominal strength improves these should be gradually removed; in this way the resistance of gravity and the range of movement are increased.

Where the diastasis is wide and where 'peaking' is demonstrated as the head is raised, Noble (1980) suggests that the mother crosses her hands over her abdomen, places her fingers outside the lateral borders of the recti muscles, and then opposes them as she raises her head and possibly her shoulders from the pillows. As soon as peaking begins she should go no further, but hold the position for 4–6 seconds and then lower slowly. Until the diastasis improves it is probably safer not to introduce strong rotational or side flexion activities – the shearing forces produced are said to increase separation (Noble, 1980). Instead, restrict early abdominal muscle re-education to 'straight' activities; single and double leg sliding and curl-downs (Polden and Whiteford, 1992) are safe and do not unduly strain a severely weakened abdominal wall. It is essential that any woman who has an initial diastasis of more than 10 cm is recalled or seen in the community 6–8 weeks postpartum to asssess her progress and to introduce stronger exercises. It is highly undesirable for a woman to begin another pregnancy before full recovery has occurred. In exceptional cases it may be helpful to suggest the temporary use of some form of abdominal support such as Tubigrip (double thickness), a roll-on or pantie-girdle.

Back pain

Back pain is a very common postnatal complaint and is not confined to women who experienced back pain during pregnancy. It can be coccygeal, lumbar, sacroiliac, thoracic and sometimes cervical in origin, and can seriously interfere with the quality of life experienced by the new mother at this very important time. Analgesics and rest will not deal with the causative factors – and every woman complaining of postnatal back pain has the right to receive a thorough assessment, and where appropriate, active treatment from a physiotherapist who is aware of her very special situation.

Treatment

Epidural site pain. It has been postulated that pain in the epidural site can be due to a tiny haematoma in the dura and epidural space. Heat, in the form of a hot pack or electric pad, can be soothing. Alternatively an ice pack can be used.

Lower back pain. This may be relieved initially with a double layered Tubigrip support (sizes K or L). Resting in prone lying, well supported with pillows that allow a space for the enlarged breasts, is helpful. Specific mobilization techniques for the sacroiliac, lumbar or lumbo-sacral regions may be appropriate if support alone is insufficient to deal with the pain.

Thoracic pain. This may respond to correction of feeding postures. The lumbar curve should be well supported, the baby should lie on a pillow on the mother's lap which should also be raised by the use of a footstool if necessary. Active movements, such as elbow and shoulder circling and pelvic tilting while sitting down, taking the back into forward flexion and then hyperextension, may give relief. Hot packs can be used and feeding in side lying should be suggested.

It cannot be stressed too strongly that during the establishment of lactation it is vitally important for a mother's back to be comfortable and pain-free, and great care must be taken to make certain that while she is feeding her back is always adequately supported.

Coccydynia. Coccydynia may be due to damaged ligaments with or without displacement of the coccyx, or aggravation of a previous injury. Occasionally a coccyx may spontaneously fracture during the second stage of labour (Brunskill and Swain, 1987). It can be a particularly painful and incapacitating condition in the early postpartum period, and can interfere with the mother-baby bonding process. Painkillers may not be sufficient to make life tolerable, and the new mother will need a great deal of help to find a comfortable feeding position – sitting can be impossible! Active physiotherapeutic measures such as ultrasound, ice or hot packs can give relief. Prone lying will be the most comfortable position, and frequent gluteal contractions are a self-help suggestion that may reduce initial pain. Gentle mobilizations may also be helpful, and TNS can be a valuable means of analgesia. It is essential that, until she is pain-free, the mother has a rubber ring to use when she has to sit. Unfortunately, the condition can persist for a long time.

Symphysis pubis pain

Pain in the region of the symphysis pubis is present in a small proportion of postpartum women. Symphysiolysis or diastasis symphysis pubis may have occurred antenatally, or may follow a traumatic delivery. This joint separation will give rise to acute pain on movement and an inability to walk without support. A milder form of this condition has been described (Driessen, 1987) where symptoms arose three days into the puerperium. This was attributed to postpartum swelling inside the intact fibrous confines of the joint.

Treatment

Initially, in severe cases, bed rest together with some form of firm circumtrochanteric support, and analgesics where necessary, are indicated; followed by gradual mobilization on crutches or a Zimmer frame. The obstetric physiotherapist will have a great deal to offer by way of treatment and advice. For example, the woman's knees should be flexed and tightly adducted when manoeuvring in bed and from bed, steps should be short, standing should be avoided, and she should be encouraged to rest as much as possible. Full-time help in caring for the baby is essential. Ultrasound and ice may speed healing and absorption of oedema, and relieve pain. In milder cases, or as the condition improves, Tubigrip may prove to be sufficient support. Where possible the woman should be encouraged to follow a modified programme of exercises to strengthen the abdominal muscles.

BLADDER AND BOWEL PROBLEMS

Because of the close relationship between the pelvic organs, alteration in urinary and faecal control can occur following difficult forceps deliveries; even a normal birth can result in voiding problems.

Retention of urine

It is most important that midwifery and medical staff are fully aware of the problem a newly delivered woman may be experiencing in initiating and completing micturition. There is some evidence to show that a single episode of bladder over-distension can produce chronic changes by irreversible damage to the detrusor muscle (Hinman, 1976). If retention of urine should occur, catheterization can be necessary and the mother may need to have an indwelling catheter for several days. Urinary retention can be caused by a prolonged second stage of labour, a large baby or an instrumental delivery. The urethra, being embedded in the anterior wall of the vagina, may be traumatized and unable to function normally. The mother may be too inhibited by pain and fear to allow voiding to commence. Apart from reassurance and simple explanation, the obstetric physiotherapist can offer practical help with this worrying and uncomfortable situation. Frequent, gentle pelvic floor contractions will reduce oedema and pain and give a feeling of normality. Running taps, whistling and calm breathing with relaxation on expiration, while sitting on the toilet, are suggestions which may prove successful. Some women find that they are able to empty their bladder while sitting in a warm bath.

Urgency and urge incontinence

Sometimes postpartum urinary control becomes difficult in a totally different way. Instead of being unable to initiate micturition, the mother may suffer sudden urgency (see p. 348) and may be unable to reach the toilet before the bladder empties spontaneously. Trauma to the detrusor and the urethral sphincter mechanism during labour or delivery are possible causes. The initial suggestion from the obstetric physiotherapist should be for frequent pelvic floor exercise, and the mother's ability to perform this movement correctly must be checked. Contraction of the levator ani muscle directly inhibits the sacral micturition centre (McGuire, 1979) and the voiding urge may be controlled.

Stress incontinence

Stress incontinence is a frequent early postnatal problem. It can be caused by distension and weakening of the pelvic floor musculature and connective tissue, and also by damage to their innervation (Snooks et al., 1985). It is essential that the mother understands the anatomy of the pelvic floor and how she may be able to help herself by pelvic floor exercising. Kegel (1951) has suggested 200 contractions per day. It is probably less overwhelming if the obstetric physiotherapist recommends the mother to contract the pelvic floor at least 20 times, say in groups of 4, at every feed. Initially the woman may find it easier to hold and relax these muscles quickly. She should continue this regimen and progress to longer 'holds' as soon as she is able. Counter-bracing these muscles when coughing or nose-blowing can prevent leakage where the muscles are strong enough. This knowledge will help to give confidence.

Anorectal incontinence

It used to be thought that this highly embarrassing and distressing condition was only due to direct sphincter division or muscle stretching. Research by Snooks et al. (1985) suggests that this incontinence can result from damage to the innervation of the pelvic floor muscles during perineal descent in the second stage of labour. It is more common in women who have experienced difficult instrumental deliveries and in multiparae. Neuropraxia normally resolves by two months, but some women will be left with a long-term problem.

Explanation, encouragement and pelvic floor exercise instruction is the role of the obstetric physiotherapist in the early treatment of a condition which most women are too ashamed to discuss. Rarely, a rectovaginal fistula following fourth-degree laceration (see p. 73) may be the cause of apparent faecal incontinence. It is essential for the obstetric physiotherapist to check if a woman suffering from this condition is in fact able to initiate a pelvic floor contraction, and to follow her up if this is not the case.

Constipation

Constipation is extremely common during the early puerperium and is probably due to several causes including weak abdominal muscles (a large diastasis recti abdominis would compound this), relaxation of the smooth intestinal muscles (p. 36), the change from home to hospital diet (lack of fibre and fluid), iron pills, and the fear of increasing perineal pain or reopening the episiotomy wound or tears. As well as a full explanation of these causes (understanding a problem is often halfway to solving it) and their remedies, the suggestion that the perineum is supported with a pad of soft toilet paper during defaecation can be a life-saver! It should be impressed on the new mother that improving the strength of her abdominal muscles will help in relieving constipation. It is important that women realize that life-long constipation can lead to the 'descending perineum' syndrome (see p. 381). Henry et al. (1982) described this, and pointed out that repeated strain can lead to urinary stress incontinence and faecal incontinence.

CIRCULATORY PROBLEMS

Varicose veins

Most women are pleasantly surprised by the appearance of their varicose veins after their babies are born, although some may experience pain along the length of the long saphenous vein. Because of this, many do not appreciate the necessity for continuing to be enthusiastic about circulatory leg care. There is an improvement in the severity of varicose veins following delivery, but, particularly in multiparae, once veins have become badly varicosed they will never recover completely.

Vigorous and frequent dorsiflexion (at least 30 'pumps' at a time) will prevent stasis. Today's new mother is rarely confined to bed, but she is not as active as normally, and she will be sitting feeding her baby for several long periods every day. Support tights or antiembolic stockings may be necessary for severe cases; advice about beneficial sitting positions with the legs raised needs to be given, and care taken to see that it is implemented.

Oedema

Although there is a massive diuresis following delivery, it can take several days (and even weeks) for the fluid retention of pregnancy to be reversed. Severely oedematous legs should be supported with antiembolic support stockings, the mother should rest with her legs in elevation (on her bed table or back support). She should be encouraged to feed her baby with her legs raised, and vigorous foot and ankle exercises should be carried out half-hourly. Occasionally swelling of the feet and legs occurs for the first time *after* the baby is born, which can be upsetting and uncomfortable. Reassurance, explanation and encouragement from her obstetric physiotherapist can turn what seems to be a major catastrophe into a transient inconvenience.

Venous thrombosis

Superficial vein thrombosis

The mother may complain of tenderness over a superficial vein which can be palpated, and there may be redness of the overlying skin. This is often associated with varicose veins. The mother should be encouraged to remain mobile and to exercise her legs frequently. She may be more comfortable in support tights or antiembolic stockings until the condition subsides.

Deep vein thrombosis

With deep vein thrombosis (DVT) the mother will complain of pain and discomfort in her calf or thigh, and swelling may be present if the vein is occluded. Homans' sign (calf pain when the foot is dorsiflexed while the knee is in extension) may be positive. The main danger to the mother is that a portion of the clot may break off and reach the chest as a thromboembolism. Anticoagulant therapy must be commenced, the mother should wear antiembolic stockings and, if the DVT is in the calf, will be able to remain mobile. The sufferer should beware of pressure on the back of her calf while feeding the baby and should do so with her legs raised, and, once again, carry out frequent, vigorous foot and ankle movements. If the DVT is in the iliofemoral region, the woman may have to remain in bed until the swelling has subsided. The foot of the bed may be raised, or the legs supported in elevation – but they should continue to be moved freely. Foot exercises, quadriceps and gluteal contractions, and hip and knee flexion and extension are all valuable aids to circulation.

Pulmonary embolus

Pulmonary embolism together with Mendelson's syndrome (inhalation of aspirated gastric contents while under general anaesthetic) constitute the two major causes of maternal mortality following delivery. In the case of a large embolus death can occur within 15 minutes; with smaller emboli the symptoms can include dyspnoea, chest pain, pyrexia and malaise.

Treatment

Where there is a massive embolus the patient, if she survives, will be nursed in an intensive care unit. Milder cases may be nursed on the postnatal ward and will receive heparin therapy. Physiotherapy must include maintenance of good circulation and clearance of any chest secretions.

Haemorrhoids

These distended and sometimes thrombosed veins in the anal passage can be a source of acute discomfort in the immediate postpartum period. They may have been a problem antenatally or may have appeared for the first time after the birth. Pushing in the second stage of labour can cause the veins to prolapse; on examination the swellings can resemble a small bunch of grapes. The pain experienced by some newly delivered mothers is often described as excruciating.

Apart from doing the utmost to ensure the comfort of the woman while feeding – the judicious use of pillows and a rubber ring will be helpful – the obstetric physiotherapist can use ultrasound (perhaps through a water-filled condom if the haemorrhoids are too tender to allow treatment in direct contact) and PEME, although Grant et al. (1989) did not find that these therapies helped. Crushed ice packs also alleviate the pain and reduce the swelling. Frequent pelvic floor contractions are probably the most helpful thing the mother can do as a self-help therapy, although resting in prone or side lying positions is also useful.

Steroid analgesic creams or foams are often prescribed, and if the piles have prolapsed a gentle attempt may be made to replace them. The mother should be encouraged to drink plenty of fluid and have a fibre-rich diet in order to produce soft, bulky stools, thus reducing the pain caused by defaecation.

'AFTERPAINS'

Many woman experience a postpartum lower abdominal pain which is probably uterine in origin. Murray and Holdcroft (1989) showed that 50% of primiparous and 86% of multiparous women in a study complained of discomfort of a severity between menstrual and labour pain on the McGill pain questionnaire. Physiotherapy exercises relieved pain in 40% of the primiparous but only 16% of the multiparous women. Sleep, oral analgesics, a change in position and passing urine were also helpful. Where afterpains are severe, TNS applied over the nerve roots innervating the uterus and perineum (T10–Ll and S2–S4) is often helpful.

BREAST ENGORGEMENT AND MASTITIS

Occasionally a woman may present with severe breast engorgement in the early puerperium which is so acute that expression of milk with a breast pump is too painful. Ultrasound, to the periphery of the breast initially and then moving the treatment head towards the nipple, plus crushed ice packs, can give speedy relief and encourage the milk to flow. Ultrasound has also been used successfully in the treatment of mastitis in the later puerperium.

Sore and cracked nipples

The latest opinion as to the cause of this common and distressing problem, which probably leads to many new mothers abandoning breast-feeding in the immediate postpartum period, is that they are directly related to the position of the baby on the breast. Sore or cracked nipples are *not* due to the mother's colouring or the 'toughness' of her skin, nor to the shape of her nipple.

The position of the baby – facing the mother's body, with neck slightly extended, mouth well open with the lower lip curled down, and the nipple extending as far back as the soft palate – is all-important. If the baby is correctly attached, there should be no friction of the tongue or gum on the nipple, and no movement of the breast tissue in and out of the baby's mouth. Thus the baby's sucking will not traumatize the nipple and there will be no soreness.

Although obstetric physiotherapists advocate – purely for the mother's postural benefit – a position where her back is fully supported, it may be necessary for her to lean forward initially in order to obtain the most favourable position of her breast for the baby to latch on and feed successfully. If the mother is lying back in bed or on a chair, the naturally pointed shape of the breast is flattened and the baby is unable to take the nipple to the back of the throat. Experimentation may be necessary before the best feeding position for each mother and baby is found, and the situation will need constant review as the baby grows.

The obstetric physiotherapist will not be directly involved in the active treatment of sore nipples, but should be aware of current thought in this field to help women experiencing problems.

1. Washing the breasts before and after each feed is no longer recommended – in fact soap and alcohol have both been shown to increase nipple soreness. Alcohol and chlorhexidine sprays, commonly seen on bedside lockers, are ineffective in preventing nipple trauma (RCM, 1991).
2. There is no evidence that any of the creams, ointments, sprays or tinctures frequently advocated prevent nipple soreness; some actually increase the incidence of nipple damage.

3. Limiting the sucking time does not prevent nipple soreness, and may have an adverse effect on the proper establishment of lactation.
4. Nipple shields may have an occasional place in the treatment of severely traumatized nipples, providing they are thin. The mother should be aware that their use will impair milk transfer, and she should compensate for this by offering the breast for longer.
5. Resting the breasts and expressing the milk until healing takes place is effective – but the milk supply will probably drop as the prolactin surge and oxytocin release produced in response to suckling will be absent. It must also be remembered that breast pumps can cause cracked nipples.
6. It seems that the most effective method of achieving pain-free, long-term and successful lactation is for close attention to be paid to the mother's feeding technique and the position of the baby on her breast. Exposing the nipples to the air and sunlight, if possible, rather than enclosing them in a brassiere with damp breast pads, is a commonly used therapy.

TIREDNESS

A frequent complaint by new mothers in the puerperium is 'Why didn't you tell me how tired I would be?' Undoubtedly the interruption in the normal eight or nine hours night-time sleep, together with the constant daytime demands of a new baby, can be exhausting physically and emotionally to very many women. This intense fatigue may not manifest itself immediately – the first two or three days following the birth are often accompanied by a 'high' which carries the woman through, although mothers who have had a long or difficult labour will react with immediate exhaustion. Even if the possibility of postnatal fatigue is discussed in antenatal classes, women will need reminding in the puerperium that they are likely to need several 'rest and relaxation' sessions daily (a few minutes will often suffice) during the early weeks. Sadly, many new mothers have little help with their household chores and family duties. Often, first-timers feel obliged to continue their domestic routines in an effort to prove that they are coping, without making allowances for the added burden of their new baby and the total change in their lifestyle. Sometimes pressure from a partner, lacking in understanding, for things to be 'like they were before' will add to their tiredness. Women who already have children will need to think about themselves as well as their families, and because advice can be forgotten, it is important continually to reinforce suggestions for dealing with postnatal fatigue.

1. Resting and sleeping while the baby sleeps – household chores can often be done while carrying the infant in a sling.

2. Asking the partner or a friend to take the baby for a long walk so that the mother can sleep.
3. Occasionally it is helpful for the new mother to go to bed after the early evening feed, following her supper, to sleep until her baby wakes for the next feed. A helpful partner could bring the baby to her – she can breast-feed in bed – and then he can change and settle their child while she goes back to sleep. If the baby is bottle-fed they can share the work.
4. The mother should try to close her eyes to the normal household chores; keeping the home tidy will often be all she has time for. A good dust and vacuum once a week or so is much less tiring than cleaning every day.

The new mother, however independent she is normally, should try to accept every offer of help with washing, shopping, cooking and cleaning. If relatives stay to help on her return home from hospital, they should understand that the mother's job is to care for the new baby, *theirs* is to do the chores and look after her!

Even a simple thing like breast-feeding lying down instead of sitting in a chair can be helpful. Many women find that it is easier to cope with a demanding baby if he sleeps with her instead of separately.

SPECIAL SITUATIONS

Assisted deliveries

As discussed on p. 74, it is sometimes necessary for forceps or ventouse vacuum extraction to be used to help deliver a baby. Almost always these techniques will be accompanied by a substantial episiotomy and frequently by postpartum bruising and oedema. Assisted deliveries have been shown to be followed by a higher incidence of pelvic floor muscle denervation than normal vaginal or caesarean section deliveries (Snooks et al., 1985). For some women a transient neuropraxia results in temporary numbness and muscle weakness, but for many the memory of their post-forceps delivery pain is worse than that of labour – it certainly lasts for very much longer! The consequent frustration felt by new mothers while they are learning to care for their baby, handicapped by constant, throbbing discomfort, can mar what should be a happy time, and may delay the mother-baby attachment with subsequent feelings of guilt and disappointment.

Making sure that adequate analgesic drugs are being taken and that the woman has sufficient aids such as pillows, a foam-rubber ring and a footstool to ensure maximum comfort while feeding is important. It is vital for active therapy aimed at reducing pain to be started as soon as possible. The physiotherapeutic techniques offered will depend on what is available in each maternity unit; ice and pelvic floor contractions cost nothing, however, and certainly reduce pain and swelling. The mother should be encouraged to exercise her pelvic floor constantly – six to eight tightenings every five to ten minutes are not too much. She should move her feet and legs freely and walk about, but should avoid prolonged sitting or standing. One of the most helpful suggestions – again cost-free – is resting in the prone position well supported by pillows. This is particularly useful if, in addition to oedema and bruising, the woman also has engorged haemorrhoids.

Whatever other modalities (ultrasound, PEME, infrared irradiation) are used, it is the duty of the obstetric physiotherapist to review regularly the relevant infection control procedures and to ensure that no organisms are transmitted from patient to patient, or from patient to physiotherapist or vice versa.

If the woman is still in pain when she goes home, she can continue with treatment herself using ice, pelvic floor contractions and brief warm baths, to assist resolution. It is important for the obstetric physiotherapist to check and record whether a woman is able to perform a voluntary contraction of her pelvic floor before she leaves hospital. Any woman who cannot achieve a pelvic floor contraction should be recalled before her postnatal check to ascertain whether the difficulty has been overcome. Any suspected problems should be reported to the obstetrician.

Caesarean section (see also p. 76)

A few years ago, in most maternity units, 5–7% of deliveries were by caesarean section. This has increased and today the national level is around 10–15%, with some high-risk centres reaching 20–25% (Lomas, 1988). Although it is a comparatively risk-free procedure (Editorial, 1988), it is not without problems for anaesthetists, obstetricians, midwives, physiotherapists and – most important of all – for the woman herself. It is the only major abdominal operation where the opportunity for an uninterrupted convalescence is nil, and where the patient has to get out of bed to start a new career within hours of surgery!

Caesarean section can be carried out under general anaesthesia or epidural analgesia. Danish research (Juul et al., 1988) compared two groups of women who had undergone this operation, one with a general anaesthetic and one with epidural analgesia, for anaesthetic complications, postoperative morbidity and birth experience. The puerperal period was less complicated, there was quicker re-establishment of gastrointestinal function, and the women mobilized more quickly and were less tired following epidural analgesia. Eighty-six per cent of women would opt for an epidural in case of a repeat caesarean. A further paper (Lie and Juul, 1988) showed an interesting result with respect to breast-feeding following an epidural caesarean section; these women breast-fed significantly more frequently and for a longer period after birth than a similar group who had general anaesthesia.

The mother's reaction to this method of delivery will depend on her own expectations and aspirations with regard to labour and birth. Whether it was a planned elective procedure or an emergency carried out during labour, whether she was awake or unconscious, and if her partner was able to share the experience with her or not, are all important factors in determining her degree of satisfaction. Her postoperative condition will be influenced by the type of anaesthetic used, the length of labour before the caesarean, and her own responses to surgery and pain. Some women, particularly those undergoing an elective operation with an epidural, will cope without difficulty and will be able to move about and look after their baby with minimal discomfort. Others, particularly those unfortunate enough to require a caesarean section following a failed forceps delivery, may be terrified to move, incapacitated by their pain and able to do very little for their baby, they will require constant help and support (Donovan, 1977).

Trowell (1988), in a study of 52 primiparous women undergoing elective or emergency caesarean section, found that 18 were left troubled and preoccupied, finding their caesarean section a difficult experience. A further 8 women found the operation to be an adverse life experience and were seriously troubled. All these 26 mothers were worried about the effect of the operation on their own bodies, found it hard to make the transition to motherhood and to take the responsibility for a dependent baby. They all needed to talk through feelings which they felt prevented them relating to their baby. At follow-up, in some cases as long as three years later, the children showed no objective differences from those born by normal vaginal delivery, yet their mothers found them difficult, had less eye-to-eye contact with them, and they had less complete immunization schedules.

As well as routine postoperative measures designed to maintain good circulation and ensure a clear chest, the obstetric physiotherapist must do her utmost to assist the woman to cough, move, care for and feed her baby, as painlessly, effortlessly and as soon as possible.

Coughing

By virtue of the special physiology of pregnancy (see p. 34) and the fact that the timing of an emergency caesarean section cannot be chosen, it is not uncommon for women postoperatively to have mild chest problems and secretions. Coughing after any abdominal operative procedure is painful, but following a caesarean section it is complicated by the exceptionally slack abdominal wall. Support is paramount, as is positioning. It is virtually impossible to cough comfortably and effectively in bed no matter what devices are used. As soon as possible the patient should be assisted to sit on the side of the bed with her feet supported on the floor or on a stool (Fig.7.10). Her legs should be wide apart, a soft pillow must be clasped to her lower abdomen and she should be encouraged to lean as far forward as possible. Coughing can be reduced to a minimum by using forced expiration or 'huffing' as an alternative or prelude.

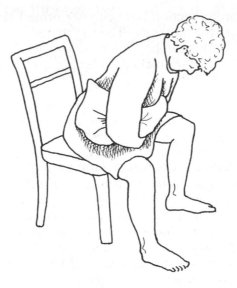

Figure 7.10 A supported coughing position.

Exercising

Apart from routine foot and leg exercises to maintain good circulation and disperse any oedema, normal postnatal exercising will have to be introduced and progressed more slowly. Three easy and comparatively pain-free movements which can be suggested are:

1. Crook lying – gentle pelvic tilting, principally using the gluteal muscles.
2. Crook lying – gentle knee rolling from side to side.
3. Half crook lying – hip hitching.

The movements have the added benefit of helping to disperse 'wind', whether it is within the anaesthetic-relaxed gut or in the form of air trapped within the abdominal cavity. Prolonged expiration with abdominal contraction, or vibrations or stroking over the 'wind' pain, may also help. Single or two-handed abdominal effleurage following the line of the colon (upwards on the right, transversely from right to left, and then downwards on the left) often gives relief from this common and extremely uncomfortable problem, and is something the mother can do for herself.

Feeding the baby

Whether the caesarean section has been performed via a Pfannenstiel or a midline incision, the mother will be frightened lest her baby kick or press on her wound. This can be avoided during feeding by positioning the baby so that the feet are tucked under her arm or by the judicious use of pillows to protect the wound (Fig.7.11).

Wound healing

Women with pendulous abdomens, whose loose flesh overhangs their wound, may experience healing problems. Their skin may become unhealthily 'soggy'. Infection may occur and healing be delayed. This situation should be pre-empted in such patients by encouraging them to rest in positions that spread the flesh and expose the wound to the air. It may even be necessary for the woman to draw the overhanging abdomen up and away for short periods. Mild infrared radiation (IRR) can be helpful prophylactically or therapeutically where infection is suspected to relieve pain, improve local circulation and encourage speedy resolution without breakdown; where wound breakdown has not occurred, an electric pad can serve the same purpose. Well equipped physiotherapy departments will have access to ultrasound or PEME.

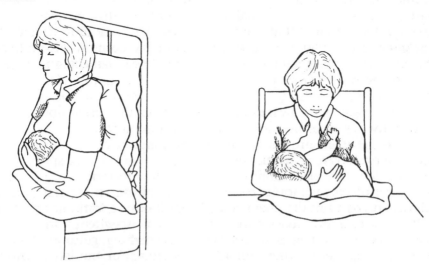

Figure 7.11 The caesarean section mother will need to be shown alternative feeding positions to reduce pressure on her wound.

Haematoma

A post-surgery haematoma sometimes occurs, giving rise to considerable discomfort. It has been suggested that PEME (Golden et al., 1981) or ultrasound can accelerate resolution.

Posture

Following caesarean section a woman needs special help in rediscovering her prepregnancy posture. The 'ship in full sail' end-of-pregnancy stance will probably have been replaced by a protective flexed position, complicated by weak abdominal muscles and possible backache. The persuasive powers of the obstetric physiotherapist may be necessary to prove to the mother that upright posture is rewarded by greater comfort.

TNS for the treatment of post-caesarean section pain

Most major surgical procedures allow for a prolonged period of convalescence on the part of the patient; this is not true for caesarean section! Mothers are often handicapped in their efforts to care for their new baby by postoperative pain, which can be intense. TNS has successfully been used for analgesia following surgery by many practitioners. Schomberg and Carter-Baker (1983) described a physical therapy trial in the use of the modality for post-laparotomy pain. TNS may be used for post-caesarean section pain and frequently gives the mother an additional source of comfort without the disorientating narcotic effects of conventional invasive postoperative analgesia. Hollinger (1986) found that TNS decreased the amount of narcotic analgesia required in post-caesarean section women; this also reduces the amount of drugs passing to the babies of breast-feeding mothers.

Two electrodes can be placed at either end of a suprapubic Pfannenstiel incision (Fig.7.12) or parallel with a vertical paramedian incision. Although women are aware of discomfort from the actual wound, they frequently describe their major source of discomfort as sited in each iliac fossa. The electrodes should be positioned over the pain, or else they can extend from just below the anterior superior iliac spine above and parallel with the inguinal ligaments. The Obstetric Pulsar can be used, and allows the mother to choose both the amplitude and mode of stimulation best suited to her needs. It also has the additional benefit of a 10% increase in intensity when the current is switched from boost mode to continuous mode – very useful for coughing, getting in and out of bed, or simply moving around when caring for the baby. Davies (1982), however, described TNS as being ineffective for post-caesarean women following epidural anaesthesia, and suggested possible causes

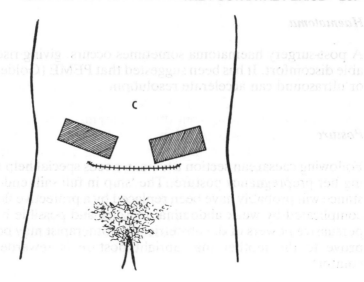

Figure 7.12 TNS electrodes may be placed slightly above the caesarean wound.

for this interesting phenomenon e.g. differential block, spinal cord and frequency-dependent effects. Once again the obstetric physiotherapist should experiment with electrode placement; two electrodes at L1 in addition to the abdominal electrodes may give greater relief.

Multiple births

Postnatally mothers of more than one baby will not only have very much weaker abdominal muscles and possibly a larger diastasis recti abdominis, they will have less time to devote to themselves because of feeding demands and will also be very tired and preoccupied with their new family. The obstetric physiotherapist will need to introduce the idea of exercising while feeding, and should point out the importance of extra help at home and plentiful rest in the early postpartum period. Where possible these women should be seen in the community once they have adjusted to their new and demanding lifestyle, so that postnatal exercises can progress (or even commence if pressure at home has been too intense initially!). Parents coping with more than one baby at a time will appreciate the help, guidance and support they can receive from local branches of the Twins and Multiple Birth Association (TAMBA – see list of useful addresses).

Postnatal emotional and psychiatric problems

In spite of the fact that postnatal mood changes have been recognized since the time of Hippocrates, who described what must have been puerperal psychosis in a mother who had given birth to twins, the emotional and psychiatric illnesses that can arise in normal, healthy women who have recently given birth, are only now being recognized as separate pathological entities. Significantly, postnatal depression was omitted from the British and American classifications of disease which appeared in 1984. Until a few years ago psychiatrists believed that women were suffering from other recognized disorders such as schizophrenia, mania or depression. Now, however, it is accepted that not only is childbirth a mighty precipitating factor in those who are genetically and constitutionally predisposed to mental illness, but that childbirth frequently brings its own mental conditions as well. Psychiatrists are very much clearer about *what* happens than *why*, and many feel that the powers of prevention are puny (Cox, 1986).

The three common manifestations of postnatal depressive illness vary in their time of onset and in their degrees of severity.

'Maternity blues'

The 'maternity', 'baby' or 'third day' blues occur in the first two to three weeks after delivery. The depression often follows a latent period of about three to four days, is usually mild and transitory but can be more intense. The mother is weepy, anxious and perhaps agitated. Maximum tearfulness and depression occur on the fifth postpartum day (Kendall et al., 1981). The condition is often aggravated by a sore perineum or breasts, fatigue from broken nights and endless visitors. A woman's sense of success or failure about her labour, delivery and baby, as well as thoughtless comments from hospital staff, can be triggering factors too.

The mother's response to her baby may not have been what she had expected; perhaps the automatic surge of love did not materialize; and the sudden realization of the never-ending responsibility for the small, new life can be overwhelming. The fact that friends, relations and hospital staff seem more interested in the baby than in her, her situation (being in hospital perhaps for the first time in her life, with strange food, bed and people), add to her sense of isolation, and maybe guilt that she is not enjoying her baby. Any or all of these can play a part in the 'blues', which are experienced by as many as 80% of newly delivered mothers. Research suggests that about 25% of mothers experiencing severe postnatal 'blues' will go on to develop postnatal depression (Cox, 1986).

Puerperal psychosis

Puerperal psychosis is a much more severe illness, which also starts in the early postnatal days. The mother may seem to lose contact with reality, have delusions or hallucinations, extreme mood swings and behave abnormally. She can suffer from intense agitation and anxiety; insomnia and very early waking are also signs of this catastrophic illness. Suicidal and infanticidal thoughts may also occur and, in its worst form, puerperal psychosis may require hospitalization – ideally in a special mother and baby unit. There is a very high likelihood of its recurrence following future pregnancies.

Postnatal depression

Postnatal depression (PND) may also begin in the early postpartum period, but it can start or become obvious much later too. It presents in a variety of ways and with varying degrees of severity. The mother may feel sad and depressed; she may worry constantly about herself and her baby, feel unable to cope and have a sense of futility and hopelessness. She may be tired to the point of exhaustion, but may be unable to sleep. She will probably suffer from a loss of libido and may have a delayed return of menstruation. Physical symptoms such as ankle swelling, loss of hair and a non-dietary weight gain may also be present. In very severe postnatal depression the mother may feel suicidal or may be frightened that she will harm her baby. Although depressive illness is the most common, other neuroses and emotional disorders can also follow childbirth; none of them is restricted to women in the affluent societies, and several authorities have described similar conditions in African women (Cox, 1979; Ebie, 1972; Oxley and Wing, 1979).

There is still considerable conflict of ideas as to the cause of these disruptive illnesses. Hormonal, neuroendocrine and even social factors are all said to play a part. Recognition of PND and its treatment is imperative for the well-being of mother, baby and family. The size of the problem can be appreciated if, based on an annual birth rate of around 700 000 births in the UK, it is realized that 50–80% of women will have the 'blues' – that is 350 000 to 550 000 women; 10% (70 000) will go on to suffer from varying degrees of PND, and about 2–3 women in every 1000 will suffer from puerperal psychosis. That constitutes a great deal of unhappiness in new mothers and their families.

Every member of the caring team has a responsibility to watch for signs of any of these disorders occurring in women in the early postnatal days, and also in the weeks and months which follow once they have returned home. The obstetric physiotherapist, who may have come into contact with a woman antenatally, during labour and on the postnatal ward, and who may continue to see her at subsequent mother and baby exercise classes, may be the one member of the team who has known the mother continuously, and will therefore be most able to recognize any changes and alert the mother's health visitor and general practitioner.

LONG-TERM POSTNATAL PROBLEMS

Although the vast majority of postnatal aches, pains and problems do resolve spontaneously after a few weeks, there are some that linger (MacArthur et al., 1991). There are also those that only become obvious once the new mother resumes her everyday routines – several months may pass before they become apparent. Prior to a woman's return home from hospital it is well worth while to draw her attention to the possibility of long-term problems and to the fact that she should not put up with these thinking that they are the 'normal' aftermath of childbirth. It is reassuring for women to know that if their local support and primary health care team – midwife, health visitor and general practitioner cannot help towards a solution (or does not seem interested), their obstetric physiotherapist is still available as an additional source of advice.

Perineal and vaginal pain

Whether perineal discomfort follows an episiotomy or a tear is immaterial – the fact that it is still there several weeks following the birth of a baby can be a serious cause of anxiety, fatigue and even depression, as well as an obstacle to the resumption of sexual intercourse. The healing rate for wounds varies from person to person, but no woman should be expected to put up with long-term perineal or vaginal pain. Causes of this include poor suturing leading to 'lumpy' scar tissue, infection, and the formation of a neuroma in regenerating nerve tissue. If self-help techniques such as warm baths, small disposable ice packs, sitting on a ring or two pillows with a space between them, repeated pelvic floor contractions or gentle self-massage with a bland vegetable oil (as long as the possibility of infection and a broken-down wound has been eliminated) do not help, then the mother must be encouraged to visit her general practitioner in the first instance, with referral back to her obstetrician or gynaecologist as the next option. She should mention the continuing pain at the six-week postnatal check and insist on a follow-up appointment. A rare source of postpartum discomfort and dyspareunia is the excessive formation of granulation tissue in the line of the episiotomy or tear (granuloma). Where this occurs it can be successfully treated by cautery. Painful scar tissue may also be helped by steroid injection. Ultrasound to external scar tissue may be useful in resolving perineal pain which is not due to infection (Fieldhouse, 1979).

Dyspareunia (see also p. 311)

Painful intercourse is possibly the most distressing long-term sequel to childbirth. Kitzinger and Walters (1981) showed that women who had an episiotomy experienced more dyspareunia, which persisted for longer than those who had lacerations. Fourteen per cent of those with lacerations had dyspareunia which lasted longer than three months, 22% of those with episiotomy, 28% of those who had a double wound and 2% of those with an intact perineum. Because fear of pain can prevent resumption of intercourse, simple advice as to the use of a lubricant, or a different position so that pressure is not an additional problem, may be all that is needed; ultrasound can also be helpful.

The mother must be encouraged to seek a second opinion if her general practitioner and gynaecologist are not able to assist in the resolution of her problem; special or family planning clinics are often good sources of help.

Backache

Good back care and posture are essential because the physiological ligamentous changes during pregnancy (see p. 38) take up to six months to reverse. In addition, changes in bone density of the lumbar spine (but not the radius) have been reported following six months' lactation (Hayslip et al., 1989). This is due to lower levels of oestrogen during this time, and it seems probable that this loss is reversed when breast-feeding ceases, although this may take some months. Before women leave hospital they should be warned that care is necessary because backache is a common problem of motherhood. A great many women of all ages feel that their backache was a direct result of childbearing and its aftermath, whether this was in fact the true cause or not. MacArthur et al. (1990) has suggested that there may be a correlation between epidural anaesthesia and long-term backache. A large proportion will put up with their discomfort because they think, or are told, that nothing can be done. The community-based postnatal 'mother and baby' group is an ideal forum for discussion about the possible causes of back pain and the ways and means by which it may be prevented and relieved. Simple exercises such as pelvic tilting in different positions and alternative resting postures (see p. 107) together with suggestions for good feeding, nappy-changing and baby-carrying habits may go a long way towards solving the problem. If these self-help techniques do not relieve the pain, women should be urged to seek further help.

Diastasis recti abdominis

The size of this intermuscular gap will reduce in most women as recovery from pregnancy and labour takes place (see p. 250); it may not disappear altogether without a careful exercise programme. Women most at risk of a continuing problem are those with multiple births, multiparae, and the very narrow-hipped who carried their babies 'all in the front'. It is most important for the correct mechanical function of the abdominal wall that the diastasis is eliminated. A great deal of encouragement may be necessary to stimulate women to keep exercising – those with multiple births will, understandably, have very little time or energy for themselves.

Mastitis and breast abscesses

These distressing problems often do not present in the immediate postpartum period. Mastitis (inflammation of the breast) may be infective, but in 50% of cases it is not (RCM, 1991) so recourse to antibiotics may not be necessary. Non-infective mastitis could arise if milk is not removed from the breast at the rate at which it is produced, or as a result of an obstruction, e.g. blocked duct, bruising following trauma or rough handling, and compression (from fingers holding the breast, or a tight brassière). Incorrect positioning of the baby could lead to ineffective breast emptying. Infection may occur externally, in the skin, and reach the inner tissue of the breast via damaged nipples. Unless mastitis is quickly treated, abscess formation requiring surgical incision and drainage can result. Apart from pain and redness, or lumpiness in the breast, the woman may become pyrexial, develop a rigor and feel quite ill. Gentle massage towards the nipple to reduce lumpiness and encourage drainage can help relieve non-infective mastitis. Ultrasound and interferential therapy have both been used beneficially in the treatment of these problems (Semmler, 1982; Maslem, 1982).

If surgery for a breast abscess is required it is not, these days, thought necessary to abandon breast-feeding. It can be continued on the affected side so long as the position of the incision allows this. The baby may continue to feed normally on the unaffected side (RCM, 1988).

Stress incontinence

There is a wide variation in pelvic floor muscle strength between nulliparous and multiparous women and from woman to woman in each category (Gordon and Logue, 1985). It has also been shown that there is a dramatic drop in the strength of the pelvic floor measured at 6 weeks' postpartum compared to before pregnancy and a slight, possibly physiological, recovery to levels still well below those prior to pregnancy by 12 weeks (Dougherty et al., 1989). Stress incontinence is probably the condition most readily accepted as 'women's lot' by sufferers of all ages and parity. Mothers and grandmothers of recently delivered women often say that bladder leakage is a 'normal' consequence of childbirth, they have suffered from it themselves since their families were born, and nothing can be done about it (bar the 'operation to repair the bladder') so it has to be lived with. Researchers have demonstrated that stress incontinence can be alleviated by a rigorous programme of pelvic floor exercises (Henalla et al., 1988; Tchou et al., 1988; Wilson et al., 1987; Bø, 1989). Dougherty et al. (1989) showed a dramatic improvement in pelvic floor strength and endurance following their programme of six weeks' intensive exercise with or without vaginal resistance. Too many women practise pelvic floor exercises intermittently ('when I think of it'), too infrequently ('ten times after breakfast') or not at all ('I haven't got time'). Before embarking on a further programme of rehabilitative exercise, it is of prime importance for a full assessment to be made of each woman's pelvic floor, including a vaginal examination – in addition a urine test to eliminate infection is advisable. A great many women are quite unable to produce a pelvic floor contraction, or are unable to maintain it for more than three seconds at best. The possibility of pelvic floor denervation (Allen, 1990) must be considered (see p. 274). The experienced obstetric physiotherapist may be able to grade the strength of the muscle contraction digitally (see p. 359). Routines of pelvic floor exercises must be tailored to each individual, and assessed and revised regularly. Progression should include the number of repetitions and the length of the 'hold'. The woman should be encouraged to exercise whenever she feeds her baby, to stop or slow urine flow and to counter-brace her pelvic floor on coughing, sneezing, laughing or blowing her nose. If frequency and urgency are also problems, a strong pelvic floor contraction should be used to inhibit detrusor activity (McGuire, 1979). If a woman is unable to produce a reasonable pelvic floor contraction, electrical stimulation is an additional method of treatment which may be useful. It is vitally important that each woman knows, on her discharge from hospital, that she has an 'open door' to her obstetric physiotherapist should urinary problems fail to resolve. Where these are long-lasting, a full urodynamic assessment will be necessary.

Faecal incontinence (see also p. 380)

This intensely humiliating and embarrassing problem does not, fortunately, affect as many women as urinary stress incontinence. However, this and other forms of dysfunction such as flatal incontinence, are known to follow perineal rupture sustained during vaginal delivery (Sørensen et al., 1988), and anal sphincter rupture (Haadem et al., 1987) and where pelvic floor denervation occurs following childbirth (Snooks et al., 1985). Factors associated with rectal injury in spontaneous deliveries include parity (multiparae were at greater risk of damage), infant birth weight (large babies caused more damage), the type of episiotomy (midline was more likely to lead to injury to the rectum) and even the place of birth (delivery room and bed were safer than a delivery table) (Green and Soohoo, 1989). Bargatta et al. (1989)

showed that the use of episiotomy and the lithotomy position with stirrups substantially increased the incidence of deep perineal tears (0.9% in women who delivered without either episiotomy or stirrups, compared with 27.0% where episiotomy and stirrups were both used). Snooks et al. (1985) showed that women who sustained third-degree perineal tears had increased pudendal nerve terminal motor latency (PNTML). This is consistent with injury to the pudendal nerves as well as direct injury to the anal sphincter. Women who had a prolonged second stage and difficult delivery (forceps are an added risk factor) and multiparae also showed increased PNTML. In addition the fibre density (FD) in the external anal sphincter muscle was increased in multiparae. An abnormal degree of perineal descent is usually present for 48–72 hours after vaginal delivery and this can persist for two months or more (Snooks et al., 1984). It is thought that this descent is sufficient to cause stretch-induced damage to the pudendal nerves (Henry et al., 1982). In 60% of women this nerve injury is reversible (Snooks et al., 1984), but 80% of all women with idiopathic anorectal incontinence have evidence of nerve damage to the pelvic floor musculature (Parks et al., 1977). It would appear that vaginal delivery alone, with or without forceps, is often sufficient to give rise to a permanently weakened pelvic floor with its attendant problems.

Where a woman has complained immediately after the birth of her baby of frank anorectal incontinence, incontinence of flatus or urgency of defaecation, it is vitally important for her future health that she be properly followed up. Some recovery of the PNTML may take place in the months following childbirth and with regular pelvic floor exercise the strength of the pelvic floor may be brought to a reasonable level. However, many women complaining of these symptoms have ineffective or non-existent pelvic floor activity – and these women will need a great deal of help if they are not to develop this form of incontinence later in life.

Although interferential therapy is often advocated as a treatment for urinary stress incontinence it has not been shown to be successful for anorectal incontinence (Sylvester and Keiltig, 1987); stimulation with an anal electrode, however, has proved to be beneficial (Sackier, 1989). It may prove to be a useful tool in the hands of physiotherapists working in this field, both as a biofeedback device to teach anal sphincter control initially, and as a method of strengthening weak, partially denervated muscle.

Diastasis symphysis pubis

Rarely, this incapacitating condition persists beyond the puerperium; it is often associated with sacroiliac problems. In most cases of pelvic relaxation the symptoms clear spontaneously or following the appropriate conservative treatment, during the weeks after delivery. The condition usually resolves after four to five months, although there is a tendency for recurrence in future pregnancies. Hagen (1974) suggested fusion of the symphysis where pain and instability continue to be a problem.

Hair loss

Hair is produced by hair follicles, which are epidermal structures. In the scalp the growing phase for hair (anagen) lasts for up to three years. The resting phase (telogen) lasts for a few weeks, after which the hair falls out. During pregnancy the number of hair follicles in telogen decreases and the woman's hair often seems thicker. After the baby is born, three to four months later, the proportion of telogen follicles increases rapidly and much hair can be lost, leading to thinning. In most women this will be temporary, and they will regain their scalp hair (Myatt, 1988).

Postnatal depression

For many women this disturbing disorder (see p. 269) may not present until the baby is several weeks old. Because it can affect 10% of all recently delivered women (Cox, 1986), carers should watch for signs of its presence in any woman who expresses strong anxieties about herself or her baby, is sad and depressed, feels unable to cope, and is overwhelmingly tired yet suffers from sleep disturbances. An obstetric physiotherapist who is meeting mothers regularly in a postnatal 'mother and baby' group is ideally placed to recognize this distressing condition, which can last for many months if not recognized and treated. It is worth noting that depression can present in different ways: physical 'aches and pains' (somatization) may in fact be a cry for help.

Carpal tunnel syndrome

Carpal tunnel syndrome occurring in pregnancy usually resolves shortly after delivery. It can, however, develop in the puerperium and appears then to be closely associated with breast-feeding. Wand (1989) described a study of 27 women who developed carpal tunnel syndrome on average three and a half weeks following delivery. In 3 women who were bottle-feeding the symptoms were mild and quickly resolved; the remaining 24 experienced painful paraesthesia, and 16 had such severe symptoms that their ability to care for their baby was affected. Complete resolution of the condition did not take place until breast-feeding had totally stopped – improvement began approximately 14 days following the beginning of weaning. Although this study shows the close association between the onset of symptoms and the establishment of lactation, and their disappearance following its cessation, the author does not offer any physiological reason for this interesting state of affairs.

Wrist splints, reassurance, diuretics, non-steroidal anti-inflammatory drugs and steroid injections have been used to treat the condition with varying results. The obstetric physiotherapist who encounters carpal tunnel syndrome in the postpartum period could use exercise, elevation, positioning, ultrasound or ice.

References

Alder E., Bancroft J. (1983). Sexual behaviour among lactating women: preliminary communication. *J. Reprod. Inf. Psychol.*, **1**,47–52.

Alder E., Bancroft J. (1988). The relationship between breastfeeding, persistence, sexuality and mood in postpartum women. *Psychological Medicine*, **18**, 389–96.

Allen R.E., Hosker G.L., Smith A.R.B., Warrell D.W. (1990). Pelvic floor damage and childbirth: a neurophysiological study. *Brit. J. Obstet. Gynaec.* **97**, 770–79.

Appelbaum R.M. (1970). The modern management of successful breastfeeding. *Ped. Clin. N. America*, **17**, 203–225

Aukett A.D. (1982) *Baby Massage*. Wellingborough: Thorsons.

Balaskas J., Gordon Y. (1987). *The Encyclopedia of Pregnancy and Birth*. London: Macdonald Orbis.

Bargatta L., Piening S.L., Cohen W.R. (1989). Association of episiotomy and delivery position with deep perineal laceration during spontaneous delivery in nulliparous women. *Am. J. Obstet. Gynecol.* **160**, 294–7.

Bewley E.L. (1986). The megapulse trial at Bristol. *J.ACPOG*, **58**, l6.

Bø K., Hagen R.H., Kvarstein B. et al. (1990). Pelvic floor muscle exercise for the treatment of female stress urinary incontinence. III Effects of two different degrees of pelvic floor muscle exercises. *Neurology and Urodynamics*, **9**, 489–502.

Boissonnault J.S., KotarinosR.K. (1988). Diastasis recti. In *Obstetric and Gynaecologic Physical Therapy* Ed. Wilder E., pp. 63–82. Edinburgh: Churchill Livingstone.

Brunskill P.J., Swain J.W. (1987). Spontaneous fracture of the coccygeal body during the second stage of labour. *J. Obstet. Gynaecol.* **7**, 270–1

Calguneri M., Bird H.A., Wright V. (l982). Changes in joint laxity during pregnancy. *Ann. Rheum. Dis.* **41**, 126–8

Cox J.L. (l979). Amakiro: a Ugandan puerperal psychosis? *Social Psychiatry*, **14**, 49–52.

Cox J.L. (l986). *Postnatal Depression*. Edinburgh: Churchill Livingstone.

Davies J.R. (1982). Ineffective transcutaneous nerve stimulation following epidural anaesthesia. *Anaesthesia*, **37**, 453–7.

DeChateau P., Wiberg B. (1977). Long term effect on mother-infant behaviour of extra contact during the first hour postpartum. *Acta Paed. Scand.*, **66** 137–151.

Donovan B. (1977). *The Caesarean Birth Experience*. Boston: Beacon Press.

Dougherty M.C., Bishop K.R., Abrams R.M. et al. (1989). The effect of exercise on the circumvaginal muscles in postpartum women. *Journal of Nurse-Midwifery*, **34**, 8–14.

Driessen F. (1987). Postpartum pelvic arthropathy with unusual features. *Brit. J. Obstet. Gynaec.*, **94**, 870–2.

Dyson M. (1987). Mechanisms involved in therapeutic ultrasound. *Physiotherapy*, **73**, 116–120.

Ebie J.C. (1972). Psychiatric illness in the puerperium among Nigerians. *Tropical Geographical Medicine*, **24**, 253–6.

Editorial (1988). Obstetric anaesthesia on report. *Lancet*, **i**, 222.

Fieldhouse C. (1979) Ultrasound for relief of painful episiotomy scars. *Physiotherapy*, **65**, 217.

Frank R. (1984). Treatment of the perineum by pulsed electromagnetic energy. *J. ACPOG*, **54**, 21–2.

Golden J.H., Broadbent N.R.G., Nancurrow J.D., Marshall T. (1981). The effects of diapulse on the healing of wounds: double-blind randomised controlled trial in man. *Br. J. Plastic Surg.*, **34**, 267–270.

Gordon H., Logue M. (1985). Perineal muscle function after childbirth. *Lancet*, **i**, 123–5.

Grant A., Sleep J., McIntosh J., Ashurst H. (1989). Ultrasound and pulsed electromagnetic energy treatment for perineal trauma. A randomised placebo-controlled trial. *Brit. J. Obstet. Gynaec.*, **96**, 434–9.

Green J.R., Soohoo S.L. (1989). Factors associated with rectal injury in spontaneous deliveries. *Obst. Gynec.*, **73**, 732–8.

Haadem K., Dahlstrom J.A., Ling L., Ohrlander S. (1987). Anal sphincter funtion after delivery rupture. *Obst. Gynec.*, **70**, 53–6.

Hagen R. (1974). Pelvic girdle relaxation from the orthopaedic point of view. *Acta Orthop. Scand.* **45**, 550–63.

Hayslip C., Klein T.A. Wray H.L., Duncan W.E. (1989). The effects of lactation on bone mineral content in healthy postpartum women. *Obst. Gynaec.*, **73** 588–92.

Henalla S.M., Kirwan P., Castleden C.M., et al. (1988). The effect of pelvic floor exercises in the treatment of genuine urinary stress incontinence in women at two hospitals. *Brit. J. Obstet. Gynaec.*, **95**, 602–6.

Henry M.M., Parks A.G., Swash M. (1982). The pelvic floor musculature in the descending perineum syndrome. *Br. J. Surg.*, **69**, 470–472.

Hinman F. (1976). Post operative overdistension of the bladder. *Surg. Gynaecol. Obstet.*, **142**, 901–2.

Hollinger J.L. (1986). Transcutaneous electrical nerve stimulation after caesarean birth. *Physical Therapy*, **66**, 36–8.

Inch S. (1987). Difficulties with breastfeeding: midwives in disarray? *Roy. Soc. Med.*, **80**, 53–8.

Juul J., Lie B., Friberg Nielsen S. (1988). Epidural analgesia vs. general anaesthesia for caesarean section. *Acta. Obstet. Gynaecol. Scand.*, **67**, 203–6.

Kegel A.H. (1951). Physiologic therapy for urinary stress incontinence. *JAMA*, **146**, 915–7.

Kendall R.E., McGuire R.J., Connor Y., Cox J.L. (1981). Mood changes in the first three weeks after childbirth. *Journal of Affective Disorders*, **3**, 317–26.

Kitzinger S.S., Walters R. (1981). *Some Women's Experiences of Episiotomy*. London: National Childbirth Trust.

Knight K.L. (1989). Cryotherapy in sports injury mnagement. *In Sports Injuries* (Grisogono V. ed.) Edinburgh: Churchill Livingstone.

Lee J.M., Warren M.P. (1978). *Cold Therapy in Rehabilitation.* London: Bell & Hyman.

Lehmann J.F., DeLateur B.J. (1982). Cryotherapy In *Therapeutic Heat and Cold* (Lehmann J.F., ed.) Baltimore: Williams & Wilkins.

Lie B., Juul J. (1988). Effect of epidural vs general anaesthesia on breastfeeding. *Acta. Obstet. Gynaecol. Scand.*, **67**, 207–9.

Lomas J. (1988) Holding back the tide of caesareans. *Br. Med. J.*, **297**, 569–70.

Low J.L. (1988). Shortwave diathermy, microwave, ultrasound and interferential therapy. In *Pain: Management and Control in Physiotherapy.* p.166. Oxford: Heinemann.

MacArthur C., Lewis M., Knox E.G., et al. (1990). Epidural anaesthesia and long-term backache after childbirth. *Br. Med. J.*, **301**, 9–12.

MacArthur C., Lewis M., Knox E.G. (1991). Health after childbirth. *Brit. J. Obstet. Gynaec.*, **98**, 1193–5.

Maslem J. (1982). Interferential therapy in the treatment of a blocked duct in a lactating breast. *National Obstetrics and Gynaecology Journal*, Australian Physiotherapy Association. April.

McGuire, E. (1979). Urethral sphincter mechanisms. Urol. Clin. N. America, **6**, 39–49.

McIntosh J. (1988). Research in Reading into treatment of perineal trauma and late dyspareunia. *J. ACPOG*, **62**, 17.

McLaren J. (1984). Randomised controlled trial of ultrasound therapy for the damaged perineum. In *Clinical Physics and Physiological Measurement*, 1984 **5**, 37–45.

Moore W., James D.K. (1989). A random trial of three topical analgesic agents in the treatment of episiotomy pain following instrumental vaginal delivery. *J. Obstet. Gynaecol.*, **10**, 35–9.

Murray A., Holdcroft A. (1989). Incidence and intensity of postpartum lower abdominal pain. *Br. Med. J.*, **187**, 1619.

Myatt A.E. (1988). Baldness. *Br. J. Sexual Med.*, August. 260–2.

Noble E. (1980) *Essential Exercises for the Childbearing Year.* 2nd edn. London: John Murray.

Oxley J., Wing J.K. (1979). Psychiatric disorders in two African villages. *Arch. Gen, Psych.*, **36**, 513–20.

Palastanga N.P. (1988). Heat and Cold. In *Pain: Management and Control in Physiotherapy.* pp. 176–179. Oxford: Heinemann.

Parks A.G., Swash M., Urich H. (1977). Sphincter denervation in anorectal incontinence and rectal prolapse. *Gut*, **18**, 656–665.

Polden M., Whiteford W. (1992). *The Postnatal Exercise Book.* London: Frances Lincoln.

RCM (1991). *Successful Breastfeeding.* 2nd edn. Edinburgh: Churchill Livingstone.

Romito P. (1988). Mothers' experience of breastfeeding. *J. Reprod. Inf. Psychol.* **6**, 89–99.

Sackier J. (1989). The anal sphincter. In *Neuromuscular Stimulation: Basic Concepts and Clinical Applications* (Rose F.C., Jones R., Vrbova G., eds.) pp. 331–349. New York: Demos.

Salariya E.M., Easton P.M., Cater J.I. (1978). Duration of breastfeeding after early initiation and frequent feeding. *Lancet*, **ii**, 1141–3.

Schomberg F.L., Carter-Baker S.A. (1983). Transcutaneous electrical nerve stimulation for post-laparotomy pain. *Physical Therapy*, **63**, 188–93.

Semmler D.M. (1982). The use of ultrasound therapy in the treatment of breast engorgement. *National Obstetrics and Gynaecology Journal*. Australian Physiotherapy Association, July.

Shepherd A. (1980). Re-education of the muscles of the pelvic floor. In *Incontinence and its Management*. (Mandelstam D., ed.) London: Croom Helm.

Slaven S., Harvey D. (1981). Unlimited suckling time improves breastfeeding. *Lancet*, **i**, 392–3.

Snooks S.J., Setchell M., Swash M., Henry M.M. (1984). Injury to innervation of the pelvic floor sphincter musculature in childbirth. *Lancet*, **ii**, 546–50.

Snooks S.J., Swash M., Henry M.M. Setchell M. (1985). Risk factors in childbirth causing damage to the pelvic floor innervation. *Br. J. Surg.*, **72**, Suppl., 515–7.

Sørensen S.M., Bondesen H., Istre O., Vilman P. (1988). Perineal rupture following vaginal delivery – long-term consequences. *Acta Obstet. Gynecol. Scand.*, **67**, 315–8.

Stanway A., Stanway P. (1983). *Breast is Best*. London: Pan.

Sylvester K.L., Keiltig S.E.J. (1987). The use of interferential therapy in the treatment of ano-rectal incontinence. *Physiotherapy*, **73**, 207–8.

Tchou D.C.H., Adams C., Varmer R.E., Denton B. (1988). Pelvic floor musculature exercises in treatment of anatomical urinary stress incontinence. *Physical Therapy*, **68**, 652–5.

Trowell J. (1989). Psychological effects of lower section caesarean. *Midwife, Health Visitor and Community Nurse*, **25**, 22–4.

Wand J.S. (1989). The natural history of carpal tunnel syndrome in lactation. *J. Roy. Soc. Med.*, **82**, 349–50.

Wilson P.D., Al Samarrai T., Deakin M. et al. (1987). An objective assessment of physiotherapy for female genuine stress incontinence. *Brit. J. Obstet. Gynac.*, **94**, 575–82.

Winnicot D.W. (1987). *Babies and Their Mothers*, p. 93. New York: Addison-Wesley.

Further Reading

Cox J.L. (1986). *Postnatal Depression*. Edinburgh: Churchill Livingstone.

Enkin M., Keirse M.J.N.C., Chalmers I. (1990). *A Guide to Effective Care in Pregnancy and Childbirth*. Oxford: Oxford University Press.

Grant B. (1989). *Multiple pregnancy*. In *Myles' Textbook for Midwives* (Bennett V.R., Brown L.K., eds.). Edinburgh: Churchill Livingstone.

Linney J. (1983). *Multiple Births: Preparation – Birth – Managing Afterwards*. Chichester: John Wiley.

MacArthur C., Lewis M., Knox E.G. (1991). *Health after Childbirth*. London: H.M.S.O.

Nielsen C.A., Sigsgaard J., Olsen M. et al. (1988). Trainability of the pelvic floor. *Acta Obstet. Gynecol. Scand.*, **67**, 437–40.

Polden M., Whiteford W. (1992). *The Postnatal Exercise Book*. London: Frances Lincoln.

Price F.V. (1990). *Report to Parents of Triplets, Quads and Quins*. Child Care and Development Group, University of Cambridge.

Price J. (1988). *Motherhood – What it Does to Your Mind*. London: Pandora.

RCM (1991). *Successful Breastfeeding*. 2nd edn. Edinburgh: Churchill Livingstone.

Renfrew M., Fisher C., Amis S. (1990). *Best feeding: getting breastfeeding right for you*. Berkeley: Celestial Arts.

Useful addresses

Association of Breastfeeding Mothers
13 Mayflower Road
London SE26

Association for Postnatal Illness
7 Gowan Avenue
London SW6 6RH

Caesarean Support Groups
81 Elizabeth Way
Cambridge CB4 1BQ

CRY-SIS (Crying babies)
BM CRY-SIS
London WC1N 3XX

Episiotomy Support Group
232 Ifield Road
West Green
Crawley, West Sussex RH11 7HY

Foundation for the Study of Infant Deaths
15 Belgrave Square
London SW1X 8PS

La Leche League (Breastfeeding)
BM 3424
London WC1N 3XX

Nippers (Premature babies)
Sam Segal Perinatal Unit
St Mary's Hospital
Praed Street
London W2 1NY

National Childbirth Trust (NCT)
Alexandra House
Oldham Terrace
Acton, London W3 6NH

Stillbirth and Neonatal Death Society (SANDS)
29-31 Euston Road
London NW1 2SD

Twins and Multiple Birth Association (TAMBA)
360 Woodham Lane
Newham
Weybridge, Surrey

CHAPTER 8

The Climacteric

The term *menopause*, is used for the last menstrual flow experienced by a woman, and can only be judged retrospectively. The menopause occurs at some time between the ages of 45 and 55 years for most women in the UK, but varies with race, economic status and nutrition. For example, a mean age of 49.8 years has been calculated for women in North America, 51.4 years for the Netherlands, 49.7 years for the Bantu, and 44 years or younger, according to nutrition, in the Punjab, New Guinea and Central Africa (Gray, 1976). In New Guinea in areas of poor nutrition it is 43.6 years, whereas in areas with better conditions it is 47.3 years. Regardless of these factors, a few women experience a very premature menopause before 40 years.

Menstruation may stop suddenly, or the menopause may be heralded by menstrual periods becoming more widely spaced. Alternatively a single menstruation, then two or three consecutive ones, may be missed, the flow may vary from cycle to cycle, or the flow may become progressively less with successive cycles. It is important for women to be enabled to discriminate between these normal variations and signs of disease. For example, bleeding that occurs more than one year after the menopause is known as postmenopausal bleeding, and may be indicative of carcinoma of the body of the uterus.

Prior to the actual menopause, when periods are erratic, a woman may be referred to as being premenopausal, and following the menopause as postmenopausal. However, in popular usage the word 'menopause' is synonymous with the phrase 'the change of life', and is a broad concept including the unpleasant symptoms some women experience around this time – the perimenopause. More correctly, the interrelated anatomical and physiological changes that occur as a woman proceeds from her fertile to infertile years are termed the climacteric (Fig.8.1). These changes occur because the ovaries become exhausted of viable follicles; they shrink and fail to produce oestrogens. The anterior pituitary gland is thus released from the cyclic inhibition of oestrogen and so continues to produce follicular stimulating hormone (FSH) and luteinizing hormone (LH). In some women some oestrogens continue to be produced in the suprarenal cortex and by synthesis of androgens in fatty tissue. Thus heavy women have higher circulating levels of oestrogens (particularly oestriol) than slender women. Following the menopause there is a gradual atrophy of all the chief target

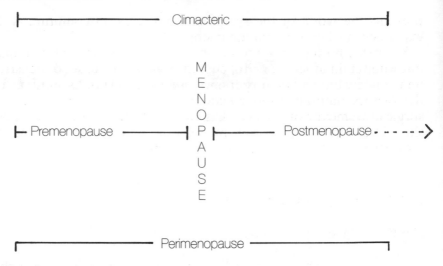

Figure 8.1 Terms used in relation to the climacteric.

organs for oestrogen. There is involution of the breast structure and a cessation of cyclic breast changes. The ovaries shrink, the uterus becomes smaller, the endometrium shows atrophic changes and becomes thinner, the cervix diminishes in size and its secretions decrease. There are atrophic changes of the vaginal wall with loss of elasticity and the fornices become shallower. There is a fall in the acidity of secretions within the vagina, making it more prone to infection. There is atrophy of the supporting structures to the genital tract and a predisposition to prolapse. The labia become flatter and infection may occur (vulvitis), and pubic hair decreases. Atrophy of the epithelium of the bladder including the trigone and the urethra, and of the supporting corrective tissue, may give rise to frequency, dysuria, stress and urge incontinence. These changes may predispose to infection, but may also present similar symptoms to an infection.

Some women pass through this stage in their lives noticing very little difference either physically or mentally. They rejoice in the cessation of premenstrual tension and menstruation, and in their new sexual freedom with no need of contraception. However, there are others who experience severe physical and mental problems, and who are distressed by their loss of fertility. They experience some or all of the following: frequent hot flushes, night sweats, vaginal soreness, dyspareunia, urinary disorders, dry skin, reduced concentration, loss of memory, inability to make decisions, anxiety, mood swings, irritability, tiredness and depression. Such unpleasant symptoms may begin premenopausally and can continue for several years after the menopause. Increasingly doctors are administering hormone replacement therapy (HRT) through the worst of the unpredictable undulations in hormonal levels, with the option of gradually withdrawing the replacement therapy when the body levels have stabilized. This theoretically prevents the worst of the symptoms, but some discomfiture will be experienced when the treatment stops.

Women who have a hysterectomy before their natural menopause but who retain at least one functioning ovary will cease to menstruate immediately but will not experience other menopausal symptoms until the ovaries naturally stop functioning. However, if the ovaries are surgically removed or a woman has therapeutic irradiation of the pelvis, she will experience an abrupt menopause, and climacteric symptoms may occur and last for 6–12 months or longer.

PHYSICAL SYMPTOMS

Hot flushes and night sweats

Flushing and sweating suddenly occur, usually over the upper chest, neck and face. Sometimes this is triggered by a stressful situation, a hot drink or hot, spicy food; often, however, there is little or no apparent reason for these embarrassing and inconvenient events which may happen occasionally or many times a day. The pulse rate rises and there may be palpitations. In addition (or alternatively) women may wake in the night soaked in perspiration, often needing to change their nightwear. These symptoms are known to be associated with low levels of oestrogens in the blood, and may also be due to temporary rises in the levels of FSH and LH. They are certainly alleviated by HRT but return as soon as it is stopped; they then disappear over time.

Vaginal soreness – atrophic vaginitis

Vaginal and cervical secretions are decreased and less acid; the vaginal lining becomes thin, dry and less elastic. This results in the vagina being more prone to infection and easily becoming sore. In addition there may be narrowing of the introitus and dyspareunia with consequent marital stress. These symptoms respond well to oestrogen given orally (systemic) or transdermally (vaginal applications of hormonal cream).

Urinary disorders

Atrophy, inflammation and infection of the vagina may have secondary effects on the urethra and bladder and there may be atrophy of the urethra, trigone and associated supportive ligaments. Oestrogen deficiency has also been shown to result in a reduction in turgidity of the cells forming the urethra. These facts should be borne in mind where women complain of cystitis, urethritis, frequency, dysuria, urgency or stress incontinence during the climacteric. Oestrogen replacement helps some women.

Dry skin

The collagen content of skin is known to be oestrogen dependent. Loss of collagen results in it becoming thinner and less elastic (Brincat et al., 1987). Oestrogen receptors have been found in sebaceous glands, which probably accounts for the dryness of skin complained of by some women and traded on by cosmetic manufacturers. This improves with HRT.

PSYCHOLOGICAL AND EMOTIONAL SYMPTOMS

Women blame the menopause for a great deal and complain of a variety of psychological and emotional difficulties. There is no doubt that low oestrogen levels do affect a woman's mental faculties and that there is improvement with HRT. However it is worth considering the other life stresses the average woman experiences through her late 40s and early 50s. For example, a mother's role has to change considerably as children go through teens and leave home, and the behaviour of some children causes huge stress; partners may seek other relationships, become ill or even die; redundancy or early retirement of self or partner alters status; and older relatives may need increasing time and support. These and other normal life events may well affect a climacteric woman. Gaining insight into the whole picture, understanding stress and having a selection of coping strategies may sometimes deal with the prime problems and obviate the need for HRT.

Sexuality in the climacteric – see p. 313

POSTMENOPAUSAL PROBLEMS

The postmenopausal population has increased rapidly in the UK over recent years; better health and medical care has resulted in a life expectancy for women of well over 80 years. With the menopause at around 50, women can now expect to be postmenopausal for more than a third of their lives.

Consequently there is increasing interest in the effects on women over time of what has until now been considered the normal and inevitable reduction in oestrogen level. Some now call this an 'oestrogen deficiency', and there is much discussion of the desirability, efficacy and associated risks of long-term HRT (Belchetz, 1989). The most critical known effects of lowered oestrogen levels are an acceleration of osteoporosis and subsequent fractures, and an increased risk of arterial disease. To combat these two potential killers women increasingly are being asked to consider long-term HRT.

Osteoporosis

The peak of a person's bone mass is achieved following adolescence, late in the second decade or in the third decade. Thereafter there is a slow, age-related fall which accelerates when the ovaries cease to function; it has been shown that following removal of the ovaries there is a 2.5% bone loss per annum for the first four years which then decreases to about 1%. Thus it can be calculated that following the menopause the average woman may lose more than 20% of her bone mass by the age of 70 years. Both trabecular and cortical bone are lost; Riggs (1987) gives 50% and 35% to be the amounts of these two components respectively that a woman may expect to lose in a lifetime, and it is suggested that 50% of postmenopausal women are seriously at risk of developing clinically significant osteoporosis. It is not only the bone mineral content but also collagen that is lost. There is a greater prevalence of osteoporosis amongst slender women and they are at greater risk for fractures; probably because androgens produced by the adrenal glands are converted to oestrogens in fatty tissue. Thus obesity may give some protection against osteoporosis by assisting oestrogen production and by the stressing effect of weight-bearing on the skeleton (Sinahi, 1989). Fractures of the femur, wrist and vertebrae predominate; in 1985 35 000 women sustained fractures of the femoral neck (Boyce and Vessey, 1985); these affect independence and can be life-threatening. Of every 100 women who fracture a femoral neck, 50 are unable to return to their own home and up to 20 die (Melton and Riggs, 1983). The peak for fractures of the wrist has been shown to be the 55–59 year age group (Winner et al., 1989), although the cause of the increase in the risk of falling remains unexplained. For women 45 years old the statistic for Colles' fracture is 0.3 per 1000; at 85 years old it is 20 per 1000. Fractures of vertebrae cause untold suffering and dependence.

How lower levels of oestrogens influence bone formation in this way has been a puzzle, but a clue has been uncovered recently with the discovery of oestrogen receptors in the nuclei of osteoblasts (Komm et al., 1988; Eriksen et al., 1988).

Prevention of osteoporosis

Table 8.1 shows the risk factors associated with osteoporosis, and prevention, it has jokingly been suggested, starts with parentage. The black ethnic groups are favoured in this respect compared to the white

Table 8.1 Risk factors for osteoporosis

White or oriental ethnic group
Slim build
Early menopause or early oophorectomy
Positive family history
Poor diet:
   low calcium
   excessive animal protein
   high phosphate
High coffee intake
High alcohol intake
Cigarette smoking
Nulliparity
Sedentary lifestyle
Disorders affecting mineral metabolism
Cushing's disease
Corticosteroid treatment

groups, and have very strong bones. Consequently the women can lose bone mass for more years before becoming vulnerable. Prevention continues in childhood by ensuring an adequate calcium intake in the first two decades of life, together with plenty of exercise in order to build up a substantial peak bone mass. Physiotherapists in obstetrics and gynaecology have an important health promotion role, educating women concerning diet and exercise not only for their children's sakes but also for their own. The inevitable bone loss through life is variable between individuals, but for a postmenopausal woman the advice is still that exercise is vital because weight-bearing and strengthening exercise has the potential to build bone mass and decrease bone loss, and decrease the frequency of falls (Sinahi, 1989; Chow et al., 1987); and nutrition is important, although the results of calcium supplementation are disappointing in reversing osteoporosis (Stevenson et al., 1988). Long-term HRT should be considered, particularly if at the menopause the newer bone screening techniques (e.g. dual photon absorptiometry) show a woman to be in the 'high loss' group. Hormone replacement has been shown to delay osteoporosis and thus offers some protection against fractures (Weiss et al., 1980; Paganini-Hill et al., 1981; Ettinger et al., 1985; Riggs and Melton, 1986; Munk-Jensen et al., 1988; Purdie, 1988).

Arterial disease

Prior to the menopause women seem to have protection from ischaemic heart disease compared to men, but after the menopause this changes. Atheroma increases, and rapid calcification of the abdominal aorta has been found (Witteman et al., 1986, 1989) indicating an increased risk of vascular damage e.g. strokes. Research has shown that oestrogen therapy protects against such disasters (Ross et al., 1981; Stampfer et al., 1985; Paganini-Hill et al., 1988).

The administration of hormone replacement therapy

When HRT was first introduced oestrogen was administered orally and daily; this caused hyperplasia of the endometrium, and the incidence of endometrial carcinoma rose from 1 per 1000 in the untreated women to 4 or 5 per 1000 after only one year of treatment. This effect was cumulative so that in a few years it quickly became a totally unacceptable risk. More recently 'opposed' oestrogen therapy has been employed, whereby progesterone is also given for 10–12 days each month. This causes a withdrawal bleed *per vaginam* which is usually brief, slight and acceptable. There has been concern that HRT may raise the risk of breast and ovarian cancer but research findings have been inconclusive; however, women on HRT are under regular medical supervision.

There are three ways in which oestrogens may be administered:

1. Orally. Tablets are taken daily; the hormone is absorbed in the intestines then passed via the portal system to the liver, where it undergoes metabolic changes that reduce its potency, necessitating a higher initial dose.

2. By implant. A small tablet or pellet is introduced under the skin (usually of the abdomen) after a local anaesthetic; it slowly dissolves and the hormone is released. This method maintains an appropriate oestrogen level for about six months. The oestrogen may be combined with cyclic oral testosterone.

3. Transdermally.
(a) Hormone creams are used for atrophic vaginitis and vulvitis; if topical application is not successful then systemic oestrogen is used.
(b) Adhesive patches impregnated with oestrogen are applied like sticking plasters to buttock, thigh or abdomen and the hormone is absorbed through the skin; one patch gives a sufficient dosage for about 2 days. In addition progesterone is taken orally for 12 days in each cycle.

References

Belchetz P. (1989). Hormone replacement treatment. *Br. Med. J.* **298**, 1467–1468.

Boyce W.J., Vessey M.P. (1985). Rising incidence of fracture of the proximal femur. *Lancet*, **i**, 150–1.

Brincat M., Moniz C.F., Kabalan S. et al. (1987). Decline in skin collagen content and metacarpal index after the menopause and its prevention with sex hormone replacement. *Brit. J. Obstet. Gynaec.* **94**, 126–9.

Chow R., Harrison J.E., Notarius C. (1987). Effect of two randomised exercise programmes on bone mass of healthy postmenopausal women. *Br. Med. J.*, **295**, 1441–4.

Eriksen E.F., Colvard D.S., Berg N.J. et al. (1988). Evidence of oestrogen receptors in normal human osteoblast-like cells. *Science*, **241**, 84–6.

Ettinger B., Gerant H.K., Cann C.E. (1985). Long-term oestrogen replacement therapy prevents bone loss and fractures. *Ann. Intern. Med.* **102**, 319–24.

Gray R.H. (1976). *The Menopause: Epidemiological and Demographic Considerations in the Menopause* (Beard R.J. ed.) pp.25–40. Lancaster: MTP Press.

Komm B.S., Terpening C.M., Benz D.J. et al. (1988). Estrogen binding, receptor mRNA and biologic response in osteoblast-like osteosarcoma cells. *Science*, **241**, 81–4.

Melton L.J., Riggs B.L. (1983). Epidemiology of age-related fractures. In *Osteoporotic Syndrome* (Avioli L.L., ed.), pp. 45–72. New York; Grune Stratton.

Munk-Jensen N., Nielsen S.P., Obel E.B., Eriksen P.B.(1988). Reversal of postmenopausal vertebral bone loss by oestrogen and progesterone. *Br. Med. J.* **296**, 1150–2.

Paganini-Hill A., Ross R.K., Gerkins V.R. (1981). Menopausal oestrogen therapy and hip fractures. *Ann. Intern. Med.* **95**, 28–31.

Paganini-Hill A., Ross R.K., Henderson B.E. (1988) Postmenopausal oestrogen treatment and stroke: a prospective study. *Br. Med. J.* **297**, 519–22.

Purdie D.W. (1988). Broken bones – a gynaecological problem. *Br. J. Obstet. Gynaec.*, **95**, 737–9.

Riggs B.L. (1987). Pathogenesis of osteoporosis. *Am. J. Obstet. Gynecol.* **156**, 1342.

Riggs, B.L., Melton L.J. (1986). Involutional osteoporosis. *New Engl. J. Med.*, **314**, 1676–86.

Ross R.K., Paganini-Hill A., Mack T.M. et al. (1981). Menopausal oestrogen therapy and protection from death from ischaemic heart disease. *Lancet*, **i**, 858–60.

Sinahi M. (1989). Exercise and osteoporosis – a review. *Arch. Phys. Med. Rehabil.*, **70**, 220–8.

Stampfer M.J., Willett W.C., Colditz G.A. et al. (1985). A prospective study of postmenopausal estrogen therapy and coronary heart disease. *New Engl. J. Med.*, **313**, 1044–9.

Stevenson J.C., Whitehead M.I., Padwick M. et al. (1988). Dietary intake of calcium and postmenopausal bone loss. *Br. Med. J.*, **297**, 15–17.

Weiss N.S., Ure C.L., Ballard J.H. et al. (1980). Decreased risk of fractures of the hip and lower forearm with postmenopausal use of oestrogen. *New Engl. J. Med.*, **303**, 1195–8.

Winner S.J., Morgan C.A., Grimley-Evans J. (1989). Perimenopausal risk of falling and incidence of distal forearm fracture. *Br. Med. J.*, **298**, 1486–8.

Witteman J.C.M., Kok F.J., van Saase J.L. et al. (1986). Aortic calcification as a predictor of cardiovascular mortality. *Lancet*, **ii**, 1120–2.

Witteman J.C.M., Grobec D.E., Kok F.J. et al. (1989). Increased risk of atherosclerosis in women after the menopause. *Br. Med. J.*, **298**, 642–4.

CHAPTER 9

Common Gynaecological Conditions

Gynaecology is the study of diseases that are peculiar to women. It is a specialty that demands of the physiotherapist a particularly mature blend of attributes which, when necessary, enable the patient confidently to disclose some of the most intimate and personal details of her life. In addition to sound theoretical knowledge and a high degree of clinical compctence, the physiotherapist must always make time to listen, be easily approachable, unshockable and non-judgemental.

GYNAECOLOGICAL HEALTH

That some gynaecological conditions may be silent in progress, some simply debilitating, others life-threatening, has been increasingly appreciated. Recent advances in the understanding of the early presentation and development of infections and malignant disease of the female reproductive organs and breasts has resulted in women in the UK being encouraged to avail themselves (once sexually active) of regular free screening by means of cervical cytology, and to learn to monitor their own breasts by monthly systematic palpation. These methods are best taught in the community-based Well Women Clinics, where early detection and treatment of disease, prevention and health promotion are the chief objectives. Visits to these clinics are increasingly seen to be the ideal opportunity for a regular physical check which may realistically include:

1 Measurement of blood pressure.
2 Breast examination.
3 Examination of perineum, vagina and cervix for signs of infection and prolapse, and cough test for stress incontinence.
4 Cervical cytology.
5 Bimanual pelvic examination, and test of pelvic floor strength.
6 Urine test for infection, sugar, etc.
7 Discussion of the woman's state of health and any problems she may be experiencing (eg. sexual problems).

Some Well Women Clinics are extending this service with seminars on health matters, and exercise classes taken by physiotherapists to encourage fitness by improving mobility and strength and to try to delay osteoporosis; attention is also being given to weight control.

Cervical cytology

As a member of the Well Women or gynaecological team it is important for the specialist physiotherapist to know the classification of cervical cytology results. Smears may be classified into five grades:

Grade 1 Normal smear.
Grade 2 Inflammation.
Grade 3 Dyskaryosis, i.e. abnormal nuclei, requiring further investigation but may revert to normal.
Grade 4 A few malignant cells.
Grade 5 Many malignant cells.

More recently the cervical intra-epithelial neoplasia (CIN) classification has been introduced:

CIN 0 Normal smear.
CIN 1 Mild dysplasia, i.e. growth of stratified epithelium disordered and proliferating, suspicious of dyskaryosis, may revert to normal.
CIN 2 Moderate dysplasia, some abnormal cells, test should be repeated.
CIN 3 Severe dysplasia, many abnormal cells, refer for colposcopy and treatment

Cervical cytology is not diagnostic but indicates when further investigation is necessary. Colposcopy (colpos = cervix or neck) enables minute inspection of the cervix through a colposcope – a binocular instrument which magnifies up to 20 times.

Some centres are able to offer minor treatments at the clinic such as cauterization, cryosurgery and laser treatment, and physiotherapy for incontinence.

GYNAECOLOGICAL DISORDERS

The most common disorders of the female genital tract can be classified as infections, cysts and new growths, or displacements and genital prolapse.

Infections

Vulva (vulvitis)

The continuous moist discharge from glands in the vulva supplemented by that from the uterus and cervix, together with traces of urine and faecal material, ensure that there is always a profusion of micro-organisms in the perineal area. Infection may track up the vagina or may have tracted from it; thus vulvitis often becomes vulvovaginitis. It is suggested by some that the recent trend to nylon tights, the fashion for the habitual wearing of tight-fitting trousers by some women and increased sexual freedom have all contributed to maintaining the incidence of infections of the perineum and pelvic organs in women at a high level against the trend of many other infections. It is important to realize that pruritus vulvae, a severe and distressing irritation of some part of the perineum, is a common experience amongst women, but it is a symptom and not a condition in its own right. It requires careful investigation to determine the precise cause, which can be as diverse in nature as lichen simplex, incontinence, liver disease or Hodgkin's disease. Pruritus ani may be part of the same problem or have an individual cause such as threadworms. It is also worth remembering that the perineum may become sensitized to cosmetic or other chemical preparations.

Infections of the vulva may be fungal, bacterial, viral or parasitic. The fungus *Candida albicans* is frequently implicated in vulvitis in pregnancy, especially if the renal threshold for sugar becomes lowered. It is commonly called 'thrush', and is characterized by irritation, acute inflammation, rawness and a curdy, white discharge; the vagina is often also infected. Staphylococcus bacteria infect sebaceous glands and hair follicles on the perineum causing little boils; gonorrhoea and syphilis are other infections that may affect this area. Vulval warts are caused by a virus. Herpes genitalis is a sexually transmitted viral infection which has been linked with cervical cancer. It is a serious problem in pregnancy, where it can cause abortion, and elective caesarean section may be indicated if the mother has active herpes at term; otherwise the fetus could become infected at delivery and subsequently die or suffer neurological damage. Parasites such as lice can be transmitted from head hair to pubic hair and can cause perineal irritation.

The duct of each Bartholin's gland is narrow, and easily becomes blocked. If this occurs mucoid secretions distend the gland, forming an often painless cyst. This may become infected forming an abscess, or an infection of the gland can occur independently of any duct narrowing; any such infection is excruciatingly painful.

Vagina (vaginitis)

The vagina can become infected by a variety of organisms similar to those found in the vulva, and 'vaginal discharge' is another symptom of which women often complain. There is a normal cycle of changes in the amount and nature of secretions within and passed *per vaginam* associated with the menstrual cycle which has been described on p. 22.

Normally all secretions are transparent or white, so any change in colour, bleeding, or any unusual odour or quantity should be a cause for consultation. Organisms that commonly cause infective vaginal discharge are *Candida albicans, Trichomonas vaginalis, Neisseria gonorrhoeae* and *Gardnerella vaginalis* (Clayton et al., 1985). It is of interest that *Chlamydia trachomatis*, which has been implicated in pelvic inflammatory disease, does not produce noticeable discharge. Vaginal organisms are transmitted sexually so, in treatment, partners must also be considered. Vaginitis may also be caused by sensitivity to spermicides and douches.

Cervix (cervicitis)

Erosions of the cervix are quite common; they can be infected but usually are not. Normally, columnar epithelium partly or completely lines the cervical canal and butts on to the stratified squamous epithelium which lines the vagina, and covers the vaginal aspect of the cervix. Where there is an erosion, columnar epithelium appears to replace some of the cervical stratified epithelium. Erosions sometimes appear in pregnancy and in women taking oral contraceptives; they are rarely seen after the climacteric and improve when oral contraceptives are discontinued. This suggests a hormonal factor. Infections of the cervix are commonly caused by sexually transmitted organisms like *Gonococcus* spp. or *Chlamydia trachomatis*, and may follow trauma such as that which can occur at childbirth, abortion or as a result of operative procedures requiring dilatation of the cervix.

Uterus (endometritis)

Infections of the uterus with resulting endometritis are less common than those of other areas of the genital tract by virtue of the protection afforded by the vagina and cervix – i.e. the length of the vagina, the downward movement of secretions, the constriction formed by the cervix and the viscosity for much of the time of its secretions – and by the cyclic shedding of the endometrium. However, infections do track upwards; it is said that sperm can act as carriers, the tails of intra-uterine devices have been implicated, and after delivery or abortion the open placental site, the lochia or retained products of conception all potentially provide a superb culture medium. Any medical procedure that opens the cervix has the potential to introduce infection.

Fallopian tubes (salpingitis)

Infection of the fallopian tubes, which is often associated with infection of the ovary (salpingo-oophoritis), may result from ascending infection but can also occur following infection of the gut or other abdominal organs. Salpingitis may be acute or chronic and can be a cause of infertility when scarring and adhesions block the tube, or damage muscle and cilia.

Pelvic inflammatory disease

The close proximity of structures particularly within the true pelvis and their interconnection via ligaments and peritoneum means that infection is able to spread to involve other organs and produce what is known as pelvic inflammatory disease (PID). In the UK a variety of bacteria can be responsible for PID, but *Chlamydia trachomatis*, *Neisseria gonorrhoeae* and *Mycoplasma hominis* currently seem to be most common. Such infections may occur independently or concurrently, and are sexually transmitted. The number of women suffering from PID appears to have risen steeply: just under 600 acute cases were hospitalized in 1960, whereas in 1981 there were 14 690, and no figures are published for sufferers treated in outpatient clinics where most are managed.

The infection causes inflammation, and the body's response in the highly vascular pelvic area is the production of adhesions (sometimes profuse) and scarring, which contort structures and glue or bind them to adjacent ones. In the acute phase women complain of pelvic or abdominal pain and of feeling thoroughly unwell; they may even be pyrexial. Sometimes there are difficulties in achieving an accurate clinical diagnosis due to the problems in obtaining a sample from the infection site and because the accuracy of tests has been poor. Consequently the condition in many women becomes chronic and results in continuing ill-health, persistent lower abdominal pain, serious internal damage and eventually infertility. It adversely affects relationships and the ability to work successfully. *Chlamydia trachomatis* is a Gram-negative intracellular bacterium and is not detected, as *N. gonorrhoeae* can sometimes be, by routine microscopy. A special, time-consuming cell culture and staining test has been necessary to detect *Chlamydia*. However, quicker, simpler and more accurate tests are being developed; in some cases a specimen will need to be collected by laparoscopy. *N. gonorrhoeae* usually responds to penicillin, but it is less well appreciated that *Chlamydia* does not; it is however usually sensitive to the tetracyclines.

Physiotherapy in the treatment of gynaecological infections

There is no role for physiotherapy in the acute phase of gynaecological infections. These must be promptly and properly diagnosed, and effectively treated with the correct chemotherapy. However in the chronic phase, where the organism is resistant to antibiotics or when adhesions are causing pain, there may occasionally be a place for physiotherapeutic measures such as continuous or pulsed short-wave diathermy. The physiotherapist can also offer coping strategies to deal with pain and stress, and advice on the promotion of good health.

Acquired immune deficiency syndrome (AIDS)

Before leaving the subject of infections, AIDS must be considered so that physiotherapists may best be able to protect themselves and their patients. AIDS is caused by a virus known as the human immunodeficiency virus (HIV). Infected persons carry the virus in body fluids, and may be fit and well for varying lengths of time. HIV is transmitted during intimate sexual contact, or through direct contact via mucous membrane or broken skin with infected blood or genital secretions from a carrier in any other circumstances. The virus can be transmitted to the fetus across the placenta and is present in the amniotic fluid of HIV carriers. The infection is diagnosed by the presence in blood samples of the appropriate antibodies. However, there is a time lag of months or years between acquiring the infection and developing antibodies. It is not yet known what determines if and when a carrier will develop the syndrome.

The physiotherapist working in obstetrics and gynaecology must take account of these facts for personal protection and to avoid cross-infection via equipment between patients. The District Infection Control Officer should be consulted regularly to ensure that precautions are based on the latest information.

Cysts and new growths

The term 'cyst' usually signifies a pathological fluid-filled sac bounded by a wall of cells. The fluid is often clear and colourless, and may be secreted by the cells lining the cyst or derived from the tissue fluid of the area. There are cysts peculiar to each organ, and these may be congenital or acquired. Congenital cysts occur in vestigial remnants of embryonic tissue; they are common in the genitourinary tract, and the broad ligament is a frequent site. Acquired cysts may be caused by obstruction to the outflow of a duct and consequent retention of secretions (e.g. Bartholin's gland). Alternatively, distension cysts form in natural enclosed spaces; they are common in graafian follicles and corpora lutea.

Benign tumours are formed by a mass of well-defined cells which are still recognizably similar to the originating tissue, and the mass is encapsulated by a layer of normal cells so the tumour cells cannot escape. Benign tumours tend not to be troublesome and do not generally threaten life. By contrast the cells of malignant tumours show varying degrees of reversion to the embryonic unspecialized state, and look less like the original cells. They seem to lose control of cell division and divide repeatedly, they are less differentiated and lose the specialist function of their parent cell. They have no containing capsule and so invade surrounding tissue. Highly malignant cells lose the mature cell's adhesiveness to its neighbours, and regain the embryonic cell's ability to detach and migrate to form secondary deposits or metastases. They also have the ability to stimulate the growth of new blood capillaries around and within the growing cell mass, ensuring an adequate supply of nutrients. Thus malignant tumours tend to be life-threatening until successfully treated.

Gynaecological cancers have been classified and clearly defined in stages by the International Federation of Obstetrics and Gynaecology (FIGO) The most recent definitions were published in detail in the August edition of the British Journal of Obstetrics and Gynaecology, 1989, pages 889–92.

Vulva

Vulvar cancer is classified in stages by FIGO:

Stage 0 Carcinoma *in situ* and intraepithelial.
Stage 1 Confined to vulva and/or perineum; lesion <2 cm in greatest dimensions, no palpable nodes.
Stage 2 As for stage 1, except that lesion is >2 cm in greatest dimension.
Stage 3 Any size tumour with spread to lower urethra and/or vagina or anus, and/or unilateral lymph node metastasis.
Stage 4 Further spread to bladder, rectum, pelvis and/or bilateral node metastasis or distant metastases.

Both benign and malignant tumours occasionally arise on the vulva, particularly in postmenopausal women. Vulvar cancers may be primary, but where there are multiple foci, they are commonly secondary growths as a result of lymphatic spread. Excision of the tumour or vulvectomy may be appropriate.

Bartholin's glands

In the sebaceous and Bartholin's glands of the perineal area benign cysts can result from blockage of the ducts but are of little significance unless they become large or infected. Cysts may be excised and the ducts opened (marsupialization).

Vagina

Cysts, and benign and malignant tumours can occur; carcinoma of the vagina is rarely primary but most commonly spreads down from or via the cervix. It may then involve the rectum and other tissues and be very difficult to treat.

Uterus and cervix

The most common benign tumour of the genital tract, found in 15–20% of women over 35 years of age, is the so-called 'fibroid' which grows on or within the wall of the uterus or cervix. In that it usually consists of unstriped muscle as well as fibrous tissue, the term 'fibromyoma' is more accurate. In the mature women one or more fibroids of the uterus, with accompanying heavy menstrual bleeding (menorrhagia), are grounds for considering hysterectomy once childbearing is complete. In less severe cases myomectomy may be sufficient. Fibroids vary hugely in size and number and may develop on a pedicle, in which case the name polyp is more appropriate. They are uncommon in those under 20 years old but then are found most often in the nulliparous, possibly because they are causes of infertility and miscarriage. They occur three times more frequently in black women than in white women, although the reason for this is unknown.

In general fibroids grow slowly, and atrophy following the menopause; they are prone to secondary degenerative changes such as hyaline degeneration, fatty degeneration and even calcification, all probably associated with gradual inadequacy of the blood supply to a particular fibroid. In pregnancy they tend to hypertrophy, may cause pain, and may be actually palpable and visible under the skin of the woman's distended abdominal wall in the third trimester. One particular type of degeneration – red degeneration – occurs most commonly in pregnancy, although it can occur at other times. This is the result of a rapidly renewed blood supply to a fibroid that has previously undergone some fatty degeneration, resulting in a degree of haemolysis and giving a local appearance of raw meat. The abdominal pain it causes can be alarming for the mother-to-be, but reassurance and palliative treatment only is required.

Malignant tumours of the cervix most commonly arise in women between 45 and 55 years of age, but are apparently increasing among younger women. Almost all sufferers will have had sexual intercourse, but there is a more potentially significant correlation with those women who began to be sexually active very early and who have had several sexual partners. Once sexual activity has been commenced a woman must be encouraged to have regular cervical smears taken. Precancerous dysplasic changes in the cervical epithelium, if recognized, can be treated and the development of cancerous changes be prevented.

Established carcinoma of the cervix is classified in stages by FIGO, as follows.

A. Preinvasive cervical carcinoma
Stage 0 *Preinvasive carcinoma or carcinoma* (CIN 3, see p. 290) intraepithelial (i.e. the basement membrane of the epithelium is intact); there is no infiltration, but the epithelial cells are undifferentiated and closely packed.

B. Invasive cervical carcinoma
Stage 1 Changes confined to the cervix and body of uterus.
Stage 2 Changes confined to cervix plus upper two-thirds of vagina and/or pelvic ligaments.
Stage 3 Changes now extended into pelvic wall or lower third of vagina.
Stage 4 Changes extending beyond the true pelvis or involving bladder or rectum.

In the UK about 4000 new cases of invasive cervical cancer are diagnosed each year. Cauterization, cryosurgery and laser treatment effectively destroy tissue, and constitute conservative treatments suitable for women with early cervical changes (CIN 1). Cone biopsy may be used for CIN2 and 3 (see p. 321).

The more serious stages of cervical carcinoma may be arrested and usually cured by radiotherapy or surgery, or a combination of the two. The surgery used is hysterectomy, extended where necessary. Surgery particularly for Stage 1 cervical carcinoma may be preceded by treatment with radioactive isotopes aimed at destroying the malignant tissue and so avoiding spread of cells at surgery.

Carcinoma of the uterine endometrium – that is of the uterine body (corpus) – is seen most commonly in women between 50 and 65 years of age, and does not have a coital correlation, as nearly 50% of the sufferers are nulliparous. The only constant symptom is irregular bleeding. Malignant changes begin in the glandular element of the endometrium. Spreading is less rapid than in cervical cancer, possibly because the myometrium forms some sort of containing barrier, but secondary growths may be found in the ovaries and liver. There is a similar FIGO classification, here given in brief:

Stage 0 Malignancy suspected but not proven.
Stage 1 Carcinoma confined to body of uterus.
Stage 2 Carcinoma extending to cervix.
Stage 3 Carcinoma further extending into pelvis.
Stage 4 Carcinoma now additionally involving bladder or rectum, or
has extended outside pelvis, e.g. to liver.

Treatment is again commonly a combination of radiotherapy and surgery.

Fallopian tubes

Despite being prone to infections, the fallopian tubes rarely support a primary carcinoma, although metastases or extensions of growths from the ovaries, uterus or gut do occur. Primary carcinoma is a relatively silent condition and therefore may either be found unexpectedly at surgery or not diagnosed until the condition is advanced.

Ovaries

There is a wide variety of possible cysts and benign or malignant tumours of the ovary. The menstrual cycle is disturbed in some cases and the patient may have pain, but often there is no obvious indication of the real cause. Follicular cysts are one of the most common types; most resolve spontaneously, others can be surgically removed. Bleeding may occur into cysts, and if present for some time the altered blood will become tar-like, making the cyst look dark. Reports of surgery or laparoscopy may refer to 'chocolate' cysts. 'Oyster' ovaries indicate that the ovaries may appear enlarged, shiny and pearly; this is a sign of polycystic ovarian disease. However, amongst women who die of cancer of the genital tract, ovarian cancer is the most common primary site, affecting about 4000 women per annum. A major problem in early detection is that it is a silent cancer, often with no symptoms until the tumour has extended into the peritoneum. In an attempt to combat this, voluntary ovarian screening by ultrasound and blood test is being offered in some centres. However unnecessary anxiety has been caused in some cases by false positive results, not least because with ultrasound scanning it is not easy to discriminate between benign and malignant structures. The FIGO categorization of ovarian cancer is briefly as follows:

Stage 1 Growth limited to one or both ovaries.
Stage 2 Growth contained within the pelvis.
Stage 3 Growth spreading to other abdominal tissue.
Stage 4 Additional secondary growths at a distance.

Treatment consist of a combination of surgery, radiotherapy and chemotherapy.

Endometriosis

Endometriosis is a mysterious condition which, although not a cyst or a tumour, has certain aspects that make it an acceptable inclusion in this section. It is a disorder in which plaques of tissue, histologically exactly similar to the lining of the uterus, are found implanted in other sites such as the ovaries, the outer surface of the uterus, bowel or bladder, and rarely much further away, e.g. in the lungs, or nasal cavity. The tissue responds to the hormonal changes of the menstrual cycle, proliferates and may bleed at the appropriate point in that cycle. The bleeding causes inflammation, may be contained and fibrose, or track, causing dense adhesions. The plaques grow, infiltrate and multiply, mimicking a malignancy. The ovaries, uterosacral ligaments and Pouch of Douglas are most commonly affected, and in severe cases adhesions mesh the pelvic structures together; Llewellyn Jones (1986) refers to such a pelvis as 'frozen'.

There are several theories as to how this condition arises:

1. *The transportation theory.* In 1921 John Sampson first used the term endometriosis. He postulated that during menstruation there was reflux of endometrial debris and blood through the fallopian tubes and into the peritoneal cavity; endometrial cells could thus be deposited outside the uterus. In 1927 Halban suggested instead that fragments of endometrium could be transported as emboli in veins and lymphatics.

2. *The metaplastic theory.* A contemporary of Sampson's named Meyer suggested that repeated irritation (for example due to recurrent infection) might cause cells derived from the same embryological tissue as the endometrium to change and differentiate abnormally. A similar theory suggests that a chemical substance, perhaps environmentally derived, acts on cells outside the uterus causing them to be transformed into endometrial cells.

3. *Autoimmune deficiency theory.* A recent hypothesis is that women with endometriosis suffer from an autoimmune deficiency so the body does not reject and dispose of endometrial cells if they become displaced elsewhere in the body, as it would normally be expected to. The fact that endometriosis runs in families supports this theory.

Whatever the cause, it has been estimated that 10 million women in the USA and 2 million women in Britain suffer with the condition, which causes a great deal of pain and suffering, menorrhagia, dyspareunia, infertility and general ill-health. Diagnosis is made by laparoscopy which enables visualization and biopsy. The only way of curing the condition is by hysterectomy and pelvic clearance, but hormone replacement risks reactivating the disease. Medical treatment is hormonal, aimed at producing a pseudopregnancy or pseudomenopausal state of no menstrual cycles. However some of the side-effects – masculinization, weight gain, hypoglycaemia, depression – are difficult to tolerate. More recently lasers have been used to destroy endometrial implants and adhesions, and so can delay the progress of the condition. Surgery may also be used to remove adhesions thought to be causing pain, or to facilitate conception where adhesions have blocked or distorted the fallopian tubes. Women with endometriosis are encouraged to start their family as early as possible (Brentkopf, 1988).

Physiotherapy in the treatment of gynaecological cysts and new growths

Physiotherapy has no place in the actual treatment of cysts or new growths, but there are important prophylactic and therapeutic roles for the physiotherapist where chemotherapy or radiotherapy, involving bed rest, or surgery is undertaken. Patients will benefit from advice and assistance to optimize their physical and mental condition before as well as after such procedures. Appropriate physiotherapeutic modalities should be considered where pain is troublesome, but the value of pulsed short-wave diathermy or ultrasound to assist in the softening and absorption of painful abdominal adhesions is unproven. However, the physiotherapist has much to contribute to the quality of life of those whose condition places heavy stresses on marital relationships and the ability to work, or who are terminally ill.

Displacements and genital prolapse

Although the uterus is free to move according to the changing volumes of bladder and rectum, its usual orientation in relation to the vagina is shown in Fig. 1.7 on p. 7. The cervix is directed backwards and the uterus is said to be anteverted. Where the uterus is further bent forwards on itself it is said to be anteflexed. If, however, the cervix is found to be pointing forwards and the fundus of the uterus is directed backwards the uterus is said to be retroverted, and where the uterus is then further bent backwards on itself it is said to be retroflexed. Twenty per cent of normal women have retroversion of the uterus; infertility, backache and dyspareunia have been attributed to it. The uterus may be drawn or held in retroversion as a result of adhesions associated with endometriosis or pelvic inflammatory disease.

As described in Chapter 1, the pelvic organs are maintained and supported in position by a combination of fascia and ligaments, and indirectly by the pelvic floor and levator ani muscles. Where these vital supportive components are congenitally weak, are weakened, elongated or actually damaged by childbirth, constipation, violent persistent coughing or a substantial abdominal tumour, or become atrophied as in the menopause and old age, then displacement and particularly descent of the organs from their normal position becomes possible. Prolapse most commonly occurs in women who have borne children, although it can occur in the nulliparous.

Occasionally, following hysterectomy, attachment of the cut ends of the uterosacral and transverse cervical ligaments to what is conserved of the vagina is not successful, and this may lead to subsequent vaginal prolapse. Figures 9.1 and 9.2 illustrate the most common types of displacement and prolapse encountered by the physiotherapist, together with a rough guide as to how they may present at perineal examination. The symptoms are variable but patients may complain of a lump, a dragging sensation, 'something coming down' or a feeling of heaviness when they are standing, and as a progressive sensation through the day. It is 'not there' when the patient is lying down. There may be complaint of backache but it is not often caused by the prolapse. Sexual intercourse may be affected by difficulty in penetration, dyspareunia (see p. 311) or lack of satisfaction on the part of one or both partners. Displacement of the bladder (cystocele) does not always affect continence but some patients complain of frequency and urgency of micturition, and of stress incontinence which may be anything from very mild to severe. A rectocele and an enterocele may result in difficulty in defaecation, constipation and haemorrhoids.

1 Cystocele

Weakness of the pubocervical fascia allows the bladder to displace downwards and backwards against the anterior wall of the vagina. If this is slack it will protrude. In more severe cases a pouch of bladder is formed which holds residual urine. Patients complain of frequency and incomplete emptying of the bladder which predisposes to infection; they may also have stress incontinence. A cystocele may occur in the absence of uterine descent, but where there is uterine descent it will be accompanied by some degree of cystocele because of the intimate fascial connections between the bladder base and the cervix.

2 Urethrocele

The urethra alone, being closely attached to the anterior wall of the vagina, may sag backwards and downwards when it receives insufficient support from the vagina or surrounding fascia; it may kink.

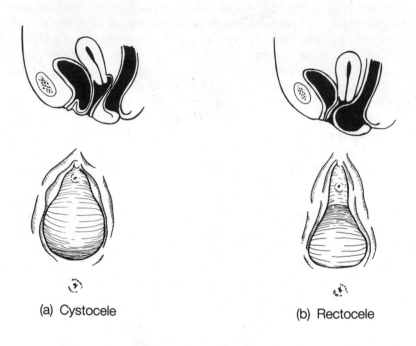

(a) Cystocele

(b) Rectocele

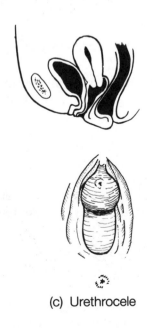

(c) Urethrocele

Figure 9.1 Three types of displacement and the associated perineal appearance.

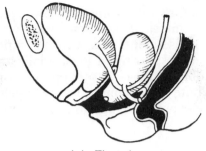

(a) First degree

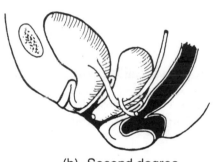

(b) Second degree

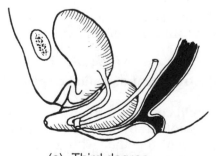

(c) Third degree

Figure 9.2 Degrees of uterine prolapse.

3 Rectocele

Prolapse of the rectum forwards against the lower part of the posterior wall of the vagina is almost always associated with damage to the perineal body and consequent loss of the support it provides. Inadequate or ineffective suturing of episiotomies and perineal tears associated with childbirth, or lack of appreciation of the damage sustained, may contribute to this condition. Rectocele is not necessarily associated with uterine prolapse because the rectum is not directly connected to the cervix.

4 Enterocele

A descent of the vaginal vault frees the upper part of the posterior vaginal wall to drop, bulge and protrude, allowing an extended pouch of Douglas to herniate. Thus an enterocele usually accompanies a uterine prolapse.

5 Uterine prolapse

When lack of adequate support allows the uterus to descend, it causes the vaginal vault to descend also and the vagina to invert. Such a prolapse will be associated with cystocele and enterocele (see above). Three degrees of uterine prolapse (Fig. 9.2) are used in clinical description:

First degree. The cervix remains within the vagina.

Second degree. The cervix appears at the perineum or protrudes particularly on straining, with the possibility of damage, infection and ulceration.

Third degree or procidentia. The entire uterus comes to be outside the body, causing total inversion of the vagina. A procidentia is almost inevitably associated with cystocele and an enterocele.

Physiotherapy in the treatment of genital displacements and prolapse

Most patients with mild conditions in any of the above five categories will benefit from physiotherapy directed at strengthening the pelvic floor muscles (see p. 366) together with attention to chest and other infections, obesity, constipation and work loads. Research suggests that exercise is a realistic alternative to surgery in patients with mild stress incontinence (Klarskov et al., 1986). Considering the cost – both human and financial – and the inherent risks associated with surgery, it makes good sense for all patients to be offered an intensive 6–8 week period of specialist physiotherapeutic treatment before surgery is mooted or once they are placed on the surgical waiting list. In any case surgery will be delayed whenever practicable until childbearing is complete; physiotherapy or a pessary may help to tide a woman over until then. For the more resistant cases, surgery in the form of a repair or hysterectomy will eventually be required (see pp. 322 and 317).

FURTHER GYNAECOLOGICAL CONDITIONS OF RELEVANCE TO THE PHYSIOTHERAPIST

Disorders associated with menstruation

For most women the onset of menstrual flow is a regular and reasonably predictable event, and the length of the menstrual cycle is individual and constant – usually somewhere between 27 and 32 days. However, there can be few women who do not, at some stage in their lives apart from pregnancy, experience irregularities and/or discomfort associated with their menstruation. The regularity of periods may change, and bleeding from the uterus may be delayed (oligomenorrhoea), may be more frequent (polymenorrhoea) or may simply be unpredictable, as is common in the menopause. The amount of menstrual flow may alter to be continuous or excessive (menorrhagia), or scant (hypomenorrhoea); additional bleeding may occur between periods (epimenorrhoea) or after intercourse.

Menorrhagia is a term used for excessive menstrual flow from the uterus. Bleeding may also arise from other organs in the tract, e.g. the vagina, and from other tracts e.g. the urinary tract; occasionally patients confuse these with menstruation. Not surprisingly it has been shown that women vary hugely in what they construe as abnormal and worthy of consultation, and reports of symptoms can be unreliable. Chimbira et al. (1980) investigated 92 women complaining of menorrhagia (defined as heavy bleeding although the periods were regular), and found no correlation between the patients' subjective assessment of blood loss and the objectively measured menstrual blood loss. Once reported, such symptoms of change in pattern are worthy of investigation in many cases, to exclude organic disease.

The menarche

Menarche is the onset of menstruation which occurs on average at the age of 13 years. An early menarche is said to correlate with an early menopause. A girl's first cycles are often irregular and are usually painless, but may be anovular and so prolonged. When menstruation has not occurred by the age of 17 years, the situation should be investigated.

Amenorrhoea

Amenorrhoea is the absence of periods, which may be total, or simply indicate the missing of one or more expected bleeds. The latter is common in girls when they leave home for the first time or experience acute stress of other kinds. Amenorrhoea or infrequent periods may occur with serious illness, starvation (e.g. anorexia nervosa, where amenorrhoea may occur before excess weight loss is obvious) and with gross obesity.

Dysmenorrhoea

The term dysmenorrhoea is used to describe pain associated with menstruation. The condition may be primary or secondary.

Primary or spasmodic dysmenorrhoea. This is the more common; there is no apparent structural abnormality or pathology. The pain is felt over the lower abdomen and sacral region in the first hours of a period, and it may be colicky. When pain is very severe, nausea, vomiting and even diarrhoea may be experienced. Pain decreases with increasing blood loss. Some gynaecologists suggest that in such patients the uterine isthmus is hypertonic, and that this results in menstrual flow debris being temporarily retained causing pressure on this highly innervated zone. Others postulate that the pain may be due to ischaemia of vigorously contracting uterine muscle.

Secondary or congestive dysmenorrhoea. This is associated with some structural abnormality or pathology, e.g. a fibroid, endometriosis or infection. The pain, which may be unilateral or bilateral, begins three days before menstruation and is relieved or temporarily exacerbated as bleeding commences. It may increase with activity.

The physiotherapist must assess every referral with care. Primary dysmenorrhoea may be managed using pain coping strategies such as relaxation, breathing awareness, TNS and distraction techniques. Where the patient's occupation and lifestyle is predominantly sedentary (as is often the case) or fitness is in question, guidance as to ways of wisely increasing physical activity may be helpful. It has been hypothesized that if the pain was caused by ischaemia this could indicate an inadequate blood supply to the uterus for vigorous contractions. Thermic treatments using continuous short-wave diathermy have been used with the aim of encouraging an increased blood supply to the area. The results have been inconclusive.

'Breakthrough bleeding'

This phrase describes intermenstrual bleeding with is associated with systemic contraceptives. An increase in the progesterone dosage or a change of preparation may be required.

Premenstrual tension

Premenstrual tension (PMT) is more common in women over 30 years of age and is a diagnosis used to describe the irritability, depression, lumbar backache, tenderness and enlargement of breasts, abdominal pain and distension, water retention, weight gain and insomnia associated with the menstrual cycle of which some women complain. Some or all of these symptoms commence up to 10 days prior to menstruation, and usually recede quickly once the menstrual flow has commenced. There is evidence in some women that their cognitive ability falls and that they are more aggressive and accident-prone at this time, which is relevant for those with demanding and responsible employment. There have been several cases in law where PMT has been used in defence. The retention of fluid is thought by some to be due to a relative lack of ovarian progesterone, but there is also an increased output of antidiuretic hormone (ADH) by the posterior pituitary gland.

Hormonal treatment may be helpful, but the physiotherapist has a role in helping women to understand the condition and to consider ways of adjusting the stress levels being placed on the body, both generally and at particular times. The Mitchell method of relaxation should be taught.

Dysfunctional uterine bleeding

Dysfunctional uterine bleeding (DUB) describes abnormal uterine bleeding not due to organic disease of the genital tract. It is one of the most frequently encountered conditions in gynaecology, can occur at any age and is not one disease but a category of diseases (Dewhurst, 1981). It is thought by some to be due to endocrine dysfunction. For example, girl infants may menstruate in the first weeks of life, probably as a result of no longer receiving placental oestrogens. All cases must be thoroughly investigated and if necessary reinvestigated; for example, anaemia may be the cause or the effect of menorrhagia, and malignant disease may become unmasked. A physiotherapist's role may simply be to encourage a further consultation or second opinion.

Backache and abdominal pain

Women with gynaecological conditions frequently assume that this is also the source of their back pain. This is not always so, and much needless additional suffering could be avoided by appropriate physiotherapeutic assessment and care. However, back and abdominal pain, particularly chronic pain of gradual onset, may have a direct gynaecological origin (Fig. 9.3); and certainly gynaecological pain may coexist with pain from the back and is a late symptom of malignant disease. Over the abdomen, true gynaecological pain rarely extends above the anterior superior iliac spines; when of uterine origin it may radiate to the anterior aspect of the thighs. Pain may be exacerbated by abdominal pressure over the site of the lesion. Posteriorly it is usually located over the upper half of the sacrum and may extend laterally to the glutei. By involving lymphatic nodes around the sacral plexus, cervical cancer may cause pain radiating down the back of the legs. Backache associated with uterine prolapse is relieved by lying down; it becomes more severe on prolonged standing and as the day progresses.

The physiotherapist can be an invaluable member of the gynaecological team in helping to analyse the cause, particularly of back pain, and treating it where appropriate. Where pain cannot be cured but must be endured, TNS may be helpful.

Chronic lower abdominal pain with pelvic congestion

Beard et al. (1984) suggested a cause for pelvic pain in women of reproductive age with no obvious somatic pathology; dilated veins and vascular congestion in the broad ligaments and ovarian plexuses were

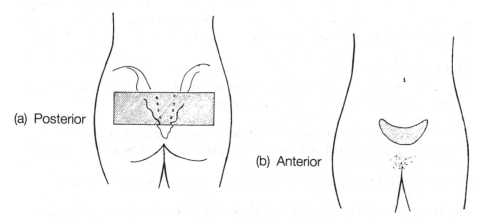

(a) Posterior

(b) Anterior

Figure 9.3 Zones of gynaecological pain.

apparent in 91% of the women in this study. When examining the clinical features in women with pelvic pain and congestion, which was demonstrable on pelvic venography, the following was found (Beard et al., 1988):

1. The women were more often multiparous.
2. The pain was dull and aching with sharp exacerbations.
3. Pain was commonly on one side of the abdomen, but could also occur on the other side.
4. The pain was made worse by postural changes and walking.
5. Congestive dysmenorrhoea, deep dyspareunia and postcoital ache were common.
6. Evidence of significant emotional disturbance was present in 60%.

Alleviating factors were lying down, analgesics, local heat and relaxation.

Although various treatments are currently under trial for this distressing condition, the obstetric physiotherapist who is working closely with gynaecological colleagues may be asked to teach relaxation and stress coping strategies to women with this diagnosis.

Psychosexual problems

The physiotherapist working in the fields of obstetrics, gynaecology and urology must be prepared for clients to want to discuss their sexual difficulties. Some of these may be direct referrals of women suffering from dyspareunia; but frequently the subject will arise following surgery, or during treatment for various forms of incontinence and weak pelvic floor muscles, and of course during pregnancy and following childbirth.

Although sex and sexuality are more openly discussed today, most people have great difficulty in exposing their very personal sexual problems to outsiders. The physiotherapist must respect their wanting to confide in her, provide a non-judgmental listening ear, and, if unable to help directly, should know of further sources of psychosexual counselling in the area.

Female sexual dysfunction is caused by many variables. Hawton (1985) mentions three causal categories:

1. Predisposing factors, which include experiences early in life.
2. Precipitants, which are events or experiences associated with the initial appearance of a dysfunction.
3. Maintaining factors, which explain why a dysfunction persists.

Broadly, sexual problems can be classified as those that are physical and are caused by physical illness, trauma at surgery and drugs; and those that have a psychological origin. Obviously physical and psychological causes will interact closely, one with the other. Sexual dysfunction is a direct cause of disharmony and stress in relationships and leads to great personal anguish; female sexuality is frequently affected by life events such as pregnancy, birth, illness and the climacteric, all of which will be encountered by physiotherapists working with women.

Various authors (Kegel, 1952; Masters and Johnson, 1966; Kline-Graber and Graber, 1975; Gillan and Brindley, 1979) have drawn attention to the role played by the pelvic floor musculature, and particularly the bulbospongiosus, ischiocavernosus and the most medial fibres of the levator ani muscles, in the achievement of female orgasm. Kegel (1952) reported that weak pelvic floor muscles were accompanied by complaints of sexual dissatisfaction, and Graber and Kline-Graber (1979) have reported that orgasmic women had better circumvaginal musculature (pelvic floor muscles) based on clinical assessment and perineometer readings. Stimulation of the pelvic floor using a vaginal electrode to treat urinary incontinence in women has produced increased coital satisfaction (Scott and Hsuch, 1979). All these findings have interesting implications for physiotherapists giving pelvic floor re-education treatments; it could be that anorgasmic women would be helped by improving the strength of their pelvic floor muscles.

Psychological causes play a large part in female sexual dysfunction (Masters and Johnson, 1970), but disease and the oral contraceptive pill may also reduce libido. Dyspareunia can certainly inhibit sexual arousal; its causes are varied (see p. 311) and should always be properly investigated and treated.

General sexual dysfunction

There is decrease in libido, leading to a lack of erotic feelings and reduced vasocongestion in the arousal phase. Vaginal lubrication and expansion will not occur.

Orgasmic dysfunction

Although erotic sensations and vasocongestion may occur, orgasm is not experienced. This may be primary (orgasm has never been achieved) or secondary (having experienced orgasm previously, a woman is unable to reach a climax).

Vaginismus

Vaginismus is spasm of the muscles surrounding the vaginal introitus and even the adductor muscles of the thigh which prevents penetration during intercourse. It is considered to be a psychosomatic condition. Phobic anxiety to vaginal penetration is said to be the most common cause – rarely, though, there will be a physical cause, and dyspareunia, for whatever reason, may play a part in the aetiology of this distressing condition.

Dyspareunia

Dyspareunia is defined as painful or difficult sexual intercourse; it is a distressing symptom and can lead to problems and conflict within a relationship. It is usually described as being superficial or deep, and can be due to infection or allergy, following trauma (such as episiotomy or perineal and vaginal tears accompanying childbirth or gynaecological surgery), postmenopausal changes, congenital defects, neoplasms and poor sexual technique.

Causes of superficial dyspareunia – usually due to a local lesion:

1. Vaginal and vulval infections with such organisms as *Candida albicans*, *Trichomonas vaginalis* or herpes simplex; Bartholin's gland infections or infected cysts.
2. Damage sustained during childbirth – a tear or episiotomy – or gynaecological surgery sometimes leaves scar tissue which can be acutely uncomfortable during intercourse, particularly that involving the posterior wall (Haase and Skibsted, 1988). Spencer (1986) has shown that women repaired with glycerol-impregnated chromic catgut following childbirth were more likely to have perineal pain at 10 days and to suffer dyspareunia at 3 months than those who were sutured with untreated chromic catgut. Grant et al. (1989) in a follow-up study of the original affected women reported that three years later persistent dyspareunia was still being experienced by a significant number of women. It is surmised that the perineal tissues reacted differently to the glycerol-impregnated catgut, possibly by increased fibrosis. Grant suggested that there is no place for the use of this material in the repair of perineal wounds.
3. Menopausal changes due to oestrogen deficiency give rise to atrophic vaginitis or narrowing of the introitus and the vagina.
4. Urethritis or a urethral caruncle.
5. Congenital conditions such as rigid hymen or vaginal stenosis, or a vaginal septum.
6. Inadequate genital lubrication – perhaps due to ineffective sexual arousal or psychological factors. This can be a problem following childbirth, surgery or the menopause, when fear of pain can inhibit the natural increase of vaginal and vulval secretions.

Causes of deep dyspareunia – commonly associated with pelvic pathology:

1. Acute or chronic pelvic inflammatory disease.
2. Endometriosis.
3. Ectopic pregnancy.
4. Retroverted uterus, prolapse of the bladder, uterus or rectum, prolapse of the ovaries into the pouch of Douglas, broad ligament, tear.
5. Postoperative scarring following vaginal repair or, occasionally, a high vaginal tear.
6. Constipation.
7. Neoplasm and its accompanying secondary infection.

Increasingly physiotherapists are being asked to treat patients, particularly postpartum, complaining of dyspareunia. Usually the patient has had an episiotomy or a considerable tear needing suture following a recent delivery; occasionally this wound has become infected and broken down. A raised and sensitive scar may be palpable in some cases, in others there is nothing obvious. Obstetricians offer to excise such a scar and resuture, with a 50/50 expectation of improvement. Understandably women are reluctant to accept further trauma at such low odds. Where the introitus has been sutured apparently 'too tightly', dilators may be suggested.

Physiotherapists are finding that they are able to treat many such patients very successfully using a combination of 'tender loving care', listening, counselling, education, ultrasound to soften scar tissue, and the teaching of self-massage and pelvic floor exercises. No scientific evaluation of these techniques has so far been undertaken but the gratitude of patients and their partners is significant.

There are a few patients who, after childbirth or pelvic surgery, will be found to have fantasies concerning their pelvic floor, fearing trauma and deformity that make intercourse impossible. Examination and reassurance by someone empathetic whom they trust, e.g. the postnatal class or clinic midwife or physiotherapist, insight into the fact that childbirth or surgery may have caused minimal changes, and guidance to self-examination using a mirror is often all that is needed.

SEXUALITY

In pregnancy and the puerperium

The physical and psychological changes of pregnancy have an effect on sexual activity which shows a progressive decline, particularly in the final trimester. Apart from physical discomfort and anxiety about the fetus, medical advice may be a reason for a reduction in coitus, although this is usually only given if there is a risk of pre-term labour, antepartum haemorrhage and premature rupture of membranes. Female sexuality is often adversely affected in the puerperium and there are probably multiple reasons for this, including perineal trauma, hormonal readjustments, fatigue, and psychological causes including anxiety and depression.

In the climacteric

The hormonal changes at the climacteric can significantly reduce sexual activity. Atrophic vaginitis, hot flushes, mood changes and possibly bladder problems can all play a part in altering a woman's sex life. Aging has also been shown to lead to a reduction in sexual interest, orgasmic capacity and coital frequency (Hallstrom, 1980). This report also showed that sexuality is affected by psychosocial as well as by biological factors; higher social class was significantly related to normal sexual activity.

In older age

More and more people of both sexes are reaching their 70s, 80s and even 90s, many are in very good health. Continued sexual activity and enjoyment will be possible for many although neurological damage and/or physical disability may effect it for some. Thus it is important that those caring for the elderly should never assume that regular intercourse has ceased, particularly when arranging accommodation.

It is logical to suppose that for a woman sexual activity with the increased blood supply of arousal and muscular contraction of orgasm can only be beneficial to the pelvic floor, and, by inference, to the maintenance of continence. This contention appears to be supported by unsolicited opinions which have been voiced to physiotherapists by recently widowed women now experiencing incontinence suggesting that it is because they are not now having regular intercourse they are 'getting weak underneath'.

Physiotherapists who become interested in this field should approach the Association of Chartered Physiotherapists in Obstetrics and Gynaecology for information regarding psychosexual counselling courses that will admit physiotherapists.

The psychological and emotional implications of gynaecological disease

Gynaecological disease strikes at the core of a woman's psyche, sapping her physical, mental and spiritual health. The effects are often covert and low grade, undermining a woman to the point that, although she goes through the motions of living, she temporarily or permanently becomes a 'second-class citizen'. In more severe cases she tires easily and may not be able to hold down a full-time job; she is often in pain and irritable; she may not want or even be able to leave the house at times, and becomes moody and depressed; her closest relationships are stressed and her fertility threatened. She finds it hard to talk about her problems and experiences rejection by most people unless they are fellow-sufferers. The partners of such women also have grave problems, for however much they give to the relationship it is never enough. Such a couple's social life is probably restricted and sexual relationships fraught – causing pain, curtailed by bleeding and certainly no source of pleasure and strength. The further psychological effects of gynaecological surgery and incontinence are discussed on pages 326 and 345. The psychological support given to such people has been largely deficient but the growth in recent years of self-help groups has been particularly noticeable in this field; a list of these will be found at the end of this and the next two chapters.

References

Beard R.W., Highman J.H., Pearce S., Reginald P.W. (1984). Diagnosis of pelvic varicosities in women with chronic pelvic pain. *Lancet*, **ii**, 946–9.

Beard R.W., Reginald P.W., Wadsworth J. (1988). Clinical features of women with chronic lower abdominal pain and pelvic congestion. *Brit. J. Obstet. Gynaec.*, **95**, 153–61.

Brentkopf L., Bakoulis M. (1988). *Coping with Endometriosis*. Wellingborough: Grapevine, Thorsons.

Chimbira T., Anderson A.B.M., Turnball A.C. (1980). Relationship between measured menstrual blood loss and patient's subjective assessment of loss, duration of bleeding, number of sanitary towels used, uterine weight and endometrial surface area. *Brit. J. Obstet. Gynaec.*, **87**, 603–9.

Clayton S.G., Lewis T.L.T., Pinker G.D., eds. (1985). *Gynaecology by Ten Teachers*, 14th ed, p.109. London: Edward Arnold.

Dewhurst J.(1981). *Integrated Obstetrics and Gynaecology for Postgraduates*, 3rd edn, p.565–6. Oxford: Blackwell.

Gillan P., Brindley G.D. (1979). Vaginal and pelvic floor responses to sexual stimulation. *Psychophysiology*, **16**, 471.

Graber B., Kline-Graber G. (1979). Female orgasm: the role of pubococcygeus muscle. *J. Clin. Psychiatry*, **40**, 348–51.

Grant A., Sleep J., Ashurst H., Spencer J.A. (1989). Dyspareunia associated with the use of glycerol-impregnated catgut to repair perineal trauma. Report of a 3-year follow-up study. *Brit. J. Obstet. Gynaec.*, **96**, 741–3.

Haase P., Skibsted L. (1988). Influence of operations for stress incontinence and/or genital descensus on sexual life. *Acta. Obstet. Gynaecol. Scand.*, **67**, 659–61.

Hallstrom T. (1980). Sexuality in the climacteric. *Clin. Obstet. Gynaecol.*, **4**, 227–39.

Hawton S. (1985). *Sex Therapy, a Practical Guide*. Oxford: OUP.

Kegel A.H. (1952). Sexual functions of the pubococcygeus muscle. *Western J. Surg. Obstet. Gynaecol.*, **60**, 521.

Klarskov P., Belving D., Bischoff N. et al. (1986). Pelvic floor exercises versus surgery for female urinary stress incontinence. *Urology Int.*, **41**, 129–32.

Kline-Graber G., Graber B. (1975). *A Guide to Sexual Satisfaction – Woman's Orgasm*, p. 21–54. New York: Popular Library.

Llewellyn-Jones D. (1986). *Fundamentals of Obstetrics and Gynaecology*, Vol 2. London: Faber.

Masters W.H., Johnson V.E. (1966). *Human Sexual Response*. Boston: Little, Brown.

Masters W.H., Johnson V.E. (1970). *Human Sexual Inadequacy* Edinburgh: Churchill Livingstone.

Scott R.S., Hsuch G.S.C. (1979). A clinical study of the effects of galvanic muscle stimulation in urinary stress incontinence and sexual dysfunction. *Am. J. Obstet. Gynecol.*, **135**, 663.

Spencer J.A., Grant A., Elbourne D., et al. (1986). A randomised comparison of glycerol-impregnated chromic catgut with untreated chromic catgut for the repair of perineal trauma. *Brit. J. Obstet. Gynaec.*, **93**, 426–430.

Further reading

Barnes J. (1983). *Lecture Notes on Gynaecology*, 5th edn. Oxford: Blackwell.

Brown A.D.G. (1982). Sexual dysfunction in gynaecological and obstetrical practice. In *Recent Advances in Obstetrics and Gynaecology 14*, (Bonnar J. ed.) pp. 283–306. Edinburgh: Churchill Livingstone.

Clayton S.G., Lewis T.L.T., Pinker G.D., eds. (1985). *Gynaecology by Ten Teachers*, 14th edn. London: Edward Arnold.

Useful addresses

Anorexics Anonymous
45a Castelnau
Barnes
London SW13

Association of Chartered Physiotherapists in Obstetrics and Gynaecology
c/o CSP
14 Bedford Row
London WC1R 4ED

Endometriosis Support Group
65 Holmdene Avenue
Herne Hill
London SE24 9LD

Herpes Association
41 North Road
London N7

National Osteoporosis Society
PO Box 10
Radstock
Bath BA3 73B

Pelvic Inflammatory Disease Support Group
Women's Reproductive Rights Information Centre
52–54 Featherstone Street
London EC1 8RT

CHAPTER 10

CHAPTER 10

Gynaecological Surgery

It is an interesting fact that of all the women considered in this book, the warded gynaecological surgery patient, in the UK, is the most likely to be seen routinely by a physiotherapist. The preoperative condition of such patients is very variable, from the relatively healthy to the severely ill. A thorough physiotherapy assessment is essential as far in advance of the surgery as possible, because treatment instituted before the surgery will pay dividends for certain women, for example those with chest conditions, poor posture, backache, weak pelvic floor or general debility. It is highly cost-effective to provide at least one preoperative preparatory assessment and treatment. Patients are generally highly motivated at this time, learn faster, remember more and practise; subsequently they are better equipped to manage themselves, and so need less attention than those who first meet their physiotherapist in a drugged and painful state postoperatively. Physiotherapists must ensure that surgeons and nursing staff are fully aware of all that a physiotherapist is able to contribute to patient care – only then will the patients' best interests be served. Some of our colleagues still see the physiotherapist's role as limited to dealing with problems once they have arisen, and they fail to use a health promotion, 'whole person' approach either before or after surgery.

This chapter considers briefly the three broad groupings of gynaecological surgery commonly encountered by the physiotherapist – excision, repair, incontinence surgery – and reviews the appropriate physiotherapy.

EXCISION OF GENITAL STRUCTURES

Hysterectomy

Hysterectomy is the surgical removal of the uterus, first successfully performed in 1853, although the mortality rate in those early days was about 80%. Today the operation is still ranked as major surgery, and although the mortality rate is now about 0.02% (Open University,

1985), other problems may be caused (see p. 320). These facts should always be borne in mind, for hysterectomy is now the most common of all forms of major surgery and is therefore the most common operation performed on women (Open University, 1985). There are, however, demographic differences in usage. Current figures show that 50% of all American women will have a hysterectomy at some time in their lives, against 20% of British women. Originally it was used as an operation of last resort; patently this is no longer so, and there have been accusations of an epidemic of surgery. What is in question is whether this increase is in the best interest of women.

Hysterectomy is performed for a variety of conditions, e.g. prolapse, menorrhagia, fibroids or carcinoma, and may be carried out by the vaginal or abdominal route:

Vaginal hysterectomy

Providing childbearing is complete and the condition of the uterus is non-malignant, a vaginal hysterectomy is often chosen particularly in cases of uterine prolapse. It is also easily combined with anterior or posterior colporrhaphy (see p. 322) should this be desirable.

Procedure. There are small differences between surgeons as to the precise order in which the stages of the operation are carried out and the approach, but the general principles are described here. Usually under general anaesthesia, the cervix is drawn down, an incision is made in the anterior wall of the vagina and extended to encircle the cervix in the vault of the vagina. This enables the uterus and cervix to be further drawn down and out. The transverse cervical and uterosacral ligaments are divided from the cervix, and the uterine blood vessels are ligated and cut.

Once the fallopian tubes, round ligaments and ovarian ligaments are tied and divided, as near to the uterus as possible, the uterus with the cervix can be removed. The uterine ends of the fallopian tubes (pedicles), the round ligaments, and the transverse cervical and uterosacral ligaments are sewn together and to the vault of the vagina which is closed with sutures – sometimes incompletely to allow drainage. This gives support to the vagina and to the pouch of Douglas so preventing a subsequent enterocele. The lower two-thirds of the vagina is retained where possible. An anterior and/or posterior colporrhaphy or perineorrhaphy are performed if necessary. Finally the vaginal wall is closed, leaving the vagina as a cul-de-sac.

Schauta's hysterectomy is a radical vaginal hysterectomy in which ovaries, tubes, most of the vagina and pelvic cellular tissue are also removed vaginally.

Postoperative condition. The vagina is packed to control bleeding; this is left in situ for 24–48 hours. A supra-pubic or urethral catheter is inserted, draining into a urine bag; micturition is difficult for the first few days due to the general trauma in the area. An intravenous drip is set up for 24–48 hours until drinking and eating are resumed.

Complications. Haematoma of the vaginal vault may occur and may become infected.

Abdominal hysterectomy

The majority of hysterectomies are performed abdominally usually via a Pfannenstiel (bikini line) incision. However, should the uterus be grossly enlarged, for example by a large uterine fibroid, then a midline or paramedian incision may be preferred. The abdominal route allows inspection of other organs and surrounding tissue. A full pelvic clearance (exenteration) can only be performed by the abdominal route. Commonly a total abdominal hysterectomy (TAH) is performed which involves just the removal of the uterus with the cervix. The procedure can be conveniently combined with the removal of one or both fallopian tubes or ovaries, if this is deemed necessary.

Procedure. The abdomen is entered to expose the pelvic organs. At the top of the broad ligament the fallopian tubes, ovarian ligament and round ligament are divided on either side, and the broad ligament is opened to expose the uterine vessels so that they can be ligated and cut. The cervix is excised from the vagina, leaving as much vagina as possible, and from the transverse and uterosacral ligaments so that the entire uterus can be removed. Great care is taken to avoid trauma to the ureters, which run forward below the uterine arteries about the level of and just adjacent to the cervix. The pedicles and ligaments are sutured together as for a vaginal hysterectomy. The upper end of the vagina is closed and attached to the ligaments for support, and the abdominal cavity is closed in layers.

Other types of abdominal hysterectomy.
1. Wertheim's hysterectomy – only carried out for carcinoma, and involves the removal of the uterus, fallopian tubes, ovaries, most of the vagina, associated pelvic lymph nodes and pelvic cellular packing material. There is particular risk to the blood supply to the ureters in this severe operation.
2. Subtotal hysterectomy – the removal of the fundus and body of uterus leaving the cervix. It is rarely performed now because of the risk of the cervix becoming subsequently unhealthy.
3. Total hysterectomy with bilateral oophorectomy – the removal of uterus, fallopian tubes and ovaries. If the patient has not reached the menopause she may be offered hormone replacement therapy.
4. Extended hysterectomy – total hysterectomy plus removal of a cuff

of vagina; a pelvic lymph node may be taken for biopsy. Used for carcinoma which has spread into cervix and vagina.

Postoperative condition. Similar to vaginal hysterectomy, except that with the more severe surgeries a wound drain and a blood transfusion may be necessary.

Complications. Following hysterectomy there is some evidence to suggest that while the operation may solve some problems, others may be generated; backache, stress incontinence, dyspareunia and depression have been cited (Gath et al., 1982; Hysterectomy Support Group, personal communication). Recent research (Taylor et al., 1989) found a highly significant association between persistently reduced bowel frequency and persistently increased urinary frequency. It is suggested that the cause may be autonomic denervation due to trauma during surgery.

Oophorectomy

Oophorectomy is the removal of an ovary. Ovarian cysts can be very big, so a substantial incision may be necessary. Where the cyst is fluid-filled it may be possible to tap it through a small incision. Where there is a benign ovarian tumour, it may be possible to shell it out leaving normal tissue behind; a 'wedge resection' indicates the removal of ovarian tissue including diseased tissue. With a malignant tumour, a decision will have to be made whether to remove other structures as well as the whole ovary, e.g. the uterus and fallopian tubes.

Ovarian cystectomy

This is the removal from the ovary of benign cysts.

Salpingectomy

Salpingectomy is the removal of a fallopian tube. This is rarely carried out on its own except for tubal pregnancy, or where an encapsulated quantity of fluid (hydrosalpinx) or pus (pyosalpinx) has collected within a tube.

Myomectomy

Myomectomy is the removal of fibroids through one or more incisions in the uterine wall. The fibroids are shelled out and the resulting cavities are closed with stitches.

Cone biopsy

Cone biopsy is the excision of a cone-shaped piece from the tissue surrounding the lower part of the cervical canal; it includes the junction between squamous and columnar epithelium, and may extend up the canal as far as the internal os. The diameter and height of the cone is determined by the exact boundaries of the affected zone. This has been used for suspicious lesions or for very localized carcinoma (CIN1 and 2), and is said to be curative in 90% of cases. However, some younger women who have undergone this treatment have been reported to have experienced difficulty with cervical dilatation in subsequent labours. Using a colposcope it is now possible to be more specific, and cauterization, cryosurgery and laser techniques are current methods of destroying tissue.

Radical vulvectomy

Radical vulvectomy is a very severe operation carried out for carcinoma of the vulva, and involves removing all the tissues of the vulva down to bone and fascia together with the superficial and deep inguinal glands and the glands associated with the external iliac vessels.

Radiotherapy prior to surgery

Where there is carcinoma, surgery aimed at excision may be preceded by treatment with a radioactive isotope such as cobalt or caesium, to kill the tissue and thus avoid spread of malignant cells during the operation. The radioactive material is introduced by means of special containers which are inserted *per vaginum*, and carefully packed against the tumour using gauze. It is important to protect the bladder and bowel, which are particularly sensitive to irradiation; the normal cervix can tolerate high doses.

The physiotherapist's role is to teach the patient simple, low-activity exercises, for the period of one or two days when she has to lie still with the radioactive material in position, in order to prevent chest and circulatory complications and to ease discomfort. Slow, deep breathing; strong, slow foot movements; slow, static contractions of large muscles; and gentle arm and head movements are all possible with care. Respiratory secretions must be removed by gentle 'huffing' (forced expiratory breathing) rather than coughing. Such exercises are not only positively important, they also help to pass the time. Because the physiotherapist is usually barred from actually treating the patient while the radioactive material is in position, careful teaching prior to treatment is imperative; and in addition, having established a relationship it is often possible to remind and encourage from a distance.

REPAIRS TO GENITAL STRUCTURES

Colporrhaphy

Colporrhaphy is an operation to repair the vagina.

Anterior colporrhaphy

A cystocele or urethrocele (see p. 301) is commonly treated by means of an anterior colporrhaphy once childbearing is complete. This operation aims to reconstitute the normal anatomy of the area as far as possible.

Approached via the introitus, the cervix is drawn down, the anterior vaginal wall over the cystocele is opened, and if the uterus is tending to prolapse downward as well, the transverse cervical and uterosacral ligaments are shortened. Otherwise the protrusion of cystocele or urethrocele is mobilized, then obliterated and supported in a more normal position by tightening and suturing available fascia, such as the pubocervical ligaments and the fascia over the bladder. The position of the urethra and the bladder, and the level of the bladder neck, are reviewed to ensure that continence is favoured. Finally a longitudinal or diamond-shaped strip of the stretched vaginal wall is excised and the vagina closed.

Posterior colporrhaphy

This procedure is used for rectocele, enterocele and repairs of the perineum. For a rectocele the posterior wall of the vagina is opened, the rectocele is obliterated and supported using available peri-rectal fascia and by approximating and suturing the medial edges of the levator ani muscles. A triangular section of the stretched excess vaginal wall is excised and the vagina closed.

An enterocele can be repaired in a similar way, but in this case excision of the enterocele's peritoneal sac is performed, and the uterosacral ligaments are sutured together to give support.

Perineorrhaphy is suturing of the perineum for example to repair lacerations caused by childbirth which may involve the anal sphincter. A colpoperineorrhaphy is a combination of a posterior colporrhaphy and a perineorrhaphy.

Fothergill or Manchester repair

This repair can be chosen to remedy a uterine prolapse and is suited to a woman who does not want a hysterectomy. Pregnancy is not impossible, although delivery would be by caesarean section. Anterior and posterior colporrhaphy are carried out together with amputation of most of the cervix, for the cervix is often an unusually elongated structure in these patients. The transverse cervical and uterosacral ligaments are also shortened.

Gilliam's ventrosuspension

This is a means of correcting retroversion of the uterus. Through a small incision, or via the laparoscope, the round ligaments are identified and shortened in order to pull the uterine fundus forward. It may well be considered where there is deep dyspareunia.

Salpingostomy

Microsurgery is being increasingly used to repair fallopian tubes.

Complications

Surgery involving the vagina, particularly the posterior wall, has been shown to predispose to dyspareunia (Haase and Skibsted, 1988).

SURGICAL TREATMENT OF STRESS INCONTINENCE

In simple terms, the operations are designed to lift the bladder neck above the pelvic floor so that, when the intra-abdominal pressure is raised, it will act as a compressive force around the outside of the upper portion of the urethra; this will reinforce the urethral closure pressure and cancel out or match the pressure also being exerted on the bladder. Elevation of the bladder neck can be achieved by:

1. Suturing tissue surrounding the urethra to the symphysis pubis, usually via the vagina.
2. Suturing tissue surrounding the urethra to the rectus sheaths or the inguinopectineal ligaments. This is performed using a suprapubic incision.
3. Producing some form of sling (natural tissue or synthetic) which loops around behind the neck of the bladder from anterior attachments to the rectus sheaths or iliopectineal ligaments.

Three possible methods are described below.

Marshall – Marchetti – Krantz urethropexy

Through a suprapubic incision, silk sutures are used to attach vaginal tissue either side of the upper part of the urethra to the pubic periosteum. Sometimes additional sutures are used to attach the bladder to the rectus sheath. Thus the vagina is used to support the bladder neck and pull up the urethra.

Burch's colposuspension

Through a suprapubic incision, four or five sutures are used to attach paravaginal and vaginal tissue on either side of the neck of the bladder and upper part of the urethra to the inguinopectineal ligaments. Thus the bladder neck is lifted.

Stamey's operation

This operation combines a vaginal approach with two small suprapubic incisions either side of the symphysis, to introduce a nylon sling which loops behind the urethra and is attached to the rectus sheaths on either side. A 90% cure rate is claimed (Stamey, 1980). The problems associated with this operation are early groin pain, which improves, and the attachment of the sling subsequently breaking loose, usually requiring reoperation. Recent research (Peattie and Stanton, 1989) reported that although the operation had minimal operative and postoperative morbidity, the success rate in the elderly was unsatisfactory.

Complications

The chief complications following surgical treatment for stress incontinence are detrusor instablity and bladder emptying problems (Cardozo et al., 1979). Sand et al. (1988), reporting on 86 women who underwent retropubic urethropexy, suggested that patients undergoing such surgery should be made aware of the possibility that the operation may cause urinary incontinence due to detrusor instability even if it cures their genuine stress incontinence, and that if they have both genuine stress incontinence and detrusor instability prior to surgery, their chances for an operative cure of both conditions is low.

DEFINITIONS OF OTHER USEFUL TERMS AND PROCEDURES

Colposcope. A low-powered microscope designed for examining the vaginal aspect of the cervix.

Colposcopy. Examination using a colposcope.

Culdoscopy. An endoscope is introduced into the pelvic cavity through a small incision in the posterior vaginal fornix.

Dilatation and curettage (D and C). The cervix is gently dilated and the uterine cavity is systematically curetted.

Hysterotomy. The termination of a pregnancy by what is essentially a mini-caesarean section; it can be carried out at any stage of pregnancy.

Laparoscopy. An endoscope which has a fibreoptic light and telescope capability is introduced into the peritoneal cavity by a small incision in the abdominal cavity, frequently at the lower border of the umbilicus. The abdominal cavity and its contents can be inspected.

Laparotomy. Inspection of the abdominal cavity through an abdominal incision.

Sterilization. Permanent methods of achieving female sterilization usually involve occlusion of the fallopian tubes, by ligature (with spring clips or Silastic bands), by diathermy, or by excision of a portion of the tube. The procedure is often undertaken by laparoscopy through a small transverse suprapubic incision.

Termination of pregnancy. If abortion is decided upon, the earlier it is done the better. It can be achieved by aspiration at less than 8 weeks' gestation, by suction combined with intravenous ergotamine up to 12 weeks' gestation, by an extra-amniotic injection of prostaglandins, by withdrawing amniotic fluid and replacing it with a sodium chloride solution or urea, or by hysterotomy.

Video pelviscopy for laparoscopic surgical procedures. Recently it has become possible for the surgeon to undertake a variety of procedures using laparoscopic techniques through two or more very small lower abdominal incisions. The laparoscope with video attachment is usually inserted just below the umbilicus, a second and occasionally a third incision is used to introduce tiny additional surgical instruments. Clearance of ectopic pregnancies, excision of ovarian cysts, oophorectomy, salpingectomy, salpingostomy and adhesiolysis (division of adhesions) are all suited to this approach.

Menorrhagia has been successfully treated by transcervical resection of the endometrium (TCRE). The whole thickness of the endometrium is stripped from the fundus and uterine body right down to the myometrium. Where a woman wishes to retain some monthly bleeding, a small portion of endometrium is retained around the endocervical canal.

The advantages of these new techniques are:

1. Small incisions.
2. Reduced surgical trauma and subsequent adhesion formation.
3. Reduced requirement for general anaesthesia.
4. Less postoperative pain.
5. Shorter hospitalization.
6. Speedier recovery and return to normal activities.

Consequently patients treated in this way are far less likely to require physiotherapy than those treated conventionally.

PHYSIOTHERAPY CARE OF PATIENTS UNDERGOING GYNAECOLOGICAL SURGERY

The amount of physiotherapy care required by such patients varies widely with the condition and age of the patient and with the severity of the surgery. In this area of surgery it is particularly important for the physiotherapist to have good communication with the surgeons and to read the operation records carefully in order to know exactly what was found and what was done – ideally physiotherapists should go to theatre regularly to keep up to date with procedures. Each operation is individual, and it is necessary to know (for example) following hysterectomy, whether the ovaries were removed as well, or following a repair, that the available fascia was rather thin and atrophic.

The psychological aspects of gynaecological surgery

The physiotherapist working in the gynaecological surgical ward needs to be particularly aware of the fact that the psychological reactions of a patient coming for surgery can vary greatly, may be very complex and may involve the deepest aspect of her relationship with her partner, and also his fears and sometimes those of her family and friends. For example, unlike the removal of an organ such as the appendix, the prospect of the loss of the uterus can be accompanied by a wide range of emotions. While there are certainly some women who welcome the operation as a relief from the troublesome symptoms of menorrhagia, the pain of endometriosis or the threat of yet another pregnancy, there will be others who see a hysterectomy as the end of their femininity and their role as a mother. If the surgery is to be carried out because of malignancy there will be the natural accompaniment of anxiety and fear affecting the whole family as to the eventual outcome. Some may fear depression which is often reported by women following hysterectomy whether the ovaries were removed or not (Gath et al., 1982).

Women who are to have repair operations for prolapse or stress incontinence will look forward hopefully to relief from the dragging discomfort or pad wearing and being socially restricted, but on the other hand will fear being 'tied too tight' or failing to regain the desired urinary control. The partners of these women may find it impossible to understand, let alone to articulate, their mixed-up feelings, and therefore they simply are unable to be the needed 'tower of strength' – as another man proposes to violate that intimate and special part of their woman. Occasionally one comes across a woman whose friends and family do not even know she is in hospital.

Postoperatively the situation is equally unpredictable; some women will be glad to have the procedure over and be content to face the consequences, others will be suddenly overwhelmed. Whatever the reaction both preoperatively and postoperatively it is often the physiotherapist who seems to be the only person with the time, sympathy and empathy to listen, talk, explain and draw out otherwise unexpressed worries and questions.

PREOPERATIVE PHYSIOTHERAPY

It is usual for women to be admitted to hospital at least one day before major abdominal surgery. To enable the physiotherapist to give the most effective care postoperatively, at least one preoperative session should be arranged to take place in a calm, unhurried environment. It will comprise assessment, instruction and, where necessary, treatment.

Assessment and treatment probably need to be made on an individual basis; they also serve to introduce the physiotherapist to the patient, and begin to build a good working relationship. However, in some units in the UK the basic instruction relating to the actual operation and the subsequent physiotherapy care is carried out where possible with a group of patients. This is more cost-effective for the physiotherapist and has considerable advantages in terms of camaraderie and support for those in the group.

Preoperatively patients are generally highly motivated, cooperate fully, appreciate the positive use of the waiting time, and welcome the opportunity for questions and sharing of their fears.

Assessment

Before seeing the patient the physiotherapist should obtain a clear impression from the notes of the patient's general medical condition and the specific reason for surgery. Where carcinoma is suspected or has already been confirmed, it is essential to be aware of the patient's level of knowledge. Assessment is directed towards establishing the patient's present physical state; for such patients this is highly variable, and the age range is very wide. It is helpful to know whether the patient has ever had surgery before.

The following check list may be useful:

1. General physical condition – any evidence of deformities, joint limitation or disease that may influence care or recovery.
2. General mobility – any joint limitation or muscle weakness that could additionally limit mobility postoperatively, any assistance needed at this stage with moving about the bed, dressing, etc.
3. Chest – quality of air entry and chest expansion, any secretions, whether the patient smokes or has recently stopped.
4. Circulation – any evidence of circulatory problems.
5. Any special potential physical problems – e.g. prolonged sitting causes backache.
6. Any special concerns of the patient – the physiotherapist is often the person to whom patients unburden themselves, questions are asked and fears expressed. There may be tears. Instant reassurance and comfort must always be given; however, within a particular gynaecological ward team there will be unwritten conventions, for example as to who discusses malignancy with a patient, so a physiotherapist will be aware of these and where necessary ensure that the patient is referred to the best person.

Given several days – or better still, weeks – the physiotherapist is able to improve the patient's physical condition for surgery as far as possible. It is important to ensure that the chest is clear and ventilating well, and that the patient is as mobile, strong and rested as they can be. Regrettably there is rarely the opportunity for this degree of preparatory treatment. However, in some units in the UK women with prolapse or continence problems on the surgical waiting list are referred for physiotherapy treatment in the interim. This enables a full assessment, instruction and appropriate treatment to take place within a realistic timetable. For some women with mild prolapse or stress incontinence, such treatment may obviate the need for surgery (Klarskov et al., 1986; Tapp et al., 1989).

Instruction and preparation

The patient should have a simple but correct impression of what is going to be done; usually this instruction is given by the surgeon or the surgeon's assistant, and the anaesthetist may also visit the patient. However, the patient's understanding should be checked and may be reinforced with an illustrated leaflet, e.g. *Hysterectomy and Vaginal Repair* (Haslett and Jennings, 1988). Patients should also be encouraged to become involved in their own recovery by having a clear understanding of the ways they can help themselves, particularly in the first two or three postoperative days.

The chest. The patient should understand the effects of a general anaesthetic, be able to perform slow, relaxed, deep lower costal, diaphragmatic and posterior basal breathing in crook half-lying without using the accessory muscles, be able to 'huff' and understand its use, be able to cough firmly and know how to position and hold an incision to cough. Patients undergoing surgery using a vaginal approach will need to support the perineum. Stopping or reducing smoking must be discussed.

Probably the most useful piece of advice will prove to be that forward lean sitting with feet and knees apart, with a soft pillow across the thighs and supporting the abdomen, and with the shoulders as near to the knees as possible, is the most pain-free position to cough. This can be achieved sitting over the side of the bed or in a chair (see Fig. 7.10, p. 264).

Circulation. The patient should understand the importance of slow deep breathing, full-range ankle movements (and later of hip and knee movements) to increase the venous return, and that lying and sitting still has the opposite effect. She should also appreciate that sitting with the full weight on the buttocks reduces circulation over the ischial tuberosities and can cause soreness, be able to perform gluteal contractions and change weight from buttock to buttock.

Following pelvic surgery there is a particular predisposition to deep vein thrombosis (DVT) and pulmonary embolism as a result of possible pressure and trauma to the pelvic vasculature, in addition to the normal enhancement of the clotting mechanism caused by the actual surgery and bleeding.

Bed mobility and independence. Movement in bed postoperatively is permitted and desirable, and there are huge advantages in being even partly independent for such needs as moving up the bed after slipping down, lying down from sitting, turning on to the side, and getting in and out of bed; the patient should practise ways of doing these things.

It is important for patients to be shown how to be comfortable in side lying, using a pillow under the top knee and under the lower abdomen for support when resting and sleeping. Most people normally sleep on the side, and sleep best in this position.

Pelvic floor contractions. The patient must understand and be able to perform pelvic floor contractions. It is always easier to learn pelvic floor contractions prior to surgery than afterwards, even when the surgery does not affect the pelvic floor.

Posture and backcare. Poor positioning and lack of support, particularly of the lumbar curve and the head, may cause aches and pains.

'Wind'. 'Wind' can cause acute pain. It may be due to air stationary in the gut because of reduced peristalsis resulting from the general anaesthetic, but may also be due to air in the peritoneal cavity, which

takes time to be absorbed. The latter may cause referred pain in the right shoulder. The patient should be taught to pelvic tilt, contract and relax the abdominal wall, rotate the trunk and massage the abdomen to relieve this pain.

Other appropriate exercises. It is sometimes possible to start the general abdominal exercises that will be appropriate a few days postoperatively.

Other patient concerns. What the patient perceives as relevant or an actual or potential problem is every bit as important as anything that concerns the physiotherapist!

Postoperative physiotherapy care

The chief objective of all postoperative physiotherapy is that the patients recover as well as they possibly can in the shortest time and without preventable complications. However, there are two particular aspects for the physiotherapist to consider:

1. The special predisposition to DVT (already discussed).
2. The possible adverse effect of raised intra-abdominal pressure (e.g. when coughing, struggling to get in and out of bed, etc.) on new supportive suturing. This is especially relevant for obese patients, patients with chest infections and elderly patients. Good communication with the surgeons enables the physiotherapist to be alerted if, for example, the fascia available in which to insert sutures tended to be atrophic. In such cases it may be worth adapting treatment and giving more assistance to reduce effort.

Where patients have received the preoperative instruction described above, it is remarkable how little help most need to achieve the required level of activity. If, however, no preoperative preparation has been given then instruction has to be much more immediate, and is slow and time-consuming. A greater degree of assistance is needed because the patient is often drowsy, does not understand or remember what she is asked to do, and is in pain. Initially all patients need repeated help to be well positioned and fully supported when sitting up in bed or in a chair; a pillow in the lumbar curve is crucial. In the interest of safety and patient comfort, getting in and out of bed should be monitored at first to see that it is being done in the best possible way and is safe; positions for sleeping and resting should be reviewed daily. Otherwise, where preoperative instruction has been given, it is often sufficient for the physiotherapist to check with the patient once or twice daily that the chest is clear, that circulatory and other movements are being performed regularly and that the patient is comfortable and as independent as possible. Encouragement, assistance and further instruction on additional activities and progression will be needed, but patients benefit from being given as much responsibility for their own care as they can handle and being given the credit for it.

Further progression

Pelvic floor exercises. Ideally all patients will have learned to contract the levator ani muscles before surgery. Following vaginal repair operations some surgeons prefer to delay formal pelvic floor exercise for a few days. However contractions should be recommenced as soon as possible, even when the operation did not involve the pelvic floor. All women should continue regular practice for life.

Abdominal exercises. Pelvic tilting and knee rolling exercises combined with static abdominal contractions in crook lying will help to ease backache, stiffness and flatulence. Where the incision was abdominal, or the patient's general condition will benefit, some simple abdominal muscle-strengthening exercises should be introduced toward the end of the first week.

Posture and back care. Abdominal surgery tends to produce a protective flexed posture; the patient must be made aware of this and encouraged to sit, stand and walk 'tall'. It is also important to check that each woman fully understands how to take care of her back.

Mobilizing. Most patients will sit out of bed in a chair after 24 hours. It is much easier to get into a reasonably comfortable position to cough once in a chair, using a pillow as previously described. Patients will then be encouraged to walk around the bed, and be helped to the toilet or washroom. The physiotherapist will monitor activity, analyse any apparent problems and assist in maintaining progress. By the third or fourth day repeated short walks are usually possible and beneficial. Stairs should be attempted before leaving hospital if the patient has steps or stairs at home.

Rest. The physiotherapist should be as concerned about the patients' rest as about their activity. It is normal to tire easily following major surgery, yet relaxing and sleeping in an open surgical ward can prove very difficult, and lack of rest can delay recovery. The importance of rest must be emphasized and comfortable resting positions be found; it may be appropriate to teach relaxation. Anxieties are a source of restlessness, and the patient may choose to discuss these with the physiotherapist if given the opportunity.

Postoperative complications

Chest infections. The patient will be given antibiotics. Where there is danger of straining newly inserted suturing, coughing should be reduced to a minimum and 'huffing' used as an alternative. Positioning, support and humidification should be considered to ease the effort of expectoration.

DVT. Prophylactic care of all postoperative patients is essential; those with a tendency to vascular problems should wear antiembolic stockings. Should a DVT occur, anticoagulant therapy will be commenced. If the DVT is in the calf the woman will probably be encouraged to mobilize, but if it is higher up the leg she may be advised to remain in bed. In either case deep breathing and leg exercises should be encouraged to aid circulation.

Wound infection. Occasionally infections of abdominal incisions occur; antibiotics are given and, where available, the use of pulsed electromagnetic energy may be considered.

Incontinence. Stress incontinence is reported (Gath et al., 1982) to be a possible product of hysterectomy, and operations for stress incontinence may not be successful or may result in urge continence. Occasionally a gynaecological patient will experience urinary retention or a urinary infection postoperatively. Patients affected in any of these ways require support and encouragement immediately in coping with such embarrassing and worrying problems. After a full assessment and consultation with the ward team, additional treatment may be appropriate.

Dyspareunia. This is a later complication often of surgery via the vaginal route resulting in lumpy and painful scarring. For further detail and treatment see p. 311.

Preparing to leave hospital

It is often the physiotherapist who is responsible for ensuring that the patient is fit to return home or go for convalescence. It is important to take time to acquire a clear picture of the basic demands that will be placed on the patient, e.g. the number of stairs and the distances between essential amenities, and to instruct the patient carefully and specifically as to what is wise and what is not. A booklet or leaflet reinforcing this cautionary advice is essential (Haslett and Jennings, 1988). Jill Mantle found one patient, following colposuspension, planning to resume full care of her heavy and dependent mother immediately on discharge; she could see no alternative! For patients who are wives, mothers or caring daughters it is a wise precaution to insist and check that the family also reads the advice leaflet, so that everyone knows the plan for the next four to six weeks and beyond.

Essential advice following uncomplicated major gynaecological surgery

1. The first two weeks should be extended hospital care, with frequent rests and someone around to prepare meals and shop at least for the first week.
2. Avoid standing, constipation, and lifting anything that weighs more than 1 kg, for four weeks.
3. Continue with the hospital exercises, gradually increasing the number of repetitions.
4. Potter about the house, do only light jobs.
5. After two to three weeks begin regular short walks, progressively increasing the distance.
6. After four to six weeks driving may be considered, providing that concentration is good and there is confidence.
7. At about six weeks return for follow-up appointment with the doctor. Have all questions written down so that none is forgotten. This appointment is a good time to discuss returning to work, and resuming sexual activity. If all is well healed, swimming would be a good, gentle way of increasing activity.

Postoperative radiotherapy

Following surgery to excise malignant disease, patients may have to return for a course of radiotherapy. Treatment in the pelvic region can result in scarring and narrowing of the vagina, disrupting normal sexual relationships.

References

Cardozo L.D., Stanton S.L., Williams J.E. (1979). Detrusor instability following surgery for genuine stress incontinence. *Brit. J. Urol.*, **51**, 204–7.

Gath D., Cooper P., Day A. (1982). Hysterectomy and psychiatric disorder I levels of psychiatric morbidity before and after hysterectomy. *Br. J. Psychiatry*, **140**, 335–342.

Gath D., Cooper P., Bond A. et al. (1982). Hysterectomy and psychiatric disorder II demographic psychiatric and physical factors in relation to psychiatric outcome. *Br. J. Psychiatry*, **140**, 342–350.

Haase P., Skibsted L. (1988). Influence of operations for stress incontinence and/or genital descensus on sexual life. *Acta Obstet. Gynaecol. Scand.* **67**, 659–61.

Haslett S., Jennings M. (1988). *Hysterectomy and Vaginal Repair*. Beaconsfield: Beaconsfield Publishers.

Klarskov P., Belving D., Bischoff N. et al. (1986). Pelvic floor exercises versus surgery for female urinary stress incontinence. *Urol. Int.*, **41**, 129–32.

Open University (1985). *Medical knowledge–Doubt and Certainty*, Ch. 7. Milton Keynes: Open University Press.

Peattie A.B., Stanton S.L. (1989). The Stamey operation for correction of genuine stress incontinence in the elderly woman. *Brit. J. Obstet. Gynaec.*, **96**, 1983–6.

Sand P., Bowen L., Ostergard D. et al. (1988). The effect of retropubic urethropexy on detrusor stability. *Obst. Gynec.*, **71**, 818.

Stamey T.A. (1980). *Surgery of Female Incontinence* (Stanton S.L., Tanagho E.A., eds.), p.77. London: Springer.

Tapp A.J.S., Hills B., Cardozo L.D. (1989). Randomised study comparing pelvic floor physiotherapy with the Burch colposuspension. *J. Neurourology and Urodynamics*, **8**, (4), 356–357.

Taylor T., Smith A.N., Fulton P.M. (1989). Effect of hysterectomy on bowel function. *Br. Med. J.*, **299**, 300–1.

Further reading

Amias A.G. (1975). Sexual life after gynaecological operations, Parts I & II. *Br. Med. J.*, **608**, 2, 608–609, 680–681.

Clayton S.G., Lewis T.L.T., Pinker G.D., eds. (1985). *Gynaecology by Ten Teachers*, 14th edn. London: Edward Arnold.

Hare J. (1987). Pelvic inflammatory disease – new approaches to an old problem, Parts 1 and 2. *Brit. J. Sexual Medicine*, 114, **6**, 164–6, **7**, 192–8.

Melzack R., Wall P.D., eds. (1984). *Textbook of Pain*. Edinburgh: Churchill Livingstone.

Parys B.T., Haylen B.J., Woolfenden K.A., Parsons K.F. (1989). Vesicourethral dysfunction after simple hysterectomy. *J. Neurol. Urodyn*, 8(4), 315–6.

Useful address

Hysterectomy Support Group
11 Henryson Road
London SE4 1HL

CHAPTER 11

Continence and Incontinence

The term 'continence' is used to describe the normal ability of a person to temporarily store urine and faeces, with conscious control over the time and place of voiding and defaecation. Infants do not have such control, but develop the neurological maturity and form the habits necessary usually by three or four years of age. In the adult there is considerable normal variation in the volume that is stored, and in the frequency of voiding and defaecation. A subtle combination of factors contribute to continence so that it is not only the condition and integrity of the specific organs involved and the immediate surrounding tissues that is important, but also the general health – both physical and mental – of the whole person. This chapter discusses continence in women.

URINARY CONTINENCE

Continence of urine is favoured by the following factors:

1. The bladder and urethra should be structurally sound and healthy; damage e.g. infection, will affect function.
2. The nerve supply to the bladder, urethra, external sphincter and pelvic floor must be intact; conditions such as multiple sclerosis and diabetes, and childbearing can cause disruption.
3. The bladder should be so positioned and tethered that its neck in particular is well supported and able to close, and the urethra is straight and not kinked. The angle made by the urethra with the bladder may also be of some importance. Childbirth can cause damage to supporting structures.
4. The bladder should be positioned and supported high enough, so that intra-abdominal pressure is transmitted both to it and to the proximal portion of the urethra. This is referred to by some as the 'pinchcock' effect, and should result in continence being relatively unaffected by changes in intra-abdominal pressure.
5. Bladder size, and therefore capacity, should be normal.
6. Pathological changes are absent in surrounding structures, e.g. fibroids causing pressure on the bladder.

7. The woman should have the ability to move quickly enough to a socially acceptable site in order to void; such conditions as arthritis may make going upstairs to the toilet too painful to contemplate.
8. The woman should be able to prepare herself for voiding and to adopt a suitable position. Where such conditions as rheumatoid arthritis of the hands are combined with inappropriate clothing, or where a person is mentally confused, this may impossible and accidents occur.
9. The woman should not suffer from faecal impaction, for this can cause urinary incontinence. An inappropriate diet, reduced fluid intake or inactivity can cause constipation.
10. The woman should be in good general physical health, alert, and free from depression or serious stress.

Urinary continence is thus multifactorial, but it would seem that there is a considerable margin of safety, in that some damage, deterioration with age or loss of several factors can occur without inevitable loss of continence.

Storage of urine

Urine is continuously being produced and passes, by means of peristalsis, into the bladder in varying amounts – more during the day and less at night – from the kidneys via the ureters. The normal, 'stable' bladder increases its volume to accommodate and store the incoming fluid without a significant rise in pressure until it is fully distended, and without involuntary contractions of the detrusor even with provocation, e.g. a cough, change of position. The actual pressure in the bladder is a combination of intra-abdominal pressure on the bladder from outside and pressure exerted by the elasticity of the detrusor muscle. Because the intra-abdominal pressure normally also causes compression of the proximal portion of the urethra, this in continence terms is cancelled out, and the effective pressure on the bladder is the detrusor pressure; in the filling phase this is usually less than 15 cm H_2O. The elastic ability of the bladder to accommodate an increasing volume of fluid is called *compliance*, and is objectively measured in ml/cmH_2O using the following formula:

$$\text{Compliance} = \frac{\text{volume change}}{\text{change in detrusor pressure}}$$

Peristaltic waves of muscular contraction pass down the walls of the ureters, and their oblique entry into the bladder which closes them when the detrusor contracts (see p. 17) discourages reflux of urine. Urine is also prevented from leaving via the urethra by a considerable closure pressure, about 50–70 cmH$_2$O in premenstrual women and 40–50 cmH$_2$O for postmenopausal women (for men the figure is between 60 and 90 cmH$_2$O), to which the following factors contribute:

1. the elastic connective tissue in the neck of the bladder and urethral wall, placed obliquely and longitudinally, closing the lumen of the urethra;
2. the adhesive force of contact of the moist epithelial lining of urethra walls;
3. the length of the urethra – it varies a little from woman to woman;
4. the steady contraction of the slow-twitch striated muscle of the external sphincter (see p. 19);
5. the support, occlusive compression and lift applied by the slow-twitch fibres and, when necessary, the fast-twitch fibres of the levator ani muscles;
6. the intra-abdominal pressure applied to the proximal portion of the urethra above the pelvic floor.

Eventually, as filling continues, the limit of distensibility of the bladder wall is reached and the pressure then begins to rise. The average bladder capacity is between 350 and 500 ml. Continence is maintained so long as the pressure within the bladder is lower than the closure pressure of the urethra; even in a normal, healthy person there is a point, as bladder pressure rises, at which urethral control could be overwhelmed and leakage occur.

Voiding of urine

The act of voiding is called micturition. It is normally achieved by voluntary, cortically mediated relaxation of the external sphincter and levator ani muscles which is followed, a few seconds later, by a detrusor contraction. In the absence of stressful environmental or other factors, e.g. obstruction, this detrusor contraction, combined with the normal slight shortening and opening up of the relaxing urethra, empties the bladder in a continuous steady stream in a short time. For young women this will be at a rate of at least 25 ml per second, but may be less in older women (Abrams and Torrens, 1979). It is important that a person has privacy and is able to relax to micturate. Lack of privacy may be stressful and result in sympathetic nerve discharges which favour storage rather than voiding. Preliminary data from research (Moore and Richmond, 1989) investigating the effect on micturition of crouching over a toilet, rather than sitting relaxed on the seat, appear to show that the crouching position reduces average flow rates and results in higher residual volumes remaining in the bladder on completion of voiding.

The detrusor muscle is able, by virtue of its intermeshed fibres, to reduce all dimensions of the bladder. This, and the fact that the pelvic floor relaxes and allows the bladder base to descend a little, results in the urethrovesicular angle being lost, so the urethra and trigone are in a straight line. Contraction of the detrusor opens up the bladder neck, and urine is funnelled into the urethra. When micturition appears to be complete a woman may or may not bear down or contract the abdominal muscles to attempt to squeeze out a final drop. Then the pelvic floor and external sphincter muscles contract and the detrusor relaxes. Many women are able to slow or stop the urine flow midstream by voluntarily contracting their pelvic floor, e.g. to collect a midstream specimen. With a strong pelvic floor contraction during urine flow it is sometimes possible to make the detrusor relax. and so terminate micturition without necessarily emptying the bladder. However, several authors (Kegel, 1948; Shepherd, 1990) claim that about 30% of parous women have no ability to contract their muscles voluntarily.

The micturition cycle

The micturition cycle (Fig.11.1) is the alternation of filling phases with emptying that enables a person to be continent of urine. During the filling phase, the detrusor pressure is usually less than 15 cmH$_2$O; at a volume of 150–200 ml the first mild desire to void is commonly felt. This desire must be postponed long enough for the completion of the necessary requirements for micturition, but can be voluntarily postponed sometimes for a considerable period. Eventually as the pressure rises, the sensation of fullness becomes more consciously apparent and persistent, and the woman selects a socially acceptable site and makes the necessary preparations to micturate. Because women have such a

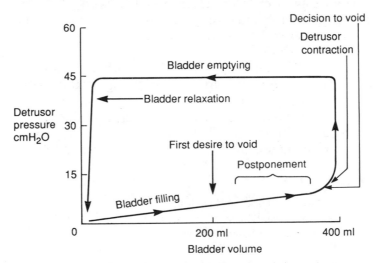

Figure 11.1 The micturition cycle.

short urethra the detrusor is not required to contract very strongly to complement gravity to achieve emptying.

The neurological control of continence

Continence is controlled neurologically at three levels – spinal, pontine and cerebral. Normally these harmoniously interact by means of a combination of somatic and autonomic pathways – chiefly parasympathetic (Fig. 11.2 a,b,c). Urine is stored and micturition occurs periodically, usually four to six times a day.

The bladder wall is richly supplied with stretch receptors whose

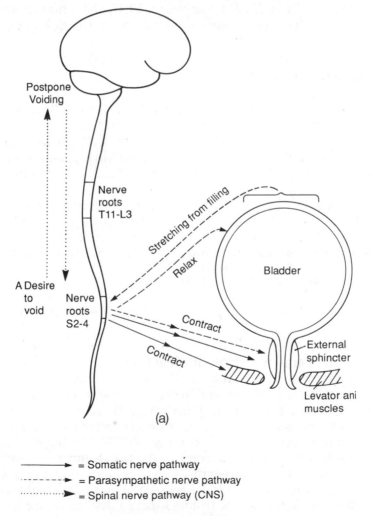

Figure 11.2 A simplified diagrammatic representation of the neurological control of urinary continence. (a) A mild desire to void.

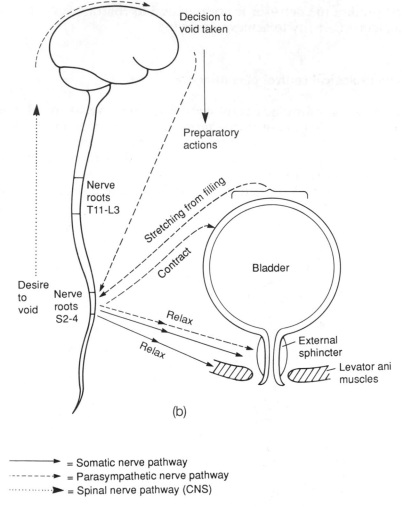

Figure 11.2 (b) Decision to void.

discharge is proportional to the intramural tension. As the bladder begins to fill, parasympathetic afferent fibres convey these impulses via the pelvic nerves to sacral roots S2–S4, to the sacral micturition centre. From there the impulses ascend in the lateral spinothalamic tracts, and are then relayed back to the pons where there are areas capable of inhibiting or exciting the sacral micturition centre. In the early stages of bladder filling, detrusor contraction is inhibited by descending inhibitory impulses to the sacral centre. As the volume of stored urine increases, so does the strength of the receptor discharges from the bladder wall, causing them to be relayed higher to several areas of the cerebral cortex including the frontal lobe, so that the desire to void may be consciously perceived. Thus the cortex now becomes involved in detrusor inhibition and, if micturition is not to take place, it is usually

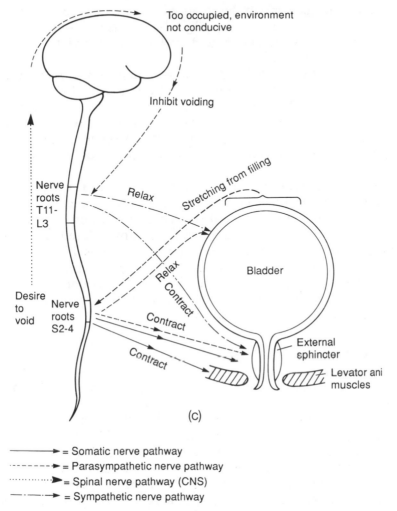

Too occupied, environment not conducive

Inhibit voiding

Nerve roots T11-L3

Relax

Stretching from filling

Bladder

Relax

Contract

Contract

Contract

Desire to void

Nerve roots S2-4

External sphincter

Levator ani muscles

(c)

──────► = Somatic nerve pathway
------► = Parasympathetic nerve pathway
············► = Spinal nerve pathway (CNS)
─·─·─► = Sympathetic nerve pathway

Figure 11.2 (c) Desire to void but environment not conducive.

possible to suppress the voiding urge to a subconscious level again and postpone bladder emptying. Also, sympathetic afferent input via the hypogastric nerves (T11–L3) from the bladder wall, trigone and smooth muscle of the urethra is able to stimulate sympathetic efferent impulses to reduce the bladder contractility and increase urethral pressure. This is probably the mechanism brought into play if the point of extreme bladder filling has been reached and a suitable site must be found quickly, and it can be complemented to advantage by conscious pelvic floor contraction (Hilton, 1989); it is also the mechanism that makes it difficult to micturate in stressful circumstances. At this point it is worth noting that Mahony et al. (1977) described a whole series of storage and voiding reflexes; one of these, the perineodetrusor inhibitory reflex, is of particular interest to physiotherapists who have used the concept quite widely, including it in the treatment of motor urge incontinence. This reflex is said to be the means by which detrusor contractility may be inhibited in response to increasing voluntary tension in the perineal and pelvic floor muscles.

When the decision to micturate is taken, descending efferent impulses are released. In addition to initiating all the preparatory activity, these impulses cause inhibition of pudendal and pelvic nerve firing, so that the pelvic floor and external sphincter relax, and inhibition of sympathetic impulses which, it is suggested, may reduce detrusor contractility and increase closure pressure of the bladder neck and urethra.

A few seconds later the cortex and the pontine centre suppress their inhibitory output to the sacral centre, and enhance excitory output to allow firing of the pelvic efferent parasympathetic nerves to cause the detrusor to contract. With suppression of any efferent sympathetic discharges the detrusor is free to contract and the sphincter to relax. The result is a marked fall in urethral closure pressure, followed by a rise in detrusor pressure and urine flow. Once emptying is complete, impulses initiated by tension in the bladder wall are no longer produced and the whole sequence begins again.

CONTINENCE OF FAECES

As food is propelled through the gut by peristalsis, digestion takes place, and finally unwanted material is delivered to the rectum where it is stored ready for periodic evacuation. The act of emptying the rectum is called defaecation or 'opening the bowels'. There is considerable variation in the frequency of defaecation; for the majority of healthy adults it occurs once a day, often after breakfast. This is because eating and physical activity stimulate fresh waves of peristaltic activity, sometimes referred to as the gastrocolic reflex. The movement passes right through the digestive tract and results in material passing into and distending the rectum. The sensation produced alerts the individual to the need for defaecation. As with micturition, preparations may be made at once to find a socially acceptable site, or the desire may be suppressed and postponed. In the event of postponement the rectum has the ability to reverse peristalsis a little, stimulated by voluntary anal sphincter and pelvic floor contractions so that the faecal material is shuffled back away from the anus.

Storage of faeces

Continence of faeces is maintained by the following factors:

1. tonic contraction of the internal anal sphincter;
2. tonic contraction of the external anal sphincter;

3. tonic contraction of the puborectalis muscle, which passes like a sling from the posterior aspect of one pubis, behind the rectum and back to the other pubis – this has the effect of forming a double right-angle bend in the rectum (see Fig. 1.7) forming a valve (this mechanism enables intra-abdominal pressure to close a section of the rectum (Fig. 11.3), and when the intra-abdominal pressure is raised for whatever reason, the closure will be all the more secure);
4. tonic contraction and absence of 'sagging' of the pelvic floor musculature (any descent of the perineum by virtue of damage or denervation will increase the angles in the rectum and compromise closure of the valve);
5. normal sensation and mental acuity to provide cortical awareness of fullness, which can then be postponed or relieved.

The consistency of faecal material is also of importance. Very liquid stools such as those occurring in infective diarrhoeas or inflammatory bowel disease may overwhelm otherwise healthy sphincter mechanisms; conversely, dry, hard stools do not respond well to peristalsis and are difficult to eliminate (constipation). The movement of faecal material is facilitated by the mucus secretions of the epithelium of the upper two-thirds of the anal canal.

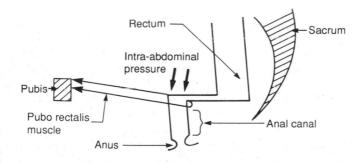

Figure 11.3 Diagrammatic representation of the anorectal flap valve.

Emptying

When the decision to defaecate is taken and a site selected, a relaxed squatting or sitting position is usually adopted. The external sphincter and pelvic floor are consciously relaxed, the latter allowing perineal descent, and so faecal material may pass through the flap valve; indeed any increasing of intra-abdominal pressure (straining) now assists the evacuation. When evacuation is complete the anus and pelvic floor including the puborectalis muscle contract again, and the sphincter mechanism is restored.

Wind or flatus

Sometimes a slightly different sensation of fullness in the lower rectum and anal canal is perceived and identified as 'wind', not faecal material. The mucosal folds of the upper two-thirds of the anal canal acquire the ability, in association with slight relaxation of the external anal sphincter, to allow this flatus through while retaining other material. In older people a reduction in control of the sphincter may result in flatus being passed at inappropriate times, particularly on changing position.

Neurological control of defaecation

The lower half (about 2 cm) of the anal canal is lined with squamous epithelium and richly supplied with sensory receptors so that flatus or faeces in the vicinity cause an immediate reflex contraction of the external anal sphincter, except when cortical mediation allows evacuation. There appear to be no appropriate receptors in the rectum to relay fullness to consciousness (Parks, 1981). It is thought that the stretch receptors within the levator ani muscle are stimulated by changes in the volume and pressure of the distending rectum and this is passed to consciousness via sacral roots S2–S4. The waves of sensation often felt in response to rectal filling are caused by the intermittent contraction of the muscle in the wall of the rectum that the increasing pressure initiates.

At first there is increased excitory efferent activity to the sphincter mechanisms, and in addition voluntary pelvic floor contractions can suppress and postpone the urge to defaecate. However, the sensation of fullness may become more insistent, increasing cortical awareness, and involuntary peristalsis may move more faecal material into the rectum and nearer the anus. Eventually the decision to empty the bowel is taken and efferent impulses, in addition to initiating preparation for defaecation, suppress the activity of the sphincters and pelvic floor musculature, and activate the breath holding and the abdominal muscles for any necessary straining; usually straining reflexly inhibits pelvic floor contraction. Further peristaltic activity often experienced in the rectum may well be in response to the actual movement of the stools and changes in pressure. Once defaecation is complete, the inhibition of the pelvic floor and external anal sphincter is lifted, sometimes with a voluntary contraction of the levator ani muscle and anus, and the closure is resumed. Regular habits of eating and rising in the morning play an important part in daily defaecation. Failure to arrange to be near a toilet at the appropriate time leads to postponement and can result in unnecessary constipation.

INCONTINENCE

Incontinence is usually defined as the involuntary leakage of urine or faeces at unsocial times and inappropriate places. At the outset it is worth remembering that this definition applies only after early childhood; and in many cases which fulfil this definition, it is a temporary state and is hardly considered as true incontinence, being associated with a specific cause, for example passing unconsciousness, infection, trauma or drug side-effects. In addition an intake of about 1 litre per day is recommended (Cardozo, 1990) but many women drink more than this. Caffeine which is found in coffee, tea, chocolate is a diuretic as is alcohol, and may exacerbate symptoms. However, for the sufferers, whether incontinence is temporary or permanent, it is humiliating, distressing, degrading and expensive. The odour and damage to property it causes militate against proper social integration and, especially in the elderly, can even result in people being ostracized and receiving insufficient care from unsympathetic or poorly informed carers. It leads to isolation, depression, loss of self-esteem, and ill health.

Surveys in Britain have shown urinary incontinence to be much more common than faecal incontinence; however, faecal incontinence is more often accompanied by urinary incontinence (double incontinence) than occurring alone. A substantial population study by Thomas et al. (1980), in two London health districts, showed urinary incontinence to be generally more common in women than men. In the population as a whole, 9% of women and 3% of men were regularly incontinent of urine, a ratio of 3:1. The percentages rise with age; for example, regular urinary incontinence was reported in 4% of women aged 15–20 years, 10% of those aged 35–44 years, 12% of those aged 55–64 years and 16% of those aged 75–84 years. This was against 1%, 1%, 3% and 8% respectively for men. No figures were given for those over 84 years old. It must be remembered, when the population is considered as a whole, that women tend to live longer than men (for example in the age group over 80 years there is a ratio of 3 women to 1 man), and this distorts the percentage of incontinence in the older sections. Hence Green (1986) suggests that 20–25% of those over 65 are incontinent of urine frequently, but he also wisely emphasizes that this means that 75–80% of older people are continent, and that in the rest the condition is not inevitably incurable. Thomas (1986) reported finding people suffering both urinary and faecal incontinence who could be cured or whose quality of life could be substantially improved with informed help.

The prospect for incontinence sufferers has greatly improved in recent years. Social mores have changed to allow freer discussion and publicity about such matters, women's magazines and chat shows have played an important part, and the caring professions are working together with greater success to seek solutions tailored to the individual sufferer. The multidisciplinary International Continence Society (ICS) was formed in 1971 and its annual conference has fostered much valuable exchange of knowledge and collaborative research. The ICS Standardization of Terminology Committee has made an important contribution by setting standards in word usage and for investigations, facilitating comparisons of results between investigators. Their latest publication (1989) *The Standardisation of Terminology of Lower Urinary Tract Function* is reproduced in Appendix III. So far the ICS has concentrated on urinary incontinence, but there is a growing body of opinion amongst its membership that it is time that faecal incontinence was also addressed. In the UK a multidisciplinary group called the Association for Continence Advice (ACA) was formed in 1981, and through this and other initiatives nurses and physiotherapists have become much more aware of their potential in the treatment and management of patients with incontinence. Post-registration courses and study days organized by the Association of Chartered Physiotherapists in Obstetrics and Gynaecology (ACPOG) have also helped physiotherapists to increase their knowledge and develop appropriate clinical skills.

Increasingly, UK health authorities are appointing nurse continence advisors whose responsibility is to plan and coordinate the services for incontinent patients and to promote continence. They are advised not to take on a personal case load, but rather 'to provide specialist input to those immediately caring for patients' (Association for Continence Advice, 1985). Many are an invaluable advisory and educational resource for other health professionals, relatives, social workers, home helps and patients. Some, however, have been specifically appointed to undertake routine urodynamic tests, instruct in intermittent self-catheterization, as well as to hold regular clinics for incontinent patients with problems and to run bladder training groups. It is to everyone's benefit for the specialist physiotherapist and the continence advisor in an area to work in the closest collaboration, with direct referral available to each other.

INCONTINENCE OF URINE

Incontinence of urine has been defined by the ICS as the involuntary loss of urine which is objectively demonstrable and is a social or hygienic problem. There is considerable individual variation in what each person classes as a 'problem', and in addition, there are still many sufferers who are too embarrassed to consult their general practitioners or any one else on the matter, or who consider their state to be inevitable. Surveys (Thomas, 1986) have shown that in the community there are those who have not sought help, whose condition could benefit from investigation and active treatment, and others for whom management measures, e.g. appliances, pads or home adaptations, would improve their quality of life. Further, gynaecologists and physiotherapists specializing in the treatment of urinary incontinence have become aware of a group of women who do seek help, but who use complaints of urinary incontinence to mask psychosexual problems. So this whole area of care is a complex one, requiring sensitive listening and caring.

Some useful definitions are given below.

Urinary incontinence is a phrase that can be used to denote a symptom or sign of a condition in its own right.

A normal desire to void is defined as the feeling that leads a person to pass urine at the next convenient moment, but voiding can be delayed if necessary.

Urgency is a strong desire to void, accompanied by fear of leakage or fear of pain.

Residual urine is the volume of fluid remaining in the bladder immediately following the completion of micturition.

Frequency is a term used to denote that a person empties the bladder very frequently. Stanton (1986) defines it as the passage of urine seven or more times during the day or the need to wake more than twice at night to void.

Dysuria is pain on passing urine.

Enuresis means any involuntary loss of urine.

Nocturnal enuresis is involuntary loss of urine during sleep.

Nocturia describes the necessity of rising from bed to pass urine at night. Technically it should be reserved for passing urine at night as a result of being roused from sleep by a strong desire to void. This is different from a habit of always waking at a certain time to void whether one needs to or not, and different from happening to wake up (or being awakened) and deciding to void without real need.

COMMON TYPES OF URINARY INCONTINENCE

Extraurethral incontinence

Loss of urine through channels other than the urethra is called extraurethral incontinence. This may be due to congenital abnormality, e.g. an aberrant ureter draining into the vault of the vagina. Fistulas between the bladder or urethra and the vagina are most commonly the result of trauma at pelvic surgery such as hysterectomy, particularly where the pelvic anatomy has been distorted by endometriosis, infection or carcinoma. In the Third World, childbirth is still a major cause of trauma (see p. 82) and it is not yet unknown in the West. Management usually includes reconstructive surgery.

Urge incontinence

Urge incontinence is the involuntary loss of urine associated with a strong desire to void. The amount lost is related to the intensity of the urgency and the amount of urine in the bladder. There are two main causes of this type of incontinence: sensory urgency due to hypersensitivity of the bladder, and motor urgency due to overactivity of the detrusor.

Sensory urgency

Sensory urgency is due to hypersensitivity of the receptors in the bladder wall, and sometimes the urethra, caused by some pathology, e.g. infection, carcinoma or stones. Thus, as the bladder fills, early and unwanted detrusor contractions are produced either spontaneously or in response to activity. Cystitis is the most common cause of this condition. The patient responds by voiding frequently in an effort to reduce leakage episodes, and this behaviour may even continue after the cause has been removed.

Management consists or removing the cause, whenever possible, and then teaching pelvic floor contractions and bladder training to regain confidence and the ability to hold reasonable volumes or urine.

Motor urgency

In patients experiencing motor urgency, involuntary detrusor contractions occur during the filling phase; these may be apparently spontaneous, or be provoked by such activities as walking or coughing. In the latter case any resulting leakage is sometimes confused with genuine stress incontinence until urodynamic assessment is made. Such contractions may indicate a neurological disorder such as multiple sclerosis, and it is known that they may occur asymptomatically, so they are only considered significant if the patient complains of the sensation or they are associated with incontinence. The term 'unstable detrusor' is used where there is no obvious neurological cause; the condition has also been called 'unstable' or irritable' bladder. It is naturally associated with frequency; it is the second most common cause of urinary incontinence in women in their middle years (Cardozo, 1984) and the most common cause in the elderly. The precise aetiology is not fully understood, but the unwanted detrusor activity can be demonstrated by means of cystometry.

Management of this simple or primary detrusor instablity consists of strong repeated pelvic floor contractions to attempt to suppress the overactive detrusor, and bladder training. Alternatively (or additionally), particularly where neuropathy is a possibility, anticholinergic drugs may be successful, but do have side-effects such as dry mouth and constipation.

Stress incontinence and genuine stress incontinence

The phrase 'stress incontinence' may be used to denote a symptom, a sign and a condition.

1. The symptom. The patient complains of incontinence on stress, i.e. when the intra-abdominal pressure is raised by coughing, sneezing or exercising. This may be due to genuine stress incontinence, but could be entirely or partly due to detrusor contractions provoked by these activities.

2. The sign. An involuntary spurt dribble or droplet of urine is observed to leave the urethra immediately on an increase in intra-abdominal pressure (e.g. when coughing). This test should be performed with a reasonable amount of urine in the bladder, and may need to be conducted standing up, rather than lying down. The patient may also be able to demonstrate how a particular activity such as jumping produces a leak.

3. The condition. Genuine stress incontinence (GSI) is the name coined to denote the condition in which there is involuntary loss of urine when, in the absence of a detrusor contraction, the intravesical pressure (pressure in the bladder) exceeds the maximum urethral pressure. Essentially the detrusor activity is normal but the urethral closure mechanism (see p. 337) is incompetent. Urodynamic assessment is the only reliable way of diagnosing GSI, and indeed urethral sphincter incompetence and detrusor instability frequently coexist.

Genuine stress incontinence

Genuine stress incontinence is often associated with urgency – which is probably a heightened awareness of any desire to void for fear of leakage – and frequency. The woman will try to keep her bladder as empty as possible by repeated voiding, and this in turn must remove the normal healthy challenge to the muscular elements of the closure mechanism, predisposing to atrophy and producing a vicious circle.

How the various factors comprising the urethra closure mechanism interact, and in what proportion, is not fully understood, nor is it known to what degree each may be compromised before GSI occurs. Prolapse of the bladder and urethra, due to damage to supporting structures or associated with uterine descent, may be a cause, possibly due to loss of the pinchcock effect of the intra-abdominal pressures. Atrophy associated with reduced oestrogen and aging presumably attacks the elastic and adhesive factors of the urethral wall. However, weakness and sagging of the pelvic floor are the factors on which physiotherapists have concentrated their attention. This weakness may result from any of the following:

1. trauma to muscle or adjacent tissue, from surgery or childbirth;
2. damage to the nerve supply to sphincter or levator ani muscle, from surgery, childbirth, stretching;
3. weakness from under use (patient may sit around all day, perhaps suffering from depression);
4. fatigue or stretching from over use, e.g. repeated coughing, straining at stool due to constipation, heavy lifting, obesity.

Management of GSI begins with its proper diagnosis, and the assessment of the precipitating factors. The treatment of a chest infection, reduction in obesity, help with a heavy dependent relative, relief of constipation, treatment for depression, encouragement to activity and other general health-promoting care may be enough to relieve symptoms. As a prophylactic measure, every woman should be encouraged from a young age to make a daily habit of pelvic floor contractions, and it is never too late to start. After that the options are surgery or physiotherapy according to the nature and severity of the condition, and to the preferences of doctor and patient. Where there is considerable prolapse with obvious bladder neck descent, surgery will probably be required, although it is not always successful and has its own morbidity (see p. 324).

A recent survey (Mantle and Versi, 1989) has shown that physiotherapists in England consider pelvic floor exercises and interferential therapy to be the most effective physical modalities in the treatment of stress incontinence. To effect the urethral closure mechanism it would seem logical that only patients who can voluntarily contract their pelvic floor and produce a reasonable closure between the two medial margins of the puborectalis muscle will benefit from vigorous pelvic floor exercises. With some machines, interferential therapy can be used to produce a contraction of the levator ani muscle, but there is no good research evidence to show that the limited number of contractions produced in a short treatment session two or three times a week are therapeutic in themselves. It may be that this therapy increases the patient's awareness and so her ability to perform an active contraction of the right muscle, as well as bringing her into contact with the encouraging, supportive and motivating influence of the physiotherapist so that she does her pelvic floor exercises more regularly. These and other modalities are described later in this chapter.

Overflow incontinence

Overflow incontinence is any involuntary loss of urine associated with overdistension of the bladder. Urine is stored in the bladder and has difficulty in escaping. Either the nerve supply to the detrusor is impaired so it does not contract, or the detrusor is so stretched it cannot contract or does so too weakly; alternatively the urethra is obstructed in some way. The result is chronic urinary retention. Eventually the pressure in the bladder rises and overcomes the urethra closure pressure, urine is passed in small amounts as a dribble or spurt, often on movement or effort, until the pressure in the bladder and the urethral closure pressure equate. This leaves a significant volume of residual urine, and the pressure then quickly builds up again.

This situation can arise from neurological damage affecting the pelvic innervation, e.g. diabetic neuropathy; some damage may result in detrusor atonia, e.g. spinal shock, cauda equina lesions. Urethral obstruction in women may be caused by faecal impaction or acute infection in the area, or can result from fibrosis following, for example, bladder neck surgery or pelvic irradiation for carcinoma.

Management consists of removing the cause where possible. Obstruction due to fibrosis may be improved by laser treatment or urethral stretching. Faecal impaction can be relieved and followed by attention to diet and bowel training. Weak detrusor activity may sometimes be enhanced by drugs. In intractable neurological cases intermittent self-catheterization may be taught, or a suprapubic catheter implanted.

Reflex incontinence

Reflex incontinence is loss of urine due to overactivity of the detrusor (detrusor hyperreflexia) or involuntary urethral relaxation in the absence of any perceived sensory desire to void and due to neurological impairment. This condition is outside the scope of this book, but is essentially the result of an uninhibited sacral micturition centre and associated reflex arc. It is seen in paraplegics, and the bladder empties incompletely and without proper conscious control.

Nocturnal enuresis

Nocturnal enuresis is incontinence during sleep, or 'bed wetting'. The vast majority of children who suffer from nocturnal enuresis are dry by puberty; of those who continue with the problem after this, most have unstable bladders (Whiteside and Arnold, 1975). The condition causes great psychological suffering and social deprivation, for example the child cannot stay with friends or go on school trips if the dreadful secret is to be kept. Recently the Enuresis Resource and Information Centre (ERIC) has been set up to assist children, parents and professionals.

Management begins with a full assessment, possibly with cystometry to detect detrusor instability. It may be necessary to change the diet to reduce caffeine intake, e.g. cola drinks. Where it is thought that the child sleeps too deeply to be aware of the desire to void, various alarm systems can be used. It is never a waste of time to teach and encourage regular practice of pelvic floor contractions, which may have some inhibitory effect on detrusor contractility.

Giggle incontinence

Girls, in particular, go through a giggling phase around puberty, if not before. A few find that this results in embarrassing leaks of urine. Where the leakage is considerable an unstable detrusor should be suspected, but it may be that the urethral closure pressure is on the low side of normal.

Management consists of first eliminating pathology; where the results are negative, time should be spent explaining exactly why the leakage occurs and teaching pelvic floor exercises. Not only should the girl practise regularly to build up strength and endurance, but she should be encouraged to develop the habit of contracting the pelvic floor before and while giggling!

Orgasmic incontinence

Because of the arrangement of the female pelvic organs, the urethra and bladder base lying immediately next to the vagina, sexual activity can cause urinary symptoms and lower urinary tract dysfunction, and can give rise to sexual problems. 'Honeymoon cystitis' or postcoital dysuria without infection, is common in young women, and dysuria, urgency and urinary tract infection are noted by postmenopausal women following intercourse. Many women also have the urge to void urine during or immediately after coitus, and some experience actual incontinence. Leakage of urine on penetration is more commonly associated with GSI, detrusor instability as well as GSI can be implicated if incontinence occurs with orgasm.

The obstetric physiotherapist is often the first person in whom the patient will confide about this embarrassing problem. Simple advice to empty the bladder prior to intercourse or to change the coital position may be helpful. Drug therapy, with imipramine or oxybutinin chloride may be prescribed for detrusor instability. The woman should exercise her pelvic floor muscles regularly.

Women who experience this distressing condition may be comforted by the realization that they are not alone; Hilton (1988) showed that 24% of 324 sexually active women referred to a gynaecology/urology clinic experienced incontinence during intercourse – two-thirds of them on penetration and one-third on orgasm.

PHYSIOTHERAPY ASSESSMENT

The patient with urinary problems should be interviewed and examined in a quiet, private and unhurried atmosphere. Fig. 11.4 shows a specimen assessement form which gives some guidance as to the principal information it will be useful to record.

History of the patient's condition and detail of present state

The initial priority is to gain insight into the problem as the patient experiences it, and the specific ways in which the condition is affecting her life. Where the patient has been referred from a consultant unit following full urodynamic testing, it should not be necessary, nor is it a cost-effective use of the physiotherapist's time, to submit the patient to yet another tedious rehearsal in minute detail of her full medical history. The professionals concerned should be encouraged to keep records in a mutually beneficial fashion. More detail is often required on referral forms, and the patient's notes must be available to the physiotherapist for the first appointment. When the patient is referred by her general practitioner, the physiotherapist may wish to construct fuller documentation. Either way, two things are worth remembering; firstly, that retrospective memory is notoriously inaccurate, and thus descriptions of childbirth should be treated with caution; and secondly, a patient's impression of such details as the volume and frequency of urinary leakage may be faulty. The former should be checked against the written record if possible; the latter emphasizes the importance of objectively measuring the present condition if this has not already been done.

Examination of the perineum and pelvic floor

An explanation is given to the woman of the examination procedure and its purposes; these are firstly to enable the physiotherapist to have an accurate knowledge of the condition of the perineum, and secondly to establish the strength of the pelvic floor muscles. It may be helpful to use a simple diagram or model of the pelvis and its contents in the explanation.

The woman's agreement to the examination is obtained and she is then helped to prepare herself on a couch under a sheet in crook lying with two pillows under her head, after removal of pants and tights. An absorbent pad is placed under the buttocks. The perineum is observed first for skin condition, haemorrhoids, prolapse and evidence of episiotomy or previous surgery. The patient is asked to cough and strain, evidence of prolapse, ballooning of the perineum or any leakage of urine or faeces is noted.

Wearing gloves and using a lubricant, the physiotherapist separates the labia; after further observation the index finger or index and middle finger of the dominant hand are gently inserted into the vagina. The texture of the walls, evidence of prolapse and any discomfort caused are noted. The woman is asked to contract the pelvic floor as if to stop leakage or stop passing wind, or to grip the therapist's fingers and prevent their withdrawal. The ability to contract or not is recorded, together with an estimate of strength and the maximum length of time the contraction can be maintained (see p. 359). With experience, judgments can be made concerning the texture of the muscle, the relative strength of the two sides of the muscle and the width between the two medial edges. The sensation over the perineum and of the anal sphincter to touch may also be tested.

Objective tests used by physiotherapists

Frequency/volume chart

The patient is asked to note the time of day and to measure the volume of urine voided each time she goes to the toilet. This is recorded on a special chart over a period of days decided between the patient and her carers (Fig. 11.5). Most conveniently the patient voids into a large measuring jug which may have to be supplied to her. However, some people find this stressful as it may involve holding the jug and crouching over the lavatory rather than sitting relaxed on the seat; this can result in a rather abnormal, interrupted or incomplete micturition sequence (Moore and Richmond, 1989). Patients may prefer to place a small washing-up bowl into the toilet, micturate into it and then pour the urine into the jug, or alternatively it is possible for some to squat over a measuring jug placed on the floor. This process can be very demanding; it may be too difficult to carry out on social outings or even at work because of the need to have the jug available. It requires agility and some dexterity, and consequently it is not suitable for all patients. However it is a test physiotherapists can use, and, for those patients who can cope, it is helpful to keep a record for two to seven days. Where incontinence is associated with a particular part of the menstrual

PHYSIOTHERAPY ASSESSMENT - URINARY INCONTINENCE

NAME   Age: Hospital No:

ADDRESS   Tel: Consultant/G.P:

                                 Date:

Occupation: Notes obtained:

Height: Weight: Target weight:

Diagnosis: Exercise activity/sport

Urodynamic findings:

History of present condition

Onset of incontinence:

Circumstances of loss: cough, sneeze, laugh, walk, lift, jump,
                          orgasm, other (specify) ....

Frequency of accidents: Pads/pants   No. of changes per day

Amount lost: few drops, spurt, complete, other (specify) ....

Type of loss: continuous, intermittent, on stress, other (specify) ....

Urinary symptoms: frequency, urgency, nocturia, nocturnal enuresis,
                         dysuria, hesitancy, post micturition dribble, haematuria,
                         straining to void, urge incontinence, stress incontinence

Frequency of voiding: day   night

Urgency: length warning time   , provocative activities/circumstances
                                          (specify) ....

Fluid intake: type of drinks:

Frequency volume chart completed: Pad test:

Midstream 'Stop Test':   stop,   slow,   no change

Faecal incontinence: Soiling:

Figure 11.4 Physiotherapy assessment form for urinary incontinence.

Obstetric history

Parity:
_____

			Duration				
Date	Type of delivery	Wt	1st	2nd	3rd	Tear/Epis	P.N. exs.
1.							
2.							
3.							
4.							

Gynae history
Menstruation: Length of cycle: No. of days:
Contraception: Menopause:
Coitus: Orgasm: Dyspareunia:
Previous surgery:

Medical history
Other surgery:
Obesity: Bowels: loose, normal, constipated
Smoking: Diabetes:
Chest condition: Blood pressure:
Cough: Depression:
Allergies, sneeze: Other (specify): ....
Drugs being taken:

Examination
Observation: perineum
                   vaginal introitus
                   effect of cough

Vaginal examination: condition
                         cystocele, rectocele, urethrocele
                         uterine descent   , grade
                         pelvic floor contraction: aware, not aware
                         pelvic floor strength: nil, min, mod, strong
                         perineal sensation:

Perineometer reading:
Urine loss without provocation:
Urine loss with provocation: cough, PF contr, head lift, standing-up, jump
General physical fitness:
Patient's assessment:
Dry   ├──────────────────────────────────────┤ Constantly very wet
No effect
on life   ├──────────────────────────────────────┤ Life intolerable

Figure 11.4 cont.

FREQUENCY/VOLUME CHART

NAME:
DAY
DATE

Time	Tick Voiding	Amount	Tick Leak	Type drink	Amount	Pad change	Comments
6 am							
7 am							
8 am							
9 am							
10 am							
11 am							
12 am							
1 pm							
2 pm							
3 pm							
4 pm							
5 pm							
6 pm							
7 pm							
8 pm							
9 pm							
10 pm							
11 pm							
12 pm							
1 am							
2 am							
3 am							
4 am							
5 am							
Totals							

Figure 11.5 Frequency/volume chart

cycle, recording over a longer period may be necessary. In addition on the same chart it is possible to record urinary accidents and the time, type and amount of drinks taken. A woman with normal control does not usually void more than six to eight times per 24 hours and does not wake from sleep to void. Normal volumes voided are 250–450 ml, with the first volume of the day often being the greatest (Warrell, 1986). From the chart it is possible to determine:

1. the actual frequency of micturition compared to the patient's subjective impression;
2. the precise degree of nocturia;
3. whether the patient has an altered circadian rhythm and is voiding more by night than by day;
4. the volumes being voided compared with bladder capacity if known;
5. the incidence of urinary accidents;
6. how much is drunk;
7. how many drinks containing caffeine are being taken per day.

The pad test

The test approved by the ICS takes one hour and comprises the following sequence:

1. The test is started without the patient voiding.
2. A preweighed absorbent perineal pad is put on and the timing begins. The patient is asked not to void until the end of the test.
3. The patient drinks 500 ml of sodium-free liquid within 15 minutes, then sits or rests to the end of the first half hour.
4. In the following half hour the patient walks around, climbs up and down one flight of stairs, and performs the following exercises: standing up from sitting (x 10); coughing vigorously (x 10); running on the spot for 1 minute; bending down to pick up a small object (x 5); washing hands under cold running water for 1 minute.

At the end of the hour the pad is removed and weighed; any difference from the starting pad weight constitutes fluid loss, and this is recorded. If the pad becomes saturated during the test then a second pad may be used. In assessment, an increase of 1 g is allowed as normal to compensate for possible sweating and vaginal discharge.

The critics of this test highlight its stressfulness and artificiality. Versi et al. (1988) showed it to be unsatisfactory as a screening test; it gave a false negative result in 32% of 311 women presenting at a urodynamic clinic, almost two-thirds of whom were subsequently shown to have genuine stress incontinence. Physiotherapists using a one-hour pad test as a quantitative monitor of response to treatment should note that patients with genuine stress incontinence may not have a positive result, and that the reproducibility of the pad test has been questioned (Christensen et al., 1984; Mundt–Petterssen et al., 1984).

Some workers have extended the test to 90 minutes, filled the bladder to a fixed volume and varied the activities (Bø et al., 1989). Recently a 24 and a 48-hour pad test have been devised whereby the patient wears preweighed perineal pads continuously for 24 or 48 hours, removing them only to void or to change to a fresh pad. Discarded pads are placed directly into individual self-sealing plastic bags, and may be weighed immediately by the patient using a supplied spring balance or returned to the clinic. The patient may also be asked to keep a frequency/volume chart, and to record fluid intake and urinary accidents. Otherwise the patient continues with her normal activities. This test has some advantages in measuring the patient in more normal circumstances and over a long period. However, it is hugely demanding and entirely dependent on patient compliance for completeness and accuracy.

Biofeedback

Signals from two electrodes mounted on a vaginal probe can be relayed to a visual display unit (VDU) and seen by the patient and physiotherapist as a brightly coloured trace against a squared graph background. The probe is introduced into the vagina with the woman in a comfortable crook half-lying position. Once the machine is switched on and adjusted, the woman is asked to contract the pelvic floor. Signals from the electrical activity of the pelvic floor muscles are shown in proportion to the intensity and duration of the contraction. This device is at an early stage of development in its use for the pelvic floor, but it is hoped that it will at least be able to confirm reliably whether or not the pelvic floor muscles are being contracted, and also serve to motivate the patient not only to practise but to work for longer, stronger contractions. It may soon be possible to send the patient home to practise, with a vaginal probe and a disc for use on a personal computer.

Manual grading of the strength of a pelvic floor muscle contraction

Attempts have been made both in the USA (Worth et al., 1986) and the UK (Laycock and Chiarelli, 1989) to devise a rating scale, similar to the Oxford scale familiar to physiotherapists. The idea is that the physiotherapist should introduce a gloved index finger (or index and middle finger) into the patient's vagina, ask the patient to contract the pelvic floor musculature, and categorize what is felt. Worth et al. (1986) used a three-point scale and measured pressure, duration of contraction, texture of muscle and whether or not the examiner's finger could be easily withdrawn. Laycock and Chiarelli (1989) proposed a six-point scale (0 = nil contraction, 1 = flicker, 2 = weak, 3 = moderate, 4 = good, 5 = strong) and also recommended measurement of duration of contraction in seconds, e.g. a grading of 2/7 would indicate a weak squeeze held for 7 seconds.

The chief criticism levelled at such methods relates to inter-rater and test–retest reliability; Worth et al. (1986) piloted a series of reliability tests, but the numbers were very small. Properly controlled research is needed here, but common sense suggests that this measure could only ever be a rather blunt tool.

Visual analogue scale

A helpful measure of the severity of symptoms of incontinence as they affect the patient may be gauged on a visual analogue scale (VAS). This technique has been used widely for pain measurement, and is useful in other fields. Such an approach makes due allowance for the variation in what individuals accept as normal or tolerable, and gives insight into the patient's perception of any problem. The patient is asked to place a cross at the appropriate point on a 10cm line, one end of which is marked, for example, 'no leakage', 'no incontinence' or 'no problem', and at the other end 'always wet', 'totally incontinent' or massive problem'. Bø et al. (1989) used a VAS before and after a course of treatment to measure ability to participate in different social activities without leaking.

URODYNAMIC, RADIOLOGICAL AND ELECTROMYOGRAPHICAL ASSESSMENT

Most patients presenting with incontinence will be asked for a midstream specimen of urine in order to be able to detect urinary tract infection, which is commonly associated with dysfunction. Patients may have both lower urinary and upper renal tract infections. Midstream specimens are inappropriate for urethral infection because the urethra is first washed through; a perineal swab may be better but is not ideal. All urine specimens should be as fresh as possible for accurate microbiological investigation. Infection by *Chlamydia* will need a special test (see p. 293). Some patients will be asked to keep a frequency/volume chart for a short time or to undertake a pad test. However, more sophisticated methods of assessing some important aspects of the micturition cycle and the factors involved in maintenance of continence are now available, and have proved helpful in diagnosis, although they are all to some degree invasive.

Cystometry

This test determines the relationship between the volume of fluid and the pressure in the bladder, both during filling and voiding. Two catheters are introduced into the bladder, one to fill it, the other to record pressure – a combination of the intra-abdominal pressure and detrusor pressure. A third catheter is introduced into the rectum to record rectal pressure, which is generally the same as intra-abdominal pressure although muscle contraction of the rectal wall will be evident. This information is interpreted electronically and is available as two continuous graphic traces or on a VDU. The rectal or intra-abdominal pressure is automatically subtracted from the total bladder pressure, and the result, the intrinsic detrusor pressure, is available as a third trace. It is therefore possible to watch and have a permanent record of the detrusor pressure as the bladder is filled with warmed normal saline (or contrast medium if radiological video-imaging is to be used). Any spontaneous detrusor contractions, or provoked contractions when the patient is asked to cough or change position, may suggest bladder instability. As filling progresses the volume at which the first desire to void is perceived and noted – usually 150–200 ml – and filling is stopped at the volume which the patient interprets as fullness. This gives evidence of bladder sensation and capacity, and the general trend of detrusor pressure is a measure of compliance – a steady low pressure is indicative of normal bladder compliance, and a rise of over 15 cm H_2O is abnormal.

Up to this point in the test the patient usually lies flat. Next the patient is tilted to the erect position, and whether this provokes detrusor contraction will be seen on the trace. Standing causes a general rise in pressure in both the bladder and rectum, but the detrusor pressure should remain as before. With radiological screening it is possible to see the outline and shape of the bladder for any hints of pathology, also the level of the bladder base and neck, and whether the neck and urethra are open or well closed. The patient is again asked to cough several times, and both provoked detrusor contractions and evidence of sphincter incompetence in terms of leakage are noted. With video-imaging it is possible, on coughing, to watch fluid being forced into the urethra and past an incompetent sphincter. The patient is then asked to commence voiding, and then to stop and restart midstream before completing voiding. The strength of detrusor contractions appears on the trace; the behaviour of the bladder neck, the rate of flow, the ability to stop or reduce flow, any effort needed to void and any residual urine can all be ascertained and visualized if necessary.

The emotional and physical stress placed on a patient by such a procedure must never be underestimated, and its artificiality must be remembered when considering the results. The test has its own morbidity in that occasionally patients develop urinary infections afterwards.

Urethral pressure profilometry

The pressure in the urethra may be measured in both the storage and voiding phases by means of a microtransducer mounted on the tip of a fine catheter, or by a fluid-filled or gas-filled catheter attached to an external transducer. The catheter is drawn down the urethra from bladder neck to the external meatus during the storage phase, with or without provocative stress, and the urethral closure pressure is measured at several points to give a urethral pressure profile (UPP). It has been suggested that although this is an invasive investigation, it might be possible to develop it to provide a repeatable, quantitative measure of the external urethral sphincter and pelvic floor increments in urethral closure pressure (Shepherd, 1990; Versi, 1990).

The procedure may be carried out during voiding (VUPP) to detect obstruction; in such cases it is necessary to measure the bladder pressure simultaneously.

Uroflowmetry

Physiotherapists have largely ignored urinary flow rate, even at the subjective question level, yet it is quite a reliable indicator of normal detrusor contraction and urethral relaxation. The patient is asked to void, in private, into a toilet in which a flow meter has been fitted. This device measures the quantity of fluid passed per unit of time.

Distal urethral electric conductance

The accurate detection of leakage of urine is obtained by inserting a short probe with two ring electrodes into the distal part of the urethra until the distal ring is 1.5 cm from the external urethral meatus. Passage of urine past the electrodes increases conductivity between them, and this can be recorded electronically, (Peattie et al., 1989).

Electrophysiological tests

For some time it has been possible to record the electrical activity associated with resting and contracting muscles. Considerable research effort has been channelled into electrophysiological studies of the levator ani muscle – particularly the puborectalis and the external anal sphincter, because it became evident that childbirth could cause not only direct division of the anal sphincter and stretching of the pelvic floor musculature, but also injury to the innervation (Snooks et al., 1984). Single fibre density (FD) and pudendal nerve and perineal nerve terminal motor latencies (PNTML and PerNTML) have been measured (Snooks et al., 1984; Swash, 1985).

Electromyography

Conventional needle electromyography (EMG) has been used to examine the puborectalis and external anal sphincter. The fine EMG needle is inserted progressively and the motor unit action potentials in the immediate vicinity of the needle can be recorded at rest and on contraction on an oscilloscope. In both these muscles activity will be expected at rest as well as on contraction. Duration, amplitude and the number of phases of the action potentials of individual motor units can be measured. Normal muscle has a typical pattern.

Single fibre density. A motor unit is comprised of an anterior horn cell and its myelinated axon which divides into a number of terminal branches, each of which serves a single muscle fibre. When the axon or any of its branches are damaged, reinnervation of the bereft muscle fibres may occur by regeneration of the axon or by collateral sprouting of neighbouring healthy motor nerve axons. In the latter case the number of muscle fibres supplied by that motor unit is greater, and the fibre density is said to be increased. In addition, the motor unit activity recorded is of greater length and amplitude, and is polyphasic. The normal fibre density in the puborectalis and anal sphincter muscles is 1.5. It is calculated by taking 20 recordings during mild contraction in various parts of a muscle, counting the components making up the 20 individual motor unit action potentials, and taking the mean (Swash, 1985).

Motor conduction tests

Pudendal nerve terminal motor latency. If a nerve is stimulated electrically, there is a delay before the muscle responds. The latency of response can be measured and is increased where a nerve passes through areas of localized injury or disease, e.g. the median nerve at the wrist in carpal tunnel syndrome, or where there is actual neuropathy. An intrarectal stimulating and recording device is introduced into the anus to stimulate the pudendal nerve and record the response of the external anal sphincter muscle. The latency of the response is measured and recorded on a graphic printout (Snooks et al., 1984).

Perineal nerve terminal motor latency. This is a similar test using a catheter-mounted recording electrode in the urethra (Swash, 1985).

Spinal motor latencies. In addition (or alternatively), transcutaneous stimulation at L1 and L4 produces motor action potentials in the pelvic muscle sphincters and the delay can be calculated (Henry and Swash, 1985; Swash, 1985).

Other tests

Measurement of perineal descent

Perineal descent is recognized clinically by ballooning of the perineum during straining effort. This is measured using a graduated latex cylinder held against the anus which moves on a frame pressed against the ischial tuberosities (Kiff et al., 1984). Using the tuberosities as a reference point, the position of the perineum can be measured at rest and on straining.

Anorectal manometry

Using a transducer, the anal sphincter pressure may be measured at rest and on maximum voluntary contraction.

Pyelogram

A radio–opaque substance is given by intravenous injection and is visible on X-ray 15 minutes later as it is being excreted by the kidney; any pathological renal damage will be apparent. Alternatively a similar material can be introduced by catheter directly into a ureter and so to the renal pelvis, and damage in this area will be seen radiologically.

Cystourethroscopy or cystoscopy

This is an endoscopic investigation of the bladder and urethra to look for pathological lesions which could explain the signs and symptoms.

UNDERSTANDING URINARY DYSFUNCTION

Following collation of the full history and the results of appropriate tests, the physiotherapist must seek to understand the patient's condition and how the signs and symptoms are being produced (Table 11.1). Only then can the best treatment be selected.

Table 11.1 Causes of urinary dysfunction

Signs and symptoms	Explanation	Cause
Storage phase		
1. Frequent desire to void, small amounts of urine passed	Bladder or urethra is hypersensitive	Infection, inflammation or other pathology e.g. fibroid,
	Neurological inhibition of the detrusor is reduced	neurological disorders; alcohol, coffee, tea or cola
	Bladder capacity is reduced Detrusor contracts spontaneously or is easily provoked, e.g. by cough, changing position, cold, water Learnt habit Woman is acutely anxious, afraid or stressed	intake
2. Frequent desire to void, normal amounts of urine passed	Woman has drunk a large amount, or eaten water-filled food Pregnancy Recent childbirth Diuretic therapy	
3. Urine leaks on physical effort	Urethral closure pressure is low Activity provokes detrusor contraction	
4. Uncontrollable urges to void, leaks	Detrusor is overactive (motor) or hypersensitive (sensory) Neuropathology present Urethra, surrounding tissue and/ or innervation has been traumatized	Recent childbirth
Voiding phase		
1. Passing urine takes a long time, flow is poor	Urethra is partially obstructed	Pressure from constipation, tumour, oedema, trauma, inflammation, urethral stricture
	Detrusor is underactive Neurological disorder	Drugs Detrusor sphincter dyssynergia (DSD)

Table 11.1 Causes of urinary dysfunction (*continued*)

Signs and symptoms	Explanation	Cause
2. Woman has desire to void, is ready but cannot start	Stress or embarrassment causes sympathetic inhibition of voiding Urethra is obstructed by a full bowel Acute urethritis with obstruction or pain inhibition	
3. Woman bears down to void	Habit See also (1)	
4. Urine dribbles after micturition apparently completed (rare)	Urine collecting in introitus Urethrocele with a 'kinked' urethra	
5. On standing up, the patient feels there is still urine in the bladder at the completion of micturition and that she may pass more if she sits down again	Residual urine Haste – woman stopped micturition prematurely Bladder so full that urine pooled in ureters and was released when the detrusor relaxed	Uterine descent, cystocele, urethrocele
6. Woman has to press pelvic floor to assist voiding	Cystocele with part of bladder hanging below the level of bladder neck	

PHYSIOTHERAPEUTIC TREATMENT

In the 1940s and 1950s physiotherapists in some UK centres were regularly involved in the treatment of urinary incontinence. They used pelvic floor exercise, often treating patients in groups, and electrostimulation which consisted mainly of faradism. Through the 1960s and 1970s doctors increasingly turned to surgery as the treatment of choice for stress incontinence, and to drug therapy for the alleviation of urge incontinence. Older surgical techniques were revised and new innovative approaches devised. In addition urodynamic and electrophysical tests developed and became more sophisticated, improving understanding of the patient's condition and the accuracy of diagnosis.

In the last decade increasing attention has been paid to the morbidity associated with surgery, and so once again some urologists and gynaecologists have shown interest in conservative therapies. These still basically consist of exercise and electrostimulation. Simple pelvic floor contractions can be taught and practised providing the patient is able to contract her pelvic floor muscles voluntarily. With care a perineometer may be used to give some guide to strength and improvement, and certainly biofeedback motivates women to practise what is unquestionably a very boring exercise. Cones, too, have their devotees; they attempt to provide intermittent and progressive resistance to the pelvic floor. An inflated Foley catheter and a simple tampon can be used to give some biofeedback, and, with tension on them, they provide some resistance. Interferential therapy is now widely used as means of producing a contraction of the pelvic floor musculature by electrostimulation. It utilizes the interference between two medium-frequency currents. An increasing range of low-frequency stimulators is being produced; some of these are cheaper and battery operated, making it a realistic future possibility for patients to treat themselves at home.

It is worth considering the implications for the affected women of the choice between surgery and conservative therapy. There is a world of difference between passively undergoing an operation 'to be put right', and being expected to cooperate over a period of three to six months in a treatment that is repetitive and boring, and that demands a high degree of discipline, perseverance and self-motivation. Many women are simply unable or unwilling to give what it takes; but many more are able and willing if only they are given the benefit of an enthusiastic and specialist physiotherapist. Whether surgical or conservative treatment is chosen, it is important for women to understand that a total cure of their incontinence may not be possible.

Pelvic floor contraction

Before instructing a woman in how to use pelvic floor contractions to increase the strength and endurance of the levator ani muscles, it is imperative to establish, beyond a shadow of a doubt, whether or not the woman is able voluntarily to activate the correct muscles. Contractions of the gluteal, hip adductor and or abdominal muscles, breath holding and even bearing down have been confused with contractions of the pelvic floor muscles. The ability to contract the levator ani muscles should ideally be established objectively by the physiotherapist, as part of the initial examination. If, following careful instruction, the woman is unable to produce a voluntary contraction, immediate steps should be taken to teach her to do so, using whatever additional means are appropriate e.g. electrical stimulation, cones, Foley catheter or perineometer. Pelvic floor contractions can be objectively confirmed by:

1. vaginal examination by physiotherapist;
2. self-examination by patient;
3. hand on perineum by physiotherapist;
4. hand on perineum by patient;
5. observation of perineum by physiotherapist;

6. observation of perineum by patient using a mirror;
7. perineometer;
8. stop and start midstream urine;
9. using a Foley catheter or tampon inserted into vagina and applying traction to detect gripping during contraction;
10. asking partner at intercourse;
11. EMG;
12. biofeedback.

Teaching pelvic floor contractions for regular practice

Teaching pelvic floor contractions, for the patient to practise regularly without aids, is one of the most difficult tasks required of the physiotherapist, probably because the muscles are not directly visible to either patient or therapist, and demonstration cannot be used.

Visualization. A large, simple diagram or model of the pelvis, pelvic organs and the levator ani muscles, is helpful to show the three openings, and the lifting and gripping effect of the muscle action.

Language. Throughout the teaching session the language must be chosen specifically for each individual patient, employing words and images that are familiar and easily understood. Ask the patient to imagine:
• stopping passing water/urine
• stopping passing/breaking wind
• stopping yourself 'blowing off'/farting
• stopping diarrhoea/shit/'poo'/'crap'
• stopping doing a 'pee'/'wee'
• stopping yourself 'having an accident'/'bursting'
• trying to stop yourself 'leaking'/'wetting your pants'
• gripping to stop a tampon falling out
• gripping your partner's penis/willy

Starting position. Pelvic floor contractions can be performed in any position, but sitting on a hard chair leaning forward to support forearms on knees, with thighs and feet apart, is a useful initial position. It is a non-threatening, unexposed position; the perineum is against the chair seat so there is some perineal sensory stimulus feedback, and a change of sensation is usually apparent over the pelvic outlet on contraction.

Concept. Women must appreciate that the pelvic floor hammock works as a single unit and that it is not usually possible to close the three openings individually. However, when teaching pelvic floor contractions it is helpful to focus attention on one opening at a time.

Example of instruction to a patient. 'Are you comfortable on that chair? Now can you sit like this? Legs apart, arms on legs. Because you are not used to trying to work your pelvic floor muscles separately you may find yourself clenching your buttocks, pulling your thighs together or drawing in your tummy and holding your breath instead, or as well. So start by trying to relax all those other muscles. Now, although the pelvic floor muscles work together, let's think first about the back passage. Imagine you want to pass wind or empty your bowels; close shut your back passage as tightly as possible. Now let go. Try twice more. What do you feel? Now let's imagine you have a full bladder, there are no toilets available and you must wait! Squeeze shut your front passage tight. Now let go. Try twice more. What does it feel like? Now think about your vagina, pretend you have a tampon slipping out and are trying to grip it. What can you feel? Try twice more then have a rest.

'Now let's try something different. Imagine your pelvic floor is like a lift standing on the ground floor. Contract your muscles underneath and take your lift up to the first floor, closing shut all three passages. What can you feel? Now let go. Try again and let go. Now try a cough; what happens to your pelvic floor? Yes, it goes down into the basement! Now pull up your pelvic floor, hold it tight and give another cough. Did it still go into the basement? That would be a good way of trying to stay dry when you cough or sneeze, or of helping you 'hold on' when you get the urge to pee.

'One more thing; there are two ways of working your pelvic floor muscles – quickly and slowly. First try a quick squeeze and let go, try that a few times. Now close all the openings tightly shut and take your pelvic floor up and in, hold that for as long as you can – now let go. Try once more, how long can you hold it before it starts to give?'

Duration and repetition of contraction. At the first session, the patient is asked to hold a contraction strongly until she feels the muscle weakening, and the duration is timed and recorded. Then long, strong contractions are repeated one after the other with a brief break between, each held for as long as possible, to see how many contractions can be performed before serious fatigue sets in, and the number is recorded. Patients should be warned that there may a little variation from day to day, according to the time of day, and even the time of the month if they are premenopausal, but that overall an increase in duration and in the number of contractions possible is the objective and is the expected reward for practising regularly.

Checking for other muscle contractions. The physiotherapist should check for the absence of contraction in the gluteal, hip adductor and abdominal muscles, and that the patient is neither holding her breath nor bearing down.

Confirmation of a pelvic floor contraction. Even when this has already been done as part of the examination procedure, it is important to repeat, perhaps by another method (see p. 367), for it is critical that the right muscles are contracting. If there is uncertainty, or where the contraction is very weak, electrostimulation should be considered. The patient should be encouraged to feel her own pelvic floor vaginally, perhaps in or just after a bath.

General advice. The patient is advised to contract her pelvic floor before any of the events which, for her, normally trigger leakage (e.g. coughing, sneezing, laughing, nose blowing, lifting, running or jumping) or a strong desire to void. This technique is called counter-bracing. The patient should also understand that it is possible to exercise the pelvic floor in a variety of situations, for example while queuing, telephoning, driving, on the bus or train, watching television or waiting for the kettle to boil.

Number of practice sessions. In discussion with the patient a plan of daily practice sessions is made. This must be realistic and attainable as well as being agreeable to the patient. Some people are happy to exercise 'a little and often' (hourly or half hourly), others prefer two or three intensive sessions per day.

Contractions. Women should be encouraged to do both fast and slow muscle contractions. Bø et al. (1989) showed improvement in patients with stress incontinence using 8–12 groups of contractions, each of which consisted of 1 contraction held for as long as possible followed by 3 or 4 short ones. This regimen was repeated three times each day and contractions were carried out in a variety of positions. The greatest improvement was found in those patients who also attended the clinic for practice sessions which included general exercise.

Reassessment and progression. Each time the patient attends for treatment a reassessment should be made. If good progress is being made a repeat examination by the physiotherapist is not necessary on each visit. If there is no improvement or there is doubt as to whether the right muscles are being used, a repeat examination is advisable.

As with all re-education the patient needs regular encouragement to increase the length, intensity and number of repeat contractions. A variety of positions should be used, working toward those in which leakage used to occur; pelvic floor contractions will be more difficult in some positions, e.g. squatting. As the woman regains reliable continence, other activities designed to develop physical fitness should be suggested, such as walking, swimming or dancing. Women must appreciate that the best hope for maintaining improvement is to continue with their programme.

Attendance for treatment

It has been suspected for many years by physiotherapists that, given such a dull, boring and repetitive programme to follow, most patients start with great enthusiasm and complete the assigned number of contractions for the first few days; but if they are left to follow the programme uncoached, the daily number of contractions drops in most cases rather than increases. Research by Thow (personal communication) seems to support this exactly, and others (Wilson et al., 1987; Bø et al., 1989) have shown that patients who are sent away to practise at home on their own experience less improvement than those who attend the physiotherapy department regularly. In response to an open question in a recent survey concerning physiotherapeutic services for stress incontinence (Mantle and Versi, 1989), physiotherapists strongly indicated that they considered the patient's motivation to be critical to outcome; yet it is difficult to maintain motivation alone. Could it be that the apparent benefit sometimes seen from the addition of regular electrical muscle stimulation to the treatment regimen has more to do with the recharging of the patient's determination to persevere with the exercises than anything else?

To derive the maximum improvement possible from a programme of pelvic floor exercises it will need to be continued for three to six months. The woman should be seen by the physiotherapist after no more than a week for a thorough check and further instruction if necessary. Initially appointments should be frequent to provide regular reinforcement and encouragement. Thereafter they can be more widely spaced in order to develop the woman's independence and responsibility for her own therapy. Group treatment sessions can be very cost-effective for the therapist as well as therapeutic and pleasant for women. A friendly telephone call periodically can be very supportive and is a valuable method of maintaining contact with women who are unable to make regular visits to their physiotherapist.

Perineometer

In 1948 Kegel described a pneumatic device which he used to measure pressure within the vagina and to motivate women to practise pelvic floor exercises. A compressible air-filled rubber portion (sensor) was inserted into the vagina by the woman and attached by rubber tubing to a manometer. The woman then contracted her pelvic floor several times and noted the highest reading on the dial and the length of time for which she could hold a contraction. Since then many attempts have been made to produce a model which reliably records vaginal pressure and is cheap, strong and acceptable to women. The Bourne perineometer is currently available in 26% of UK health authority areas (Mantle and Versi, 1989), but is expensive so patients are rarely able to have one at home. The reading tends to be influenced by changes in the patient's position and in intra-abdominal pressure, so test–retest and inter-test reliability is uncertain. Further, heightened public awareness of the risks of cross-infection have made some women reluctant to use the communal perineometer, despite the fact that the vaginal sensor is covered with a fresh condom for each use, and that it is also soaked in glutaraldehyde after each use.

So at the moment an instrument that reliably records pelvic floor muscle strength has not been marketed, but those devices that are available are useful for biofeedback, to provide motivation. They should not be used for women with very weak muscles who may find the results of their efforts depressing. Use needs expert supervision to ensure that intra-abdominal pressure is not being measured rather than a pelvic floor contraction; as many factors as possible should be held constant at each use (e.g. position, time of day), and increases or decreases in the readings on the dial should be interpreted cautiously.

Foley catheter or tampon

An inflated cuffed catheter is used by some physiotherapists, apparently successfully (Laycock and Green, 1988), as a means of providing a woman with biofeedback for pelvic floor contractions. The suggestion is that not only is there stimulus from the presence of the catheter in the vagina and threat of withdrawal, but that gentle traction can be applied to weight and stretch the pelvic floor muscles, and be correlated with a voluntary contraction to act as a resistance. An inflated cuffed catheter (e.g. Foley catheter) is inserted into the vagina, preferably by the woman herself. She is then instructed to tense her pelvic floor muscles to resist withdrawal of the catheter by the physiotherapist. Traction is gentle at first but is increased according to the tension the patient is able to develop. In addition attempts may be made to retain the catheter in position during those activities that might cause urinary leakage, e.g. coughing, bending or lifting, thus reinforcing the advice to contract the pelvic floor prior to such activities.

If this approach is effective, it has the advantage of there being a realistic possibility for each patient to have her own catheter for practice at home. Women can be taught to apply their own traction, and there is no doubt that for some the technique will motivate practice. To avoid infection the catheter must be kept clean; in the home it should be washed with soap or detergent, rinsed very thoroughly under running water, and dried with great care after each use. The catheter cuff needs to be inflated to the right degree for each individual: this is a personal judgement, there are no precise guidelines; air or water may be used, water making it a little heavier.

A tampon has been used in a similar way, reportedly to good effect, and has the additional advantages of being a familiar item to most women, and a fresh one can be used for each practice.

Vaginal cones

In the rehabilitation of muscle, resistance in the form of weights has long been used to increase strength and endurance. Attempts to find a means of applying graded resistance to the pelvic floor musculature led to the development and marketing of cones in 1988. These consist of a series of five to nine small, progressively weighted cylinders, ranging from 10 g to 100 g. They are made of lead coated with plastic, and are about the size of a tampon with a nylon string attached to one slightly tapered end. The manufacturers claim that 'the cone acts by forcing downwards on the pelvic floor muscles, and this feeling of losing the cone makes the muscles contract around it to keep it in' (Femina, 1989). Presumably the intention is first to apply weight to the superior surface of the pelvic floor to attempt to activate more motor units to support the cone, and secondly to increase a woman's awareness of her ability to contract the pelvic floor muscles voluntarily to constrict the lower end of the vagina.

Selecting the appropriate cone. The lightest cone is inserted into the vagina by the woman while in the semi-squatting or half lying position, or standing with one foot up on a chair, with the cone's pointed end and string downwards. The cone must be inserted far enough to stand vertically above the level of the pelvic floor. Once the cone is in position the patient walks around. If the cone can be retained for one minute, the patient progresses on to the next cone which is slightly heavier, and so on until a cone slips out in under one minute. The heaviest cone that can be retained for one minute is used for exercise.

Treatment sessions. Twice a day the patient inserts a cone and walks around for 15 minutes. If the cone slips down it is pushed back up. Once the cone can be retained for 15 minutes without slipping, progress is made to the next cone. A course of one month is recommended.

Discussion. The publicity promoting this product suggests that each woman should have her own set of cones to avoid cross-infection; because of the plastic coating, temperatures above 60°C must not be used (which prohibits autoclaving), and the effect of chemical sterilization on the plastic is uncertain. However, if cones are to be re-used on other women it is now being suggested that cleaning with soap and water followed by disinfection in 1000 ppm or C12 Na DCC or sodium hypochlorite or 2% glutaraldehyde followed by thorough rinsing will be an effective bactericidal and virucidal disinfection process (Colgate Medical, 1989). The promoters recommend that cones should be used in all patients as first-line treatment for genuine stress incontinence, complementary to surgery (Peattie et al., 1989). There is no facility for the supply of cones free within the UK National Health Service, so women must buy their own. To avoid women purchasing cones which they find they cannot use, each should be carefully assessed, advised as to whether they are really likely to benefit, and instructed as to use. The following factors should be borne in mind:

1. Cones are of one size – larger women may have proportionately more difficulty in retention than smaller women.
2. If the width between the medial edges of the levator ani muscles is very wide, congenitally or as a result of trauma at deliveries, retention may be impossible.
3. If the innervation to part of the pelvic floor has been permanently damaged the potential for improvement may be very small.
4. Multiparous women may be too stretched to retain even the lightest cone, or it may tilt sideways and lodge rather than weight the pelvic floor.
5. The vagina is normally a very moist and slippery tube and any one of the following will increase this: recent intercourse, spermicides, lubricant jelly or vaginal secretion in mid-cycle. This may make cone retention impossible.
6. A full rectum may make retention easier.

General exercise

In assessing the patient referred with incontinence, it is important for the physiotherapist to determine to what extent joint stiffness or lack of strength and endurance in muscles other than the pelvic floor may be actually contributing to the incontinence or aggravating it. Consideration should also be given as to how far general lack of fitness is responsible for weakness of the pelvic floor musculature. An example of joint stiffness as a contributory factor to incontinence would be osteoarthritic knees which make standing up from sitting a breath-holding struggle, resulting in leakage either because the raised intra-abdominal pressure provokes detrusor contractions or because it overwhelms the urethral closure mechanisms. In addition (or alternatively) it could result in the woman taking so long to reach the toilet that accidents occur. In such a case one solution would be specific treatment to relieve pain, mobilize joints and strengthen the leg muscles, while another would be to change the environment (Muir Gray, 1986).

Another possibility is that the inactivity and social withdrawal caused by the incontinence leads to generalized weakness including the perineal muscles. The pelvic floor musculature is active in its urethral closure role and its supportive role to a variable extent round the clock, the degree of muscle activity being related to what the woman is doing. A gradient of activity might be represented by lying, sitting, standing, walking, bending, lifting. Such activities as talking, laughing and shouting interact with the others. The amount of work done by the pelvic floor in a day is governed by what a woman does. Reduced activity, if she is sitting at home a great deal, will reduce the daily work of the pelvic floor and lead in time to many muscles (including the pelvic floor) becoming less strong. Gordon and Logue (1985) writing of post partum women reported that any form of muscular exercise improved perineal muscle function. They went on to comment that pure perineal exercises were not extensively practised either because women were not convinced of the benefit or because they found them tedious, and that perhaps more emphasis should be placed on exercise that women find interesting and fulfilling.

It seems possible that general exercise may have a place in the treatment of some incontinent women in tandem with pure pelvic floor exercise. It would attempt to combat the common scenario of incontinence undermining confidence, leading to reduced activity and social interaction. Activities that are known to cause leakage should be excluded at the start of such a programme; and being able once again to achieve them without leakage could be used as an objective test of improvement. Bø et al. (1989) used this approach, which also included group general exercise sessions. The physiotherapist is the only professional who is able to assess the patient in this holistic way and decide firstly whether specific exercises or more general exercises are required, and if so, to plan and implement the right programme for the individual.

Bladder retraining

Bladder retraining or drill is used in the management of frequency, urgency without leakage and urge incontinence (Jeffcoate and Francis, 1966; Frewen, 1978). Patient selection is very important for this form of treatment. It is particularly well suited to women who, through years of leakage, have developed a habit of going to the toilet 'just in case' at every available opportunity so that should an accident occur there is little in the bladder. The patient must be mentally able to understand the instructions, and be willing to cooperate. After appropriate urodynamic assessment the woman is first required to keep a frequency/volume chart or diary for one week which establishes her voiding pattern – how often and how much, plus 'accidents' – and it can also be arranged to include what and how much is drunk, for some patients drink a great deal, others too little. After joint appraisal of the record by the physiotherapist or continence advisor and patient, the patient is instructed in ways of delaying voiding:

1. repeated maximal pelvic floor contractions when she feels the urge to void;
2. perineal pressure;
3. distraction – companionship, games, television, music.

The average duration between voids is deduced from the record (e.g. half an hour), and daily goals are set. Then, while drinking adequate and regular amounts, the patient is encouraged to delay voiding by increasing periods until she voids only every two to four hours. Delay even at the final point on the toilet may be assisted by perineal pressure, by sitting on a chair with a firm pad or sandbag between the legs, or on the edge of the toilet. In this way the ability of the bladder to tolerate greater volumes of urine is increased, and each success develops the woman's confidence.

When this approach to treatment was first devised, a 10-day inpatient stay enabled the patient to be thoroughly supported and encouraged in her efforts, as well as giving her time to come to understand her condition. Today, with the shortage of hospital beds, women are given instructions as outpatients by the physiotherapist or continence advisor and are expected to implement them alone. Bladder training groups are cost-effective for staff and helpfully supportive for sufferers.

Interferential therapy

Medium-frequency currents in the region of either 4000 Hz (4 kHz) or 2000 Hz (2 kHz) are currently being used therapeutically in the treatment of urinary incontinence. In a survey of English physiotherapists (Mantle and Versi, 1989), 77% of the respondents put interferential therapy (IT) as either their first or second choice of modality for the treatment of stress incontinence, and they considered it to be 63% effective. This therapy is also used for patients with urge (motor) incontinence, and mixed stress and urge incontinence. Two slightly different medium-frequency currents, e.g. 4000 Hz and 4100 Hz, are arranged to crossfire and interfere with one another. A low-frequency current is produced in the area of interference, equal to the difference between the two initial frequencies, i.e. 100 Hz. If one of the medium-frequency currents is programmed to vary, then the low-frequency current will vary accordingly to produce pulses or surges of one frequency or sweeps of frequencies. At the point of application to the patient, medium-frequency currents have the major advantage over low-frequency currents that the skin resistance to them is less, and consequently there is less sensory stimulation for a given intensity. This, it is argued, makes IT a much more comfortable way of producing a contraction of innervated pelvic floor muscle than the usual low-frequency therapies, and reduces the current intensity required.

For genuine stress incontinence

The purpose of IT for patients with GSI is usually said to be the production of contractions of the pelvic floor musculature as a means of increasing the patient's cortical awareness, thus facilitating the ability to perform voluntary contractions. Some patients find it difficult to understand which muscles to contract, and it has even been suggested that cortical alienation may occur and persist following trauma such as childbirth. If the objective is an electrically produced contraction, it is vital that a contraction is obtained. Each physiotherapist is advised to test electrode placings and machines on her own pelvic floor – on the arm is not sufficient – to ensure that a contraction is obtainable with the machine available and using the proposed technique. It is unwise to rely on the patient's impression, for, to the uninitiated, the 'buzzing' sensation may be mistaken for the real thing.

Most IT machines enable medium-frequency carrier waves in the region of 4000 Hz to be selected; a few permit 2000 Hz, and there is some subjective evidence supporting the logical hypothesis that the longer pulse widths (0.25 milliseconds) of carriers in the region of 2000 Hz will be more effective than the 0.125 ms of the 4000-Hz carrier wave. It is said that muscular urethral closure is most effectively achieved at a pulse duration of 0.1–1.0 ms. Some machines enable the patient to control the intensity and/or surging. Neurons serving slow-twitch muscle fibres discharge at frequencies of about 10–20 per second, while those to fast-twitch fibres discharge at 30–60 per second. So a frequency sweep of 10–40 Hz for 15 minutes using a 2000-Hz carrier wave and the maximum tolerable intensity is favoured for GSI. Some clinicians precede or follow this with 40 Hz for 15 minutes surged, or follow it with 1 Hz or less constant – which produces quick, repetitive contractions. Some claim benefit to striated muscle via the neuron from pulsed frequencies of about 10 Hz or sweeps of 5–10 Hz, to avoid habituation, at intensities that do not produce a contraction. However the survey by Mantle and Versi (1989) showed considerable variation between clinicians – 62 different combinations of frequencies, sweeps, etc. were reported – and there is an urgent need for competent multicentre research to deduce what is most effective.

Claims that artificially produced contractions of the pelvic floor muscles, often given for only 15–20 minutes two or three times a week, in themselves strengthen the muscles must be questioned; but in that the patient practises vigorously during the treatment session, is encouraged to join in with the machine, is motivated to practise at home, is able to discuss her condition, and gains further insight, reassurance and fresh ideas for coping, this regular contact is usually very beneficial. It would not be surprising if it were found that daily treatment was even more successful, but it is very expensive in health-care terms. Providing a contraction is produced it would be reasonable to suppose that the venous and lympatic drainage is assisted, although it must be doubtful how often this is therapeutic in such a highly vascular area. It is also conceivable that any adhesions and scarring might be loosened, leading to improved function.

For urge incontinence, and symptoms of frequency and urgency

There is normally a complex reflex interaction between the detrusor and the pelvic floor musculature whereby when one is contracted the other relaxes. The objective in the treatment of urge incontinence is inhibition of the unwanted detrusor contractions, and it is suggested that repeated contraction of the pelvic floor muscles may be successful in this. It has also been shown that electrical stimulation of the pudendal afferent nerve pathways has inhibitory effects on the detrusor (Erlandson et al., 1977). Sweeps of 5–10 Hz for 30 minutes using the longer pulse with a 2000-Hz carrier wave and maximum intensity are recommended (Laycock and Green, 1988).

Application of treatment

The patient is usually treated in the half-lying position with the hips and knees slightly flexed (McQuire, 1975; Dougall, 1985), but Hendriks (1988) maintains that the patient should be treated in the supine position with the legs fully extended and abducted. Whichever position is selected, the electrode position is critical as with any other electrostimulating technique, so that interference occurs in the vicinity of the pudendal and pelvic nerves. This should enable a contraction of the pelvic floor muscles to be obtained within intensities tolerable to the patient and without too much spread to other muscles. Either four electrodes or two electrodes may be used, consequently the methods employed are described as being four-pole or two-pole methods. Where four electrodes are used, two carry each current and may be denoted as A1, A2, B1 and B2. Vacuum electrodes are available with some machines.

Four-pole methods. Several four-pole methods have been described:

1. Two electrodes on the abdomen just above the lateral portion of the inguinal ligament (A1 and B1); two electrodes high on the internal medial aspect of the thigh near the origin of the adductors (A2 and B2) (Savage, 1984), 'below the inferior border' (perhaps the medial border is meant) of the femoral triangle (Dougall, 1985) or under

the gluteal fold toward the medial side of the posterior aspect of the thigh (Hendriks, 1988).
2. Two electrodes medial to the ischial tuberosities, i.e. either side of the anus (A1 and B1); two electrodes (A2 and B2) lateral to the symphysis pubis as nearly over the obturator foramen as possible (Laycock and Green, 1988).

Two-pole methods. One medium-sized electrode is placed over the anus, covering the posterior fibres of the levator ani muscle, and a small electrode is positioned centrally immediately below the symphysis pubis (Laycock and Green, 1988).

Maximum tolerable intensity is used and most clinicians seem to consider the course of 8–12 treatments to be successful (Mantle and Versi, 1989).

Low-frequency muscle stimulation

Faradism, an unevenly alternating current, was used more than forty years ago in the treatment of the pelvic floor of both men and women suffering with incontinence. The Smart-Bristow faradic battery, in use then although temperamental, allowed the fine control of hand surging which enabled the physiotherapist and patient to integrate their efforts towards the goal of good voluntary control. The faradic battery was superseded by increasingly sophisticated electronic devices which give many varieties of surged and pulsed wave forms and lengths. To stimulate innervated striated muscle a pulse width of 0.1 to 1 ms and 0.5–40 Hz may be selected and surged.

Usually physiotherapists have employed electrostimulation in the rehabilitation process to assist patients who have difficulty in producing a voluntary contraction of the pelvic floor. This treatment might only be given once or twice, and always in a physiotherapy department. Recently work by Farragher et al. (1987) on the facial muscles of patients who have had Bell's palsy, some for many years, has introduced physiotherapists treating incontinence to trophic stimulation and to the possibility of a woman having a small electrostimulator to use at home. This latter battery-operated device, the size of a cigarette packet, with simple controls, leads and electrodes, enables patients to give themselves daily treatment, usually for about one hour. The production of such units has become a growth industry.

It is claimed that by the application of the correct electric signals it is possible to take over the normal control that exists between nerve and muscle in a motor unit. This control has two parts, one involving postural slow-twitch fibres, the other fast-twitch fibres. Postural fibres need tonic feeding by continuous impulses of low intensity at the rate of 10 Hz for an hour or more per day to preserve or restore bulk, capillary bed density and the ability to utilize oxygen (Farragher et al., 1989).

This hour of treatment may be divided into shorter sessions. Fast-twitch fibres, which give power to movement, need phased impulses of about 30 Hz sufficiently intense to produce a gentle contraction applied for shorter periods.

It seems that the pelvic floor muscles may have much physiologically in common with the facial muscles. Slow-twitch fibres when damaged or partially denervated suffer from disuse atrophy; they appear to become more fast twitch in their characteristics by losing their ability to contract for lengthy periods, and they fatigue quickly.

Superficial or internal electrodes may be used with these machines; the superficial electrodes may be very difficult for a patient to adjust to the best position. There is some evidence that recognizable levator ani muscle contraction is most satisfactorily obtained using a vaginal or anal electrode.

FAECAL INCONTINENCE

Faecal incontinence is the unintentional or uncontrolled passage of faeces. At its least severe, there may be minimal soiling of clothing sometimes associated with inadvertent passing of flatus. At its most severe, there is uncontrollable complete emptying of the bowel with little or no warning and in inappropriate places. The faecal material varies between being very liquid and very hard. Faecal incontinence seems to be less common than urinary incontinence, but it is difficult to determine accurately the prevalence of the condition because many sufferers are so embarrassed and ashamed that they hide their problem in the best way they can. Brocklehurst (1975) considered that 1 per 1000 of the UK population was affected. Thomas (1984) reported the prevalence of recognized faecal incontinence, including double incontinence, in women under 65 years old to be 0.2 per 1000, and 2 per 1000 over 65 years; but a far higher figure was reported in her postal survey and confirmed by sample interviews. From this she estimated that 1.7 per 1000 women under 65 yers old and 13.3 per 1000 over 65 years were affected. Snooks et al. (1985) confirmed that faecal incontinence is more common in women than men in a ratio of 8:1, and that most of the affected women had had children, and often had a history of a prolonged or difficult labour.

Faecal incontinence is devastating for the individual concerned, even when it is just a temporary problem, for example associated with infective diarrhoea or inflammatory bowel disease. Snooks and Swash (1986) classified faecal incontinence into two main groupings, according to whether the sphincters and pelvic floor were normal or abnormal.

Normal sphincters and pelvic floor. In this group perfectly normal closure mechanisms become overwhelmed, for example by diarrhoea, or there is a fault in another part of the system, such as a fistula. Rectovaginal fistula can result from childbirth.

Abnormal sphincters and pelvic floor. Parks (1981) expressed the opinion that the most important factor in the maintenance of faecal continence is the integrity of the anorectal angle and the flap valve (see p. 343). It follows that damage to muscle itself or to the innervation of the pelvic floor musculature, which affects the puborectalis, could cause faecal incontinence, and the same would be true of the external anal sphincter. Snooks et al. (1985) reported an increase in PNTML in women with third-degree tears at delivery. Such damage appeared to be cumulative, subsequent deliveries causing further damage, for the external anal sphincter fibre density was increased in multiparae (see p. 273). Examples of conditions or events that could cause abnormal functioning of sphincters and pelvic floor are:

1. Constipation or a history of habitual straining, encouraging stretching and perineal descent, particularly in those who have been allowed to develop faecal impaction. In this latter state the rectum is distended with hard faeces which cannot be passed by the patient. Anatomy is distorted, the flap valve is lost, and more proximal liquid faeces seep down past the blockage.
2. Prolonged or difficult labours, forceps delivery (Snooks et al., (1984), third-degree perineal tears or rupture of the external sphincter. Some women experience mild problems postpartum, such as difficulty in holding flatus and slight soiling, which then improves.
3. A history of low back pain, sciatica, laminectomy or cauda equina lesions.
4. Trauma involving the perineum or the sacral nerve roots, e.g. fractures, surgery.
5. Rectal prolapse, which causes stretching of rectal tissue.
6. Sexual abuse, possibly in childhood.
7. Brain damage or dementia, preventing awareness of the urge to defaecate.

Prevention

Chronic constipation is a major long-term cause of faecal incontinence, and the physiotherapist as a member of the health promotion team needs to be aware of this when caring for patients. Unavoidable periods of bed rest or enforced inactivity, reduced mobility, pain, hand and arm injuries which make undressing difficult, and many other situations can make it easier for even quite young people to ignore the call to stool rather than struggle to the toilet. The close rapport frequently built up between patient and physiotherapist may result in confidences concerning defaecation problems being shared. These must be treated seriously, and sensitively investigated with advice from other disciplines where needed.

Assessment

Assessment is not the task of a physiotherapist, but requires an appropriate selection of the following procedures: taking a careful history; examination of the perineum; digital examination of the anus for resting tone and for active contraction of the external sphincter; abdominal examination; proctoscopy (fibreoptic examination of the rectum); sigmoidoscopy (fibreoptic examination of the inside of the rectum and sigmoid colon); anorectal manometry; single-fibre electromyography, and nerve conduction tests.

Treatment

This consists of medical and surgical treatment.

Medical

Management. Where stools are too loose, management is directed toward curing any underlying infection or disorder, and if necessary administering simple constipating agents. Where faecal impaction is the cause, the rectum must be professionally cleared, under anaesthetic if necessary, and then education and assistance given on diet and bowel management to avoid recurrence.

Physiotherapy. Both pelvic floor contractions and electrostimulation have been used with mixed success. Recently, interest has been aroused by the new battery-operated low-frequency stimulators referred to on p. 379, and the apparently highly successful work of Sackier (in press) using two ring electrodes on an anal plug. Stimulation was applied for 20 minutes, two or three times per day and (after an inpatient period of instruction and supervision) was administered by the patient. The results of interferential therapy have been disappointing (Sylvester and Kielty, 1987).

Surgical

Division of the external anal sphincter can be repaired, either directly or by muscle grafts, e.g. from the gracilis or sartorius muscles.
  Loss of the anorectal angle may be improved by means of a posterior

repair such as that devised by Parks (1975). This involves suturing the pelvic floor together behind the rectum, which pushes the anorectal angle forward and restores it.

MANAGEMENT OF PERSISTENT URINARY AND FAECAL INCONTINENCE

Where, despite exhaustive and repeated assessment and the best of team care, a patient is still left with some degree of incontinence of urine or faeces, efforts should be directed towards management. The continence advisor can give invaluable help to all concerned in finding the best care solutions for each individual case which will maintain dignity and social integration, while reducing the work load and keeping costs down. The physiotherapist may be able to contribute toward these goals with treatment that produces just a little more strength or range of movement to enable a patient to become independent by coping with manoeuvres such as self-catheterization or pad changing, or to make it possible for the patient, in spite of all the problems, to get out and about and enjoy life. Incontinence, immobility, social deprivation and depression are a lethal cocktail.

References

Abrams P.H., Torrens M.J. (1979). Urine flow studies. *Urol. Clin. N. America*, **6**, 71–9.

Association of Continence Advisors (1985). Guidelines on the role of the District Continence Advisor. In *Incontinence and its Management* (Mandelstram D., ed.). London: Croom Helm.

Bø K., Hagen R., Jørgenson J. et al. (1989). The effect of two different pelvic floor muscle exercise programs in treatment of urinary stress incontinence in women. *J. Neurourology and Urodynamics*, **8(4)**, 355–6.

Brocklehurst J.C. (1975). Management of anal incontinence. *Clin. Gastroenterol.*, **4**, 479–487.

Cardoza L. (1984). Detrusor instability. *Clinical Gynaecological Urology* (Stanton S.,ed.). Toronto: C.V. Mosby.

Cardoza L. (1990). Medical and surgical treatment In *Micturition*, (Drife J.O., Hilton P., Stanton S.L. eds.) London: Springer-Verlag.

Christensen L., Colstrup H., Hertz J. et al. (1984). Inter- and intradepartmental variations of the urine-pad weighing test. *Proceedings of the International Incontinence Society*, **14**, 99–100.

Dougal D.S. (1985). The effects of interferential therapy on incontinence and frequency of micturition. *Physiotherapy*, **71**, 135–6.

Erlandson B.E. Fall M., Carlsson C.A. (1977). Intravaginal electrical stimulation in urinary incontinence. *Scand. J. Urol. Nephrol.*, Suppl. 44.

Farragher D., Kidd G., Tallis R. (1987). Eutrophic electrical stimulation for Bell's palsy. *Clinical Rehabilitation*, **1**, 267–71.

Farragher D. (1989). Electrostimulation Study Day ACPOG London Workshop Group July 27th – Personal Communication.

Femina (1989). Instruction leaflet. Colgate Medical Ltd, Dedworth Road, Windsor, Berks.

Frewen W.K. (1978). An objective assessment of the unstable bladder of psychosomatic origin. *Brit. J. Urol.*, **50**, 246–249.

Gordon H., Logue M. (1985). Perineal muscle function after childbirth. *Lancet*, **ii**, 123–5.

Green M.F. (1986). Old people and disorders of continence. In *Incontinence and its Management*. (Mandelstam D., ed.). London: Croom Helm.

Hendriks O. (1988). Review of the physiological mechanisms involved in electrical stimulation for urinary incontinence. *Physiotherapy Ireland*, **9**, (1) 3–9.

Henry M., Swash M. (1985). *Coloproctology and the Pelvic Floor*. Oxford: Butterworth Heinemann.

Hilton P. (1988). Urinary incontinence during sexual intercourse. *Brit. J. Obstet. Gynaec.*, **95**, 377–81.

Hilton P. (1989). Mechanisms of urinary continence. *Proceedings of the First International Congress on the Pelvic Floor*, Cannes p. 17–21.

Jeffcoate T.N.A., Francis W.J.A. (1966). Urgency incontinence in the female. *Am. J. Obstet. Gynecol.*, **94**, 604.

Kegel A. (1948). The non-surgical treatment of genital relaxation. *Ann. West. Med. Surg.*, **2**, 213–16.

Kiffe S., Barnes P.R.H., Swash M. (1984). Evidence of pudendal neuropathy in patients with perineal descent and chronic constipation. *Gut*, **25**, 1279–1282.

Laycock J., Chiarelli P. (1989). Pelvic floor assessment and re-education. *Proceedings of the International Continence Society*, **(99)**, 206–7.

Laycock J., Green R.J. (1988). Interferential therapy in the treatment of incontinence. *Physiotherapy*, **74**, 161–8.

Mantle M.J., Versi E. (1989). English physiotherapeutic practice: stress incontinence 1989. *J. Neurourology and Urodynamics*, **8(4)**, 352–3.

Mahony D.T., Laferte R.O., Blaise J.D. (1977). Integral storage and voiding reflexes. *Urology*, **9**, 95–106.

McQuire W.A. (1975). Electrotherapy and exercises for stress incontinence and urinary frequency. *Physiotherapy*, **61**, 305–7.

Moore K.H., Richmond D. (1989). Crouching over the toilet seat: prevalence and effect upon micturition. *J. Neurourology and Urodynamics*, **8(4)**, 422–4.

Muir Gray J.A. (1986). Incontinence in the community. In *Incontinence and its Management* (Mandelstam D., ed.). London: Croom Helm.

Mundt-Petterssen B., Mathiasson A., Sundin T. (1984). Reproducibility of the 1-hour incontinence test by the ICS Standardization Committee. *Proceedings of the International Continence Society*, **14**, 90–1.

Parks A.G. (1975). Anorectal incontinence. *Proc. R. Soc. Med.*, **68**, 681.

Parks A.G. (1981). Faecal incontinence. In *Incontinence and its Management* (Mandelstam D., ed.). London: Croom Helm.

Peattie A.M., Plevnik S., Stanton S. (1989). Distal urethral conductance (DUEC): a screening test for incontinent females. Paper presented to the Blair Bell Research Society, RCOG, 25 April.

Sackier J. (In press). Neuromuscular stimulation. In *Basic Concepts and Clinical Application* (Clifford Rose F., Jones R., Vrbora G., eds.). New York: Demos.

Savage B. (1984). *Interferential Therapy*, pp.95–98. London: Faber.

Shepherd A. (1990). The conservative treatment of genuine stress incontinence, Ch 13 In *Micturition* (Drife J.O., Hilton P., Stanton S.L. eds.). London: Springer Verlag.

Snooks S.J., Swash M. (1986). Adult faecal incontinence. *Hospital Update*, March, 227–32.

Snooks S.J., Swash M., Henry M.M., Setchell M. (1985). Risk factors in childbirth causing damage to the pelvic floor innervation. *Br. J. Surg.*, **72**, suppl. (5), 15–17.

Snooks S.J., Swash M., Setchell M., Henry M. (1984). Injury to innervation of pelvic floor sphincter musculature in childbirth. *Lancet*, **ii**, 546–50.

Stanton S.L. (1986). Gynaecological aspects. In *Incontinence and its Management* (Mandelstam D., ed.). London: Croom Helm.

Swash M. (1985). Anorectal incontinence: electrophysiological tests. *Br. J. Surg.*, **72**, suppl. S14–20.

Sylvester K.L. Keilty S.E. (1987). A pilot study to investigate the use of interferential in the treatment of ano-rectal incontinence. *Physiotherapy*, **73**, 207–8.

Thomas T.M. (1986). The prevalence and health service implications of incontinence. In *Incontinence and its Management* (Mandelstam D., ed.). London: Croom Helm.

Thomas T.M. Plymat K.R., Blannin J., Meade T.S. (1980). Prevalence of urinary incontinence. *Br. Med. J.*, **281**, 1243–5.

Thomas T.M., Egan M., Walgrove A. et al. (1984). The prevalence of faecal and double incontinence. *Community Medicine*, **6**, 216–20.

Thow M. (1989). Personal communication. Physiotherapy division. Queens College. Glasgow.

Versi E. (1990). Relevance of urethral pressure profilometry to date Ch 6 In *Micturition* (Drife J.O., Hilton P., Stanton S.L. eds.) London: Springer Verlag.

Versi E., Cardozo L., Anand D. (1988). The use of pad tests in the investigation of female urinary incontinence. *Brit. J. Obstet. Gynaec.*, **8**, 270–3.

Wall L.L., Davidson T.G. (1992). The role of muscular re-education by physical therapy in the treatment of genuine stress urinory incontinence. *Obstetrical and Gynecological Survey*, **47**, **(5)**, 322–31.

Warrell D.W. (1986). Prolapse and urinary incontinence. In *Integrated Obstetrics and Gynaecology for Postgraduates*. (Dewhurst D., ed.). Oxford: Blackwell.

Wilson P.D., al Samarrai T., Deakin M. et al. (1987). An objective assessment of physiotherapy for female genuine stress incontinence. *Brit. J. Obstet. Gynaec.*, **94**, 575–82.

Whiteside C.G., Arnold E.P. (1975). Persistent primary enuresis. *Br. Med. J.*, **1**, 364–7.

Worth A.M., Dougherty M.C., McKey P.L. (1986). Development and testing of the circumvaginal muscles rating scale. *Nursing Res.*, **35**, 166–8.

Further reading

Drife J.O., Hilton P., Stanton S.L. eds. (1990). *Micturition*, London: Springer-Verlag.
Swash M., Henry M., Snooks S. (1985). Unifying concepts of pelvic floor disorders and incontinence. *J. Roy. Soc. Med.*, **78**, 906–11.

Useful addresses

Association for Continence Advice
c/o The Disabled Living Foundation
380–384 Harrow Road
London W19

Enuresis Resource and Information Centre (ERIC)
65 St Michael's Hill
Bristol BS2 8DZ

International Continence Society
Hon. Sec. Paul Abrams FRCS
Consultant Urologist
Southmead Hospital
Bristol BS10 5NS

CHAPTER 12

Early Paediatric Problems

Barbara Whiteford and Diana Kverndal

ROUTINE EXAMINATION OF THE NEWBORN

All babies are routinely examined at delivery by a doctor or midwife, again in more detail within the first 24 hours and once again before they are discharged from hospital.

Routine examination at delivery

At one minute and again at five minutes after delivery the neonate is assessed using the Apgar scale (Table 12.1).

Table 12.1 Apgar a score for neonatal assessment

	0 points	1 point	2 points
Colour	blue, pale	pink body, blue extremities	pink
Respiratory effort	absent	slow, irregular	regular, crying
Heart rate	absent	less than 100 beats/min	more than 100 beats/min
Response to stimulus (nasal catheter)	absent	grimace	cry, sneeze
Muscle tone	low	some limb flexion	active movement

A normal baby should have recorded a score of 8–10 by one minute after delivery and a score of 10 by five minutes. If there is concern for the baby the test will be repeated at ten minutes. This test is essential for identifying high-risk infants both in the short and long term.

Before the mother and baby are taken to the postnatal ward, the baby is given its first examination; the following are usually checked:

1. weight and length;
2. head circumference and fontanelles;

3. temperature and pulse;
4. any obvious abnormalities, e.g. spina bifida, imperforate anus, fractures, hypospadias;
5. heart and lung sounds;
6. the presence of two arteries and one vein in the umbilical cord.

The placenta and membranes are also checked.

Routine examination within the first 24 hours

Within the first 24 hours the baby should have a full examination by a paediatrician who will check the following:

Head. The fontanelles are palpated to evaluate intracranial tension (to detect hydrocephalus, spina bifida or cephalhaematoma); the head circumference is usually plotted on a graph with weight and length; any dysmorphic features are noted.

Eyes. The eyes are checked for appearance and slant, discharge or inflammation and response to light.

Ears. The ears are checked for the presence of an auditory meatus.

Nose. The patency of the nasal passages is checked (for choanal atresia).

Mouth. The presence of cleft lip and palate is excluded using a spatula or finger.

Neck. The neck is palpated for cysts or swellings.

Upper limbs. These are checked for equality of length, number of fingers, palmar creases (Down's syndrome), asymmetry and lack of movement (e.g. in Erb's palsy, hemiplegia, fractured clavicle or humerus, etc.).

Heart. Chest and heart sounds are assessed to exclude respiratory problems and congenital heart lesions. Many babies have a heart murmur for the first two or three days which disappears spontaneously. The baby is observed for excessive respiratory effort (tachypnoea, sternal recession, etc.).

Abdomen. The abdomen (liver, spleen and kidney) is palpated for tumour or excessive distension, and the bladder percussed for size.

Spine. The spine is checked for spina bifida lesions and obvious vertebral anomalies, e.g. scoliosis.

Genitalia. Male babies are checked for hypospadias and descent of testes; female babies are checked for incomplete opening of vagina, clitoral enlargement and any vulval discharge.

Lower limbs. These are examined for instability of hip, talipes equinorvarus and calcaneovalgus, equality of leg lengths and correct number of toes. Femoral pulses are checked to exclude coarctation of the aorta.

Neurological examination

Muscle tone and head control are assessed during general handling and by the baby's response to ventral suspension and when pulled gently by the arms towards sitting from supine. The following neonatal reflexes may be tested and should be present in the normal baby at term. (If there is doubt about the baby's gestational maturity, the gestational assessment using the Dubowitz score will be used.)

Grasp

Palmar. The examiner's little finger is placed in the baby's palm from the ulnar side (avoiding simultaneously touching the dorsum of the hand): the baby's fingers grasp tightly.

Plantar. The examiner's little finger is placed on the sole of the baby's foot behind the toes: the toes curl.

Moro reflex

The baby is held in two hands just above a soft surface; support is withdrawn momentarily from the head, allowing it to fall back a few degrees, into the open hand of the examiner. The baby will respond by abduction and extension of both arms with spreading of the fingers, followed by adduction of the arms and usually crying. An asymmetrical response could indicate the present of a hemiplegia, Erb's palsy or fractured clavicle.

Placing

The anterior aspect of the leg or dorsum of the foot or hand is brought against the edge of a table. The baby lifts the leg up to step onto the table, or lifts the arm to place the hand on the table.

Positive supporting reaction and automatic stepping

When the baby is held upright with the feet on a firm surface, the legs and body straighten in a standing posture. If the baby's body is inclined forwards, this initiates a few steps of reciprocal walking. 'Scissoring' of legs or excessive plantar flexion of feet may be indicative of hypertonus and possible cerebral palsy.

Sucking and rooting

If the cheek is stimulated by a finger, the baby will automatically turn towards the stimulus and will attempt to suck.

Metabolic screening

A blood test (the Guthrie test) is done between 6 and 14 days to detect phenylketonuria or hypothyroidism.

Routine examination at six weeks

The baby is examined again at six weeks by a paediatrician in the mother's presence. Essentially the examination is the same as before, but it also includes an assessment of the baby's growth and development.

Motor development is assessed by observation of posture, muscle tone, symmetry and head control; vision by assessing the ability to fix and follow; hearing by observation of response to mother's voice and of a startle to a loud noise; social development by smiling and general alertness.

NORMAL DEVELOPMENT

As obstetric physiotherapists may be dealing with mothers and babies in postnatal classes for up to six months, they should have a basic knowledge of normal development to enable them to detect the abnormal.

Normal full-term babies lie in an attitude of flexion and relative adduction and will be variably asymmetrical. They are able to see, hear, smell and taste. They show a variety of normal primitive reflexes (see above).

Although they have little head control they are able to turn their heads to free the nose for breathing. Gradually the baby develops extension, beginning at the head and moving down the trunk to the legs over the first six months. Babies at this age roll (rotation of trunk) in both directions and are beginning to achieve sitting balance.

Over the same period of time eye and hand coordination are developing. These initially develop separately but by six months are beginning to be combined. At first, the grasp reflex predominates and the hands are held closed, but as this reflex diminishes over the next three months the baby's hands become mostly open and attempts are made to grasp objects. By four months the baby can bring two hands together and a month later can grasp objects purposefully. By six months the baby can transfer objects from hand to hand and by nine months is beginning to develop a pincer grip, uses fingers rather than the palm of the hand to hold and explore objects, and is able to release toys voluntarily.

This is only a brief outline of development and the obstetric physiotherapist must have access to a book specifically on this subject. A list of recommended reading is given at the end of this chapter.

NEONATAL ABNORMALITIES

Cerebral palsy

Cerebral palsy is a non-progressive disorder caused by irreversible damage to the developing brain. The causative factors are many and may be antenatal (e.g. congenital rubella, cytomegalovirus infection), perinatal (e.g. hypoxaemia) or postnatal (e.g. meningitis, head trauma, etc.) The severity and distribution of the neurological signs vary according to the stage of gestation at which the insult occurred and to the site and extent of the lesion; motor disorder will result and may be complicated by sensory disturbances, mental handicap, visual and hearing defects, epilepsy and developing orthopaedic deformities. The following signs in the early days may indicate neurological disorder:

- poor feeding and sucking;
- abnormal muscle tone – hypotonia, hypertonia;
- obligatory or persistent asymmetry of posture;
- excessive, abnormal or persistent primitive reflexes, e.g. obligatory asymmetrical tonic neck reflex;
- absent or excessive grasp reflex;
- poor eye contact;
- parental concern (often mothers of cerebral palsy children report concern for their baby in the first few days, even when no signs are obvious to medical staff);
- excessive irritability;
- poor head control.

As the child matures, the diagnosis of cerebral palsy becomes more certain due to the delay or abnormality of motor development, the persistence of primitive reflexes beyond the normal age and the more obvious evidence of abnormal reflexes.

If any of the above signs is detected by the obstetric physiotherapist and cerebral palsy is suspected, it is essential to report this to the paediatrician who can coordinate further diagnostic tests and arrange the essential support and counselling for the parents, without delay. Early referral to the therapy team is imperative for treatment to stand the best chance of success. The mother should be reassured of the help that is available for her child, and if possible introduced to an experienced paediatric physiotherapist and other members of the child development team who will be able to give her and her family the advice and support that she will need. The emphasis of treatment is now directed towards teaching the parents and carers that appropriate handling, positioning and play should be an integral part of the child's day.

Congenital dislocation of the hip

Congenital dislocation of the hip occurs more commonly in female babies, breech presentation, first-born babies and in babies whose family have a history of the condition. It is more common in the left hip. Early diagnosis and orthopaedic referral is essential for good results. The modified Ortolani–Barlow manoeuvre should be performed by a paediatrician within the first 24 hours, as some affected hips may temporarily lose the signs of instability shortly after birth (DHSS, 1986). Other suggestive signs which may be noticed by a physiotherapist are limited hip abduction, leg length discrepancy and asymmetrical skin creases. (Many babies have hip instability at birth and will need careful monitoring; however, of these a large percentage will recover spontaneously.)

This condition can also be associated with other congenital abnormalities e.g. spina bifida and arthrogryposis.

Initial management

Radiographs may be taken, but in the early stages these are not always helpful in the diagnosis. Recently, ultrasound scans have been found to be useful diagnostically, particularly when early signs are no longer evident.

Once diagnosis is established a variety of treatment regimens may be used. Most newborn babies will be left for a few weeks before splinting is considered, as some hips stabilize spontaneously. Prone is the position of choice for these babies. Care should be taken during handling to avoid forced extension and adduction of the hips, as this may encourage dislocation of an unstable hip, and tight swaddling should be avoided. For the baby whose hip is easily reducible, a hip abduction splint (e.g. a Von Rosen or Pavlek harness) will be used for about three months or until the hip is stable. Abduction splints should not be used on a dislocated and unreducible hip. To reduce the dislocation, a period on traction (with or without a closed bilateral adductor tenotomy) may be necessary. This will aim at gradually taking the hips into wide abduction. After the period in traction the child may then be placed in a 'frog' plaster for approximately six weeks followed by a hip abduction splint for a minimum of eight weeks or until the child is trying to walk out of it. If full reduction is not achieved by the above methods, further surgery will be necessary.

The role of the obstetric physiotherapist in the care of these babies is limited to application of splinting, and explanation to the parents of everyday handling and treatment programmes. Advice may be given regarding practical management of the babies in their splints, and if possible referral made to a paediatric occupational therapist for help with adaptions to home equipment.

Arthrogryposis multiplex congenita

This condition is characterized by joint stiffness and deformity, generally caused by abnormalities of the muscles or nerve supply to them. Resulting contractures are often influenced by the intrauterine position. The severity and distribution of the deformities are extremely variable. Treatment will involve early passive movements, splints and prostheses, stimulation of motor development and functional activities, including 'trick' movements, and probably surgery. These children usually have the normal range of intelligence and are generally well motivated to overcome their handicaps.

Talipes equinovarus

Talipes equinovarus is the most common congenital deformity of the foot. It may often be bilateral, with one foot more affected than the other. There is plantar flexion at the ankle and inversion at the subtalar and talocalcaneonavicular joints, with adduction and inversion of the forefoot. The deformity may occur in isolation or be associated with other congenital deformities such as spina bifida or arthrogryposis. It may be postural with no bone or joint abnormality, but in more severe cases it is structural with misalignment of the bones, and affects the joints and soft tissues. In the more severe cases, surgery may eventually be necessary as full correction may not be achieved by conservative methods, or regression may occur. All cases should be seen by an orthopaedic specialist who should oversee the management of the child. Some consultants choose to plaster the affected foot (or feet) immediately, and therefore the baby will not be referred to the physiotherapist. Many others, however, prefer a plan of stretching and strapping the feet and these babies will be referred immediately to the physiotherapist.

Physiotherapy management

The mother should be shown the passive movements and stretching exercises as soon as the baby is diagnosed and referred for treatment. This allows her to be involved actively in the treatment of her child and will relieve her anxiety while awaiting an orthopaedic appointment and a firm plan of management.

Stretching technique. With the knee and the hip flexed, grip the heel firmly in one hand and support the whole of the foot with the other. Pull the heel down into the midline position, then gently push the foot into abduction and eversion. Holding this position, dorsiflex the whole foot to complete the manoeuvre. Maintain this stretch and slowly extend the knee to achieve full correction. It can be suggested to the parents that these stretches are done at each nappy change.

Stimulation. Active movement should be encouraged by tickling the outer border of the foot, (toe towards the heel), and front of the lower leg.

Strapping. The orthopaedic consultant will probably request corrective strapping for six to eight weeks (Fig. 12.1). This strapping will normally be changed weekly, with overstrapping done two or three times in the interim, and all felt and strapping left off for one day before reapplication, to rest the skin. The materials used are compound benzoin tincture, cotton wool, 5 mm thick zinc oxide self-adhesive felt, 25 mm wide zinc oxide strapping (or Micropore for sensitive skins). The strapping is applied as follows:

1. Apply compound benzoin tincture liberally over the parts to be covered with felt or strapping.
2. Measure and then apply a strip of felt around the forefoot, distal edge level with the base of the toes. The join should be at the midline on the dorsum of the foot (Steps 2 and 3 in Fig.12.1).
3. Measure and apply a longer strip of felt from 25 mm above the lateral malleolus, up over the flexed knee and down the medial side to 25 mm above the medial malleolus (Steps 2 and 3).
4. To apply the tape (Steps 4 and 5), start at the midline of the base of the foot, coming laterally to the dorsum of the foot, over the medial border and back to the lateral border. Keeping the knee flexed, continue the strapping up the lateral border of the leg, exerting a

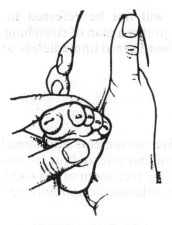

1 Position of operator's hands

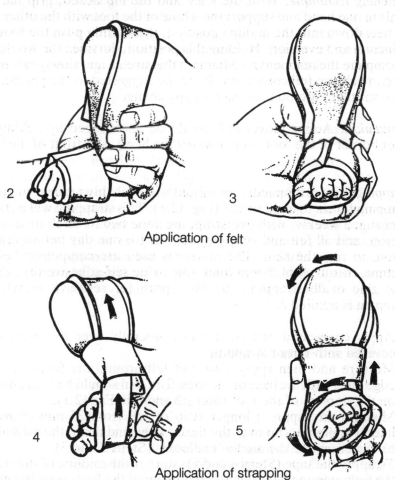

2

3

Application of felt

4

5

Application of strapping

Figure 12.1 Application of corrective strapping for talipes equinovarus (courtesy of the Hospital for Sick Children, Great Ormond Street).

pull on the foot into dorsiflexion and eversion. Continue the strapping over the knee and down the medial border to the end of the felt. A separate piece of tape is applied to the lower end of the felt to anchor the two sides.

Before the baby leaves, peripheral circulation must be checked ten minutes after application of the strapping. Parents must be alerted to signs of impaired circulation, and instructed to remove the strapping immediately, seek advice if concerned and to arrange restrapping.

Surgery

If conservative management fails, full corrective surgery is often performed, followed by plastering, then night splints and stretching as before. However, some surgeons feel that a better result may be obtained either by delaying surgery, or performing only a proximal lengthening of the tendo achilles and tibialis posterior muscle at the early stage and deferring the more extensive surgery until the child is ready to stand.

Talipes calcaneovalgus

This less common and often milder deformity of the foot is usually postural and results in the foot being held in a position of dorsiflexion at the ankle and eversion at the subtalar joint. Conservative treatment, consisting of regular passive stretchings and stimulation of the plantar-flexor and invertor muscles, is usually very successful if no structural abnormality is present. The parents must be taught the appropriate management, and the routine of stretches at each nappy change may be recommended as before. Night splints or serial plastering may be advisable as adjuncts to stretching, particularly when the condition is more severe.

Torticollis and sternomastoid tumour

In a neonate, this is a condition of uncertain origin but is thought to be due to a tear and resulting haematoma in the sternomastoid muscle following birth trauma (e.g. breech or forceps delivery). The baby generally presents at about two weeks with a benign, unilateral tumour of the sternomastoid muscle. The head is held in side flexion towards the side of the tumour with rotation towards the opposite side.

When making a diagnosis it is important to exclude other conditions which also produce head asymmetry such as congenital hemivertebra, plagiocephaly and cerebral palsy.

Physiotherapy management

Physiotherapy treatment must begin immediately, and should include reassurance to the parents of the benign nature of the tumour and its usually good prognosis. Ideally the baby should be seen daily by the physiotherapist, and the stretchings taught to one or preferably both parents until they are competent in the technique. The importance of correct positioning is also emphasized. A full description of treatment techniques is included in *Physiotherapy in Paediatrics* by Roberta Shepherd (1980).

Surgery

If conservative methods do not resolve the condition satisfactorily, surgery may be necessary to lengthen the shortened muscle.

Spina bifida

Spina bifida is a defect in the spinal column with possible protrusion of the meninges alone, or of the meninges and spinal cord. There are three classifications of this disorder.

1. Spina bifida occulta. There is incomplete formation of the vertebral arch, usually in the lumbrosacral region, but no abnormality or protrusion of the spinal cord or meninges. A tuft of hair or skin abnormality may be the only clinical manifestation and no intervention is required at this stage. Occasionally neurological problems may present later.

2. Meningocele. There is incomplete formation of the vertebral arch accompanied by protusion of the meninges. The spinal cord is usually normal and there may be no neurological signs. These children have a good prognosis following surgery.

3. Myelomeningocele. The meninges and the abnormal spinal cord protrude through the incomplete vertebral arch, usually causing ortho-paedic and neurological defects. These are the babies whom a pae-diatric physiotherapist will be required to help. The condition may be complicated by other abnormalities such as hydrocephalus, sight defects, orthopaedic problems such as talipes equinovarus, dislocated hips and scoliosis, and sphincter disorders causing urinary and faecal retention.

Physiotherapy management of myelomeningocele

Babies with myelomeningocele are generally referred to a specialized paediatric unit soon after birth. The physiotherapist may be asked to do a muscle and sensation level chart of the baby to help determine the extent of the damage, and as a baseline for postoperative management. This can only be expected to be an approximation of muscle group function and root sensory input. Various factors will be taken into consideration to determine the child's expected prognosis and quality of life before surgery is undertaken (Lorber, 1981).

After surgery, passive movements are necessary; they should be taught to parents, and appropriate skin care advice given. These children and their families will need continuing advice and support from their local paediatric therapist.

Hydrocephalus

Hydrocephalus is an increased accumulation of cerebrospinal fluid (CSF) within the intracranial cavity, causing enlargement of the baby's head and pressure on the brain. It may be due to a partial or complete obstruction of the fluid (e.g. by neoplasm, meningitis, Arnold–Chiari malformation in spina bifida, trauma), reduction in absorption, or rarely to excessive production of CSF.

In some cases there is spontaneous arrest of the disease; in many others, surgery will be required to insert a shunt which will allow the CSF to drain into the right atrium or peritoneal cavity.

As there may be delayed motor development due to the mechanical difficulties of lifting a heavy head and to possible impaired cortical function, these babies should be referred to their local paediatric physiotherapy department for monitoring.

Brachial plexus lesions

Erb's palsy

Erb's palsy is due to damage to the upper nerve roots C5, C6 of the brachial plexus and is caused by excessive traction to the neck and head during delivery, for instance after breech presentation or cephalic presentation with shoulder dystocia. The resulting flaccid paralysis generally affects the deltoid, brachioradialis, supraspinatus and infraspinatus, biceps, brachialis and the forearm supinator muscles. The arm characteristically hangs limply by the baby's side in medial rotation with an extended and pronated forearm.

Klumpke's paralysis

Less commonly, damage of the lower nerve roots C7, C8, T1 of the brachial plexus occurs – this is known as Klumpke's paralysis. The muscles principally affected are the flexors of the wrist and fingers and the intrinsic muscles of the hand, resulting in wasting and weakness of these muscles and usually some loss of sensation over the medial border of the forearm and the ulnar side of the hand.

Recovery depends on the extent of the damage to the nerves, which is effectively assessed by electromyogram and not by the initial clinical picture. In neurapraxia, full recovery may be expected within the first two months. In axonotmesis, recovery (at about 1 mm per day) can occur gradually over 18 months but may be incomplete. In neurotmesis little or no recovery can be expected unless surgery is performed. At some centres, nerve repair at around 9 weeks is now attempted, although the prognosis remains uncertain.

Physiotherapy management

A careful assessment of muscle power and tone should be made and baseline joint ranges measured. If pain or swelling is obvious, the presence of an associated fracture of the humerus or clavicle should be excluded. The possibility of a hemiplegia should also be considered.

Once the diagnosis is certain, gentle passive movements should be started after two or three days and demonstrated to the parents. In Erb's palsy the most important movements to perform are the full range of abduction, elevation and external rotation of the shoulder, flexion and supination of the forearm. During these passive movements, and also during other activities such as dressing, care should be taken not to exceed normal ranges of movement, as with the flaccid limb there is danger of dislocation. In Klumpke's paralysis, appropriate passive movements should be taught, concentrating on hand, wrist and forearm, and a cock-up splint may be recommended.

During the recovery period the baby should also be encouraged to make active-assisted and when possible active movements of all affected joints, e.g. hand to mouth, reaching up to the mother's face and reaching for toys.

These babies will need regular follow-up into childhood by an orthopaedic or neurosurgeon and a paediatric physiotherapist.

RESPIRATORY PROBLEMS IN THE PRE-TERM AND TERM INFANT

The following are the most common conditions to be encountered or treated by an obstetric physiotherapist:

1. Respiratory distress syndrome (hyaline membrane disease).
2. Meconium aspiration.
3. Pneumonia.
4. Pneumothorax.
5. Any condition requiring prolonged ventilation of the baby.

Before treating any of these conditions, the physiotherapist should be aware of the normal ranges of heart rate (120–160-beats per minute – less than 100 beats per minute indicates significant bradycardia; more than 200 indicates significant tachycardia), respiratory rate (pre-term 60–70 breaths per minute, – full term 45–60 breaths per minute) and blood gases (Pao_2 7–10 kPa, $Paco_2$ 4.5–6 kPa). Each unit will have different monitoring systems and the physiotherapist should become familiar with their workings.

Respiratory distress syndrome

Respiratory distress syndrome occurs in premature babies, and is more common in a second twin and in infants of diabetic mothers. It is due to an inadequate amount of surfactant in the lungs. Surfactant is identifiable in the foetal lung between 20–24 weeks, with secretions increasing throughout gestation, a surge occuring at the time of labour. It is a mixture of phospholipoproteins which reduces the surface tension in the lung and therefore allows adequate expansion of the gas-exchange area. Dexamethasone may be given to a mother in pre-term labour (26–32 weeks) to induce an increase in surfactant production in the foetus. Post-natal surfactant replacement therapy is now being used successfully, following administration, endotracheal suction and physiotherapy treatment should be withheld for as long as possible, unless tube obstruction is identified.

The severity of the syndrome varies with the maturation of the lungs. The baby may appear normal at birth with good Apgar scores, but over the next few hours may develop tachypnoea (in excess of 60 breaths per minute), expiratory grunting and sternal secretion. However, some babies are so severely affected (with cyanosis and little or no respiration), that they require immediate resuscitation and ventilation.

The management of these babies varies with their physical state and they may require:

1. Full ventilation via an endotracheal tube or intermittent mandatory ventilation (IMV).
2. Continuous positive airways pressure (CPAP) via a face mask, endotracheal tube or nasal prongs.
3. Humidified oxygen via a headbox.

Physiotherapy treatment

Handling should be kept to a minimum and therefore initiation and frequency of treatment will depend on the baby's stability and the amount of secretions. Treatment should always coincide with nursing care times and should be given with careful attention to the baby's state, observing temperature, respiration, heart and oxygen monitors throughout. The baby may need increased oxygen cover during physiotherapy treatment but care should be taken to return this to the correct level when the baby has stabilized. There is a danger of retinopathy if the immature retina is exposed to high arterial oxygen tensions.

Before 34 weeks these babies must not be tipped head down and postural drainage will anyway be modified by the baby's poor state. If there is no specific area of collapse, treatment is done side to side and/or supine and prone and the baby may be raised up to treat the apical lobes. A very sick baby, however, may not even tolerate turning and may have to be treated solely *in situ*.

Percussion with a small (size 1 or 2) Bennett face mask is thought now to be the most efficient way of loosening secretions (Tudehope and Bagley, 1980). Gentle vibrations given on expiration can only be done effectively if the breathing rate is sufficiently slow. Careful suction of the endotracheal tube, oropharynx and nasopharynx is done to complete the treatment. It is important to select the smallest catheter possible without compromising effective clearance of mucus. If secretions are plentiful it is often beneficial to suction after treating one side, and before turning, to prevent the loosened secretions blocking off airways or the endotracheal tube. A 'wash out' of the endotracheal tube is often incorporated into the physiotherapy regimen using saline solution or a mucolytic agent, e.g. acetylcysteine.

Meconium aspiration

Meconium aspiration is a common complication of fetal distress, where the baby passes meconium prematurely and may aspirate it into the lungs. This results in areas of collapse and overinflation of the lung; if secretions increase due to the development of chemical bronchitis, physiotherapy treatment may be required. These babies will be nursed in oxygen and will usually be prescribed antibiotics.

Pneumonia in the neonate

Neonatal pneumonias are commonly caused by bacteria associated with maternal amnionitis and may arise from inhalation of meconium, blood or infected secretions at birth; aspiration of fluids via a tracheo-oesophageal fistula or in association with a cleft palate, or contact with any of the bacterial and viral organisms carried by adults and children and transferred to a high-risk baby, particularly one receiving endotracheal care.

The baby may present with any of the following clinical signs; high or low temperature, apnoeic episodes, increased respiratory rate, respiratory distress, cough and poor feeding.

If the baby's lungs are producing excessive secretions, physiotherapy should be commenced. Treatment will depend on the maturity and general health of the baby, and is aimed at loosening secretions and clearance by suction. The physiotherapist should use palpations, stethoscope and chest X-ray findings in planning treatment.

Pneumothorax

Pneumothorax is due to rupture of one or more terminal air sacs into the pleural space and is usually seen in resuscitated or ventilated babies. If it is severe and the baby has respiratory distress, the air will need to be aspirated by needle followed by a fixed underwater seal drain.

Physiotherapy treatment is not indicated unless the baby has excessive or infected secretions. If treatment is considered appropriate the positioning and percussion of the baby will be influenced by the site of the drain and by the baby's tolerance to lying on the unaffected side. As before, the baby's maturity and general health should be taken into account.

Further reading

Brunner L.S., Suddarth C. (1986). 2nd edn. *The Lippincott Manual of Paediatric Nursing*. London: Harper & Row.

Catzel P. (1984). 2nd edn. *A Short Textbook of Paediatrics*. Seven Oaks, Kent: Hodder & Stoughton.

DHSS (1986). Screening for the Detection of *Congenital Dislocation of Hip*. London: HMSO.

Dinwiddie R. (1991). *The Diagnosis and Management of Paediatric Respiratory Disease*. Edinburgh: Churchill Livingstone.

Halliday H.L., McClure G., Reid M. (1989). *Handbook of Neonatal Intensive Care*. London: Bailière Tindall.

Illingworth R.S. (1987). *The Normal Child*. 9th edn. Harlow: Churchill Livingstone.

Jolly H. (1986). *Book of Child Care*. London: Unwin Paperbacks.

Kelner C.J.H., Harvey D. (1986). *The Sick Newborn Baby*. London: Bailière Tindall.

Lorber J. (1981). *Your Child with Spina Bifida*. London: ASBAH.

Shepherd R. (1980). *Physiotherapy in Paediatrics*. Oxford: Heinemann.

Tudehope D., Bagley C. (1980). Techniques of physiotherapy in intubated babies with respiratory distress syndrome. *Austr. Paed. J.*, **16**, 226–8.

Useful addresses

Association of Chartered Physiotherapists in Respiratory Care
c/o Chartered Society of Physiotherapy
14 Bedford Row
London WC1
Tel. 071–636 5020

Association of Orthopaedic Chartered Physiotherapists
c/o Chartered Society of Physiotherapy
14 Bedford Row
London WC1
Tel. 071–636 5020

Association of Paediatric Chartered Physiotherapists
c/o Chartered Society of Physiotherapy
14 Bedford Row
London WC1
Tel. 071–636 5020

Association of Spina Bifida and Hydrocephalus
(A.S.B.A.H.)
Tavistock House North
Tavistock Square
London WC1 H9HJ
Tel. 071–388 1382

British Paediatric Association
23 Queens Square
London WC1
Tel. 071–837 8253

Spastics Society
12 Park Crescent
London W1N 4EQ
Tel. 071–636 5020

Disabled Living Foundation (equipment advice)
380–384 Harrow Road
London W9
Tel. 071–289 6111

Bobath Centre (Cerebral palsy treatment and therapist training centre)
5 Netherall Gardens
London NW3
Tel. 071–435 3896

'Talking Through' Contractions in Antenatal Classes

EARLY FIRST STAGE

'Here's a contraction and it's starting now. Breathe out and relax. Its getting stronger – breathe slowly and comfortably, lean forwards if it helps. It's pulling your cervix up, drawing it against your baby's head. You're feeling it low down in your abdomen, perhaps in your back. It's getting weaker – dying away – and it's gone. Take a breath in, out and relax.'

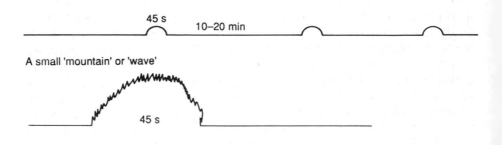

Figure 1 Early first stage.

MID FIRST STAGE

'Here's a contraction and it's starting now. Find a comfortable position – breathe out and relax. This is a stronger, longer one. Try to keep your breathing slow and calm. It's working hard – pulling your cervix up over your baby's head, easing it open, stretching it and guiding your baby down through your pelvis. You're feeling it across your abdomen and back – a deep, biting pain. You may find you're breathing becoming faster, and lighter to help you ride the "crest of the wave" – try and keep it as easy as possible. Go with it, stay with it – rock your pelvis if it helps, stroke your tummy if it eases the pain. Back and tummy massage can help too. It's getting weaker, but it's still there – your breathing will become slower and deeper again – relax as you breathe out – it's almost

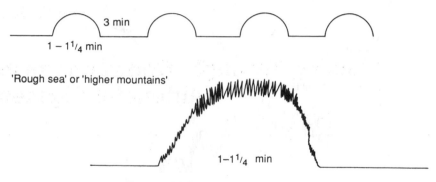

Figure 2 Mid first stage contractions.

gone – and it's gone. Take a deep breath in, out and relax. Breathe easily and change your position if you want to.'

END OF THE FIRST STAGE

'Here's a contraction and it's starting now. Breathe out and try to relax – now breathe as easily and comfortably as you can. Your uterus is working harder than ever – your cervix is nearly open and your baby is really low down in your pelvis – its head is pressing into your back passage. There's tremendous pressure – it's overwhelming. Breathe lightly at the peak of the contraction, use your voice to help you ride the powerful wave – sigh and groan if it helps. Say "I – won't – push" if you get the urge – go with your contraction, let it happen – each one is bringing you nearer to the birth of your baby. Cup your hands over your nose and mouth if you being to feel dizzy or have 'pins and needles' in your fingers. It's getting weaker, beginning to fade away – it's going, nearly gone and it's gone. Take a deep breath in and then let it out and relax. Keep breathing easily.'

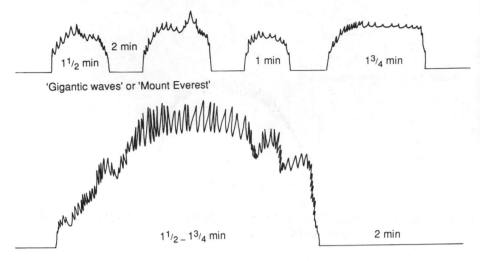

'Gigantic waves' or 'Mount Everest'

Figure 3 End of first stage contractions.

SECOND STAGE

'Here's a contraction and it's starting now. Get into a comfortable position for pushing – take at least one deep breath in and out before you breathe in to push. Your pushing urge tends to come in waves – work with your uterus – push when it tells you. Sometimes you'll hold your breath to bear down and ease your baby out – sometimes you'll find yourself pushing and breathing out at the same time. Try to relax your mouth and let your pelvic floor "give way" and stretch. It feels as if you're burning, stretching, maybe even splitting in half – don't hold back – relax your pelvic floor – let it unfold around your baby's head. Listen to your midwife – she'll tell you when to push and when to gently pant as your baby is being born.'

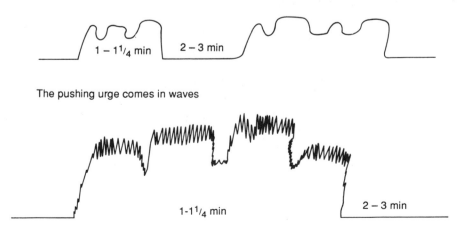

The pushing urge comes in waves

Figure 2 Second stage contractions.

LABOUR SEQUENCE

Stage	Physical signs	Mother's sensations	Mother's emotions	Self-help techniques	Companion's support
Last few days of pregnancy	Cervix may ripen, efface and even dilate a little. There may be an increase in vaginal secretions; the cervical plug of mucus, the 'show', may be released. The baby's head may engage if this has not already occured, although this often only happens in labour in multiparous women	Braxton Hicks contractions will be much stronger, more frequent and uncomfortable; could seem to be labour. Loose bowel movements may occur. Fetus may not be as active as usual. Mother may feel energetic and want to deal with last-minute chores. May experience low backache	Ambivalent: some women are fed up with their pregnancy and long for their baby to be born; others are fearful of their impending labour and their new, forthcoming responsibilities. Others look forward with excitement to the coming event	Make sure everything is ready. Eat regularly, do not give in to the surge of energy and be tempted to complete major tasks that will lead to starting labour exhausted. Get as much rest as possible. Take some exercise; walking can be helpful	Encourage and reassure her. Be readily available if possible. Give extra household help

Appendix 2 Labour Sequence (*continued*)

Stage	Physical signs	Mother's sensations	Mother's emotions	Self-help techniques	Companion's support
Early first stage – latent phase	Regular, uncomfortable contractions with cervical effacement and dilatation – 1–3 cm. A 'show' may occur. Rupturing of membranes – a sudden gush of liquor indicates forewater rupture, a continuous trickle – hindwaters – although this can happen at any time during labour	Crampy discomfort, like period pains, felt in the lower abdomen or back, lasting 35–45 seconds, 10–20 minutes apart. Contractions become stronger, last longer, and come more quickly	May be excited and confident, or apprehensive if the sensations are very strong. Becomes more serious as time passes	Continue with normal routine as far as possible to help pass the time. Have a light meal. Try to rest if it is night-time. Relax in a warm, deep bath or take a long shower. Begin using slow, calm breathing if necessary	Provide calm atmosphere; chat in between contractions. Suggest distractions such as music, a video, games. Encourage use of breathing through contractions, moving around and changes of position. Make sure she is comfortable

| First stage – active phase | Very strong, intense and painful contractions lasting up to 60 seconds and coming at 2–3 minute intervals. A 'show' may occur. Membranes can rupture. Cervix dilates slowly to 8–9 cm. Fetus descends through pelvis | Fierce, intense abdominal and/or low back pain – possibly also leg cramps or thigh pain. The pain areas will increase in size. May feel nauseous or be sick | Concentrates well initially; tires as time goes by. Aware that a process has begun that must continue – there seems to be no time to rest – can feel trapped. Can be apprehensive, may be distressed by pain and feel discouraged | Breathe out and relax as a contraction begins. Continue with slow, calm breathing over each 'mountain peak' or 'wave'; concentrate. Try lighter breaths for 'crest of wave' or 'mountain summit'. Take a deep breath in and out at the end of each contraction and relax. Change position from time to time – move around or rest as seems comfortable. Use gentle abdominal massage during contractions. Try to empty bladder every 2 hours if possible | Give loving encouragement. Watch for signs of tension – soothe with rhythmical stroking. Use deep, firm back massage if necessary. Gently stroke over area of abdominal pain if she finds this helpful. 'Talk her through' contractions – do not impose your rhythm but try and keep her breathing slow, deep and calm. Give sips of water or ice cubes to suck in between contractions. Sponge her face with a cool face-cloth. Help her change position and move around if this helps |

Appendix 2 Labour Sequence (continued)

Stage	Physical signs	Mother's sensations	Mother's emotions	Self-help techniques	Companion's support
Late active phase – the transition to the second stage	Cervix dilates fully. Fetus continues to rotate and descend	Tremendously powerful and overwhelming contractions – intensely painful – pain now covers very wide areas. Contractions last 60–90 seconds; come very rapidly, peak quickly, may have double peaks. May be aware of rectal pressure. May shake or tremble; feel sick or vomit, have hiccups, belch, grunt, hold breath, groan – anticipating bearing-down urge	May feel as if her body has been 'taken over'. Feels she cannot go on – her body is not able to give birth. Can be desperate for pain relief, irritable, exhausted, depressed and weepy. May doze between contractions and wake feeling she can no longer remain relaxed and cannot keep her breathing calm	Try to relax totally at the beginning of each contraction, then use whichever technique gives most help; slow, calm breathing; lighter breaths; saying 'I won't push' with a breath for each word; concentrating on a poem or song. Change to knee-chest position if there is an anterior lip of the cervix. Rest and relax between contractions	Keep her informed of progress – tell her how well she is doing. Give constant strong support and encouragement. Tell her the first stage is nearly over. Massage her legs between contractions, support or massage her back. Refresh her with a cool sponge, wiping her face, neck, chest and arms. Give sips of water – put cream on her lips if they become dry. Use eye contact to help her concentrate through contractions. It won't be long now!

Although the cervix is now fully dilated there is often a lull at this point – contractions can fade away for a time. If the baby's head is high, the attendants will want pushing to be delayed until the vertex reaches the pelvic floor	Contractions become weaker and more widely spaced – they may stop altogether	She may welcome this short respite or she may begin to feel anxious because labour has apparently stopped	Rest and relax, even have a short sleep if possible. If attendants ask her to begin pushing she should explain that she does not have a bearing-down urge as yet	Rest too. Encourage the mother to make the most of this 'space' in her labour. Reassure her that all is well

Appendix 2 Labour Sequence (continued)

Stage	Physical signs	Mother's sensations	Mother's emotions	Self-help techniques	Companion's support
Second stage	Contractions may be more widely spaced than in the first stage. Fetus reaches the pelvic floor which begins to distend and bulge, and the vagina is stretched open as the head emerges. There may be a small bowel movement	The urge to push becomes stronger as the head reaches the perineum. There may be tremendous rectal pressure – like a large grapefruit in the anus. Some women feel as if their baby is emerging through the wrong opening! There will be a burning, stretching sensation that mounts as the head crowns; then there may be a feeling of numbness. Some women notice symphysis pubis and sacroiliac discomfort	She may suddenly find reserves of energy and be excited and happy. Some women are frightened by the intensity of the experience and hold back from pushing in case the pain becomes worse or they defaecate. She may feel exhausted and unable to summon the energy to push	Only push when the urge is present – there may be 3 or 4 surges of the pushing urge with each contraction. Prolonged pushing is inadvisable: steady 8–10 second pushes are probably what the body will produce – follow the uterus. Find the most comfortable and efficient position for pushing – squatting is useful if the pushing urge is weak or absent	Help her into a position which suits her – support her if necessary. Help her change position between contractions if the one she has been using is unsatisfactory. Refresh her with a cool, moist sponge in between contractions – offer sips of water

The baby's head is born, followed by the shoulders and body

For some women the pushing urge is overwhelming and amazing – their body seems to take over and work as a giant piston; others may not experience this at all

Intense perineal stretching – she feels as if she is on fire or bursting!

Exhilaration, relief, disbelief, delight, exhaustion

Go with the contraction – some women will hold their breath to push – others will push while blowing air out.
Relax the pelvic floor – let it 'give' around the baby's head.
Feel the baby's head – use a mirror to see it if this is helpful.
Listen to the midwife's directions; try to do exactly what she asks. Use slow, gentle panting to 'breathe' the baby's head out

Cuddle baby

Encourage and reassure her.
Hold a mirror if she wants to see the baby's head.
Repeat the midwife's instructions if necessary

Welcome baby – cuddle and kiss mother and baby.
Hold the baby if she is tired or needs to change position

Appendix 2 Labour Sequence (continued)

Stage	Physical signs	Mother's sensations	Mother's emotions	Self-help techniques	Companion's support
Third stage	Uterus contracts gradually with physiological third stage, or rapidly if it is actively managed. Placenta separates and is expelled or drawn out by midwife. There will be some blood loss. If the baby is put to the breast and sucks well, oxytocin will be released which stimulates uterine contractions	Milder, comparatively painless contractions, more widely spaced; or a very strong, painless contraction if syntometrine was used with anterior shoulder delivery. May shake and tremble uncontrollably	Sense of amazement and joy – intense relief that labour is over, she may be overwhelmed by her experience and need time to recover; she may weep. She can be utterly enthralled and fascinated by the baby – or may prefer her partner to hold him until she has revived	Hold baby to the breast; the baby may be ready to suck soon after birth or this may not happen until 20 minutes or so later. Once the placenta is delivered, enjoys a quiet time with her partner, getting to know the new baby. Savour the wonderful moment when the baby first opens its eyes and inspects mother!	Share the feeling of wonder and exhilaration you are experiencing with your partner – enjoy cuddling your new baby while the mother is made comfortable. Make phone calls to the family to announce the birth (don't forget telephone money!) Relax with partner and baby – enjoy the experience of your new role

The Standardization of Terminology of Lower Urinary Tract Function

Reproduced with permission of the International Continence Society Committee on Standardization of Terminology
Members: Paul Abrams, Jerry G. Blaivas, Stuart L. Stanton and Jens T. Andersen (Chairman)

CONTENTS

1. INTRODUCTION

The International Continence Society established a committee for the standardisation of terminology of lower urinary tract function in 1973. Five of the six reports (1-5) from this committee, approved by the Society, have been published. The fifth report on 'Quantification of urine loss' was an internal I.C.S. document but appears, in part, in this document.

These reports are revised, extended and collated in this monograph. The standards are recommended to facilitate comparison of results by investigators who use urodynamic methods. These standards are recommended not only for urodynamic investigations carried out on humans but also during animal studies. When using urodynamic studies in animals the type of any anaesthesia used should be stated. It is suggested that acknowledgement of these standards in written publications be indicated by a footnote to the section "Methods and materials" or its equivalent, to read as follows:

'Methods, definitions and units conform to the standards recommended by the International Continence Society, except where specifically noted'.

Urodynamic studies involve the assessment of the function and dysfunction of the urinary tract by any appropriate method. Aspects of urinary tract morphology, physiology, biochemistry and hydrodynamics affect urine transport and storage. Other methods of investigation such as the radiographic visualisation of the lower urinary tract is a useful adjunct to conventional urodynamics.

This monograph concerns the urodynamics of the lower urinary tract.

2. CLINICAL ASSESSMENT

The clinical assessment of patients with lower urinary tract dysfunction should consist of a detailed history, a frequency/volume chart and a physical examination. In urinary incontinence, leakage should be demonstrated objectively.

2.1 History

The general history should include questions relevant to neurological and congenital abnormalities as well as information on previous urinary infections and relevant surgery. Information must be obtained on medication with known or possible effects on the lower urinary tract. The general history should also include assessment of menstrual, sexual and bowel function, and obstetric history.

The urinary history must consist of symptoms related to both the storage and the evacuation functions of the lower urinary tract.

2.2 Frequency/volume chart

The frequency/volume chart is a specific urodynamic investigation recording fluid intake and urine output per 24 hour period. The chart gives objective information on the number of voidings, the distribution of voidings between daytime and nighttime and each voided volume. The chart can also be used to record episodes of urgency and leakage and the number of incontinence pads used. The frequency/volume chart is very useful in the assessment of voiding disorders, and in the follow-up of treatment.

2.3 Physical examination

Besides a general urological and, when appropriate, gynaecological examination, the physical examination should include the assessment of perineal sensation, the perineal reflexes supplied by the sacral segments S2-S4, and anal sphincter tone and control.

3. PROCEDURES RELATED TO THE EVALUATION OF URINE STORAGE

3.1 Cystometry

Cystometry is the method by which the pressure/volume relationship of the bladder is measured. All systems are zeroed at atmospheric pressure. For external transducers the reference point is the level of the superior edge of the symphysis pubis. For catheter mounted transducers the reference point is the transducer itself.

Cystometry is used to assess detrusor activity, sensation, capacity and compliance.

Before starting to fill the bladder the residual urine may be measured. However, the removal of a large volume of residual urine may alter detrusor function especially in neuropathic disorders. Certain cystometric parameters may be significantly altered by the speed of bladder filling (see 6.1.1.4).

During cystometry it is taken for granted that the patient is awake, unanaesthetised and neither sedated nor taking drugs that affect bladder function. Any variations should be specified.

Specify
a) Access (transurethral or percutaneous).
b) Fluid medium (liquid or gas).
c) Temperature of fluid (state in degrees Celsius).
d) Position of patient (e.g. supine, sitting or standing).
e) Filling may be by diuresis or catheter. Filling by catheter may be continuous or incremental; the precise filling rate should be stated.
   When the incremental method is used the volume

increment should be stated. For general discussion, the following terms for the range of filling rate may be used:
i) up to 10 ml per minute is slow fill cystometry ('physiological' filling);
ii) 10-100 ml per minute is medium fill cystometry;
iii) over 100 ml per minute is rapid fill cystometry.

Technique
a) Fluid-filled catheter - specify number of catheters, single of multiple lumens, type of catheter (manufacturer), size of catheter.
b) Catheter tip transducer - list specifications.
c) Other catheters - list specifications.
d) Measuring equipment.

Definitions
Intravesical pressure is the pressure within the bladder.

Abdominal pressure is taken to be the pressure surrounding the bladder. In current practice it is estimated from rectal or, less commonly, extraperitoneal pressure.

Detrusor pressure is that component of intravesical pressure that is created by forces in the bladder wall (passive and active). It is estimated by subtracting abdominal pressure from intravesical pressure. The simultaneous measurement of abdominal pressure is essential for the interpretation of the intravesical pressure trace. However, artifacts on the detrusor pressure trace may be produced by intrinsic rectal contractions.

Bladder sensation. Sensation is difficult to evaluate because of its subjective nature. It is usually assessed by questioning the patient in relation to the fullness of the bladder during cystometry. Commonly used descriptive terms include:
First desire to void.
Normal desire to void (this is defined as the feeling that leads the patient to pass urine at the next convenient moment, but voiding can be delayed if necessary).
Strong desire to void (this is defined as a persistent desire to void without the fear of leakage).
Urgency (this is defined as a strong desire to void accompanied by fear of leakage or fear of pain).
Pain (the site and character of which should be specified). Pain during bladder filling or micturition is abnormal.

The use of objective or semi-objective tests for sensory function, such as electrical threshold studies (sensory testing), is discussed in detail in 5.5.

The term 'Capacity' must be qualified.

Maximum cystometric capacity, in patients with normal sensation, is the volume at which the patient feels he/she can no longer delay micturition. In the absence of sensation the maximum cystometric capacity cannot be defined in the same terms and is the volume at which the clinician decides to terminate filling. In the presence of sphincter incompetence the maximum cystometric capacity may be significantly increased by occlusion of the urethra e.g. by Foley catheter.

The functional bladder capacity, or voided volume is more relevant and is assessed from a frequency/volume chart (urinary diary).

The maximum (anaesthetic) bladder capacity is the volume measured after filling during a deep general or spinal/epidural anaesthetic, specifying fluid temperature, filling pressure and filling time.

Compliance indicates the change in volume for a change in pressure. Compliance is calculated by dividing the volume change (ΔV) by the change in detrusor pressure ($\Delta Pdet$) during that change in bladder volume ($C=\Delta V/\Delta Pdet$). Compliance is expressed as mls per cm H_2O (see 6.1.1.4).

3.2 Urethral pressure measurement

It should be noted that the urethral pressure and the urethral closure pressure are idealised concepts which represent the ability of the urethra to prevent leakage (see 6.1.5). In current urodynamic practice the urethral pressure is measured by a number of different techniques which do not always yield consistant values. Not only do the values differ with the method of measurement but there is often lack of consistency for a single method. For example the effect of catheter rotation when urethral pressure is measured by a catheter mounted transducer.

Intraluminal urethral pressure may be measured:
a) At rest, with the bladder at any given volume.
b) During coughing or straining.
c) During the process of voiding (see 4.4).
Measurements may be made at one point in the urethra over a period of time, or at several points along the urethra consecutively forming a *urethral pressure profile* (U.P.P.).

Storage phase
Two types of U.P.P. may be measured:
a) Resting urethral pressure profile - with the bladder and subject at rest.
b) Stress urethral pressure profile - with a defined applied stress (e.g. cough, strain, valsalva).
In the storage phase the *urethral pressure profile* denotes the intraluminal pressure along the length of the urethra. All systems are zeroed at atmospheric pressure. For external transducers the reference point is the superior edge of the symphysis pubis. For catheter mounted transducers the reference point is the transducer itself. Intravesical pressure should be measured to exclude a simultaneous detrusor contraction. The subtraction of intravesical pressure from urethral pressure produces the *urethral closure pressure profile*.

The simultaneous recording of both intravesical and ultra-urethral pressures are essential during stress urethral profilometry.

Specify
a) Infusion medium (liquid or gas).
b) Rate of infusion.
c) Stationary, continuous or intermittent withdrawal.
d) Rate of withdrawal.
e) Bladder volume.
f) Position of patient (supine, sitting or standing).

Technique
a) Open catheter - specify type (manufacturer), size, number, position and orientation of side or end hole.
b) Catheter mounted transducers - specify manufacturer, number of transducers, spacing of transducers along the catheter, orientation with respect to one another; transducer design e.g. transducer face depressed or flush with catheter surface; catheter diameter and material. The orientation of the transducer(s) in the urethra should be stated.
c) Other catheters, e.g. membrane, fibreoptic - specify type (manufacturer), size and number of channels as for microtransducer catheter.
d) Measurement technique: For stress profiles the particular stress employed should be stated e.g. cough or valsalva.
e) Recording apparatus: Describe type of recording apparatus. The frequency response of the total system should be stated. The frequency response of the catheter in the perfusion method can be assessed by blocking the eyeholes and recording the consequent rate of change of pressure.

Definitions (Fig. 1; referring to profiles measured in storage phase).
Maximum urethral pressure is the maximum pressure of the measured profile.
Maximum urethral closure pressure is the maximum difference between the urethral pressure and the intravesical pressure.
Functional profile length is the length of the urethra along which the urethral pressure exceeds intravesical pressure.
Functional profile length (on stress) is the length over which the urethral pressure exceeds the intravesical pressure on stress.
Pressure 'transmission' ratio is the increment in urethral pressure on stress as a percentage of the simultaneously recorded increment in intravesical pressure. For stress profiles obtained during coughing, pressure transmission ratios can be obtained at any point along the urethra. If single values are given the position in the urethra should be stated. If several pressure transmission ratios are

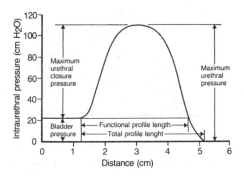

Fig. 1. Diagram of a female urethral pressure profile (static) with I.C.S. recommended nomenclature.

defined at different points along the urethra a pressure 'transmission' profile is obtained. During 'cough profiles' the amplitude of the cough should be stated if possible.

Note: the term 'transmission' is in common usage and cannot be changed. However transmission implies a completely passive process. Such an assumption is not yet justified by scientific evidence. A role for muscular activity cannot be excluded.

Total profile length is not generally regarded as a useful parameter.

The information gained from urethral pressure measurements in the storage phase is of limited value in the assessment of voiding disorders.

3.3 Quantification of urine loss

Subjective grading of incontinence may not indicate reliably the degree of abnormality. However it is important to relate the management of the individual patients to their complaints and personal circumstances, as well as to objective measurements.

In order to assess and compare the results of the treatment of different types of incontinence in different centres, a simple standard test can be used to measure urine loss objectively in any subject. In order to obtain a representative result, especially in subjects with variable or intermittent urinary incontinence, the test should occupy as long a period as possible; yet it must be practical. The circumstances should approximate to those of everyday life, yet be similar for all subjects to allow meaningful comparison. On the basis of pilot studies performed in various centres, an internal report of the I.C.S. (5th) recommended a test occupying a one-hour period during which a series of standard activities was carried out. This test *can* be extended by further one hour periods if the result of the first

one hour test was not considered representative by either the patient or the investigator. Alternatively the test can be repeated having filled the bladder to a defined volume.

The total amount of urine lost during the test period is determined by weighing a collecting device such as a nappy, absorbent pad or condom appliance. A nappy or pad should be worn inside waterproof underpants or should have a waterproof backing. Care should be taken to use a collecting device of adequate capacity.

Immediately before the test begins the collecting device is weighed to the nearest gram.

Typical test schedule
a)   Test is started without the patient voiding.
b)   Preweighed collecting device is put on and first one hour test period begins.
c)   Subject drinks 500 ml sodium free liquid within a short period (max. 15 min), then sits or rests.
d)   Half hour period: subject walks, including stair climbing equivalent to one flight up and down.
e)   During the remaining period the subject performs the following activities:
  i)   standing up from sitting, 10 times;
  ii)   coughing vigorously, 10 times;
  iii)   running on the spot for 1 minute;
  iv)   bending to pick up small object from floor, 5 times;
  v)   wash hands in running water for 1 minute.
f)   At the end of the one hour test the collecting device is removed and weighed.
g)   If the test is regarded as representative the subject voids and the volume is recorded.
h)   Otherwise the test is repeated preferably without voiding.

If the collecting device becomes saturated or filled during the test it should be removed and weighed, and replaced by a fresh device. The total weight of urine lost during the test period is taken to be equal to the gain in weight of the collecting device(s). In interpreting the results of the test it should be born in mind that a weight gain of up to 1 gram may be due to weighing errors, sweating or vaginal discharge.

The activity programme may be modified according to the subject's physical ability. If substantial variations from the usual test schedule occur, this should be recorded so that the same schedule can be used on subsequent occasions.

In principle the subject should not void during the test period. If the patient experiences urgency, then he/she should be persuaded to postpone voiding and to perform as many of the activities in section (e) as possible in order to detect leakage. Before voiding the collection device is removed for weighing. If inevitable voiding cannot be postponed then the test is terminated. The voided volume and the duration of the test should be recorded. For subjects not completing the full test the results may require separate analysis, or the test may be repeated after rehydration.

The test result is given as grams urine lost in the one hour test period in which the greatest urine loss is recorded.

Additional procedures
Additional procedures intended to give information of diagnostic value are permissible provided they do not interfere with the basic test. For example, additional changes and weighing of the collecting device can give information about the timing of urine loss. The absorbent nappy may be an electronic recording nappy so that the timing is recorded directly.

Presentation of results
Specify
a) Collecting device.
b) Physical condition of subject (ambulant, chairbound, bedridden).
c) Relevant medical condition of subject.
d) Relevant drug treatments.
e) Test schedule.
In some situations the timing of the test (e.g. in relation to the menstrual cycle) may be relevant.

Findings
Record weight of urine lost during the test (in the case of repeated tests, greatest weight in any stated period). A loss of less than one gram is within experimental error and the patients should be regarded as essentially dry. Urine loss should be measured and recorded in grams.

Statistics
When performing statistical analysis of urine loss in a group of subjects, non-parametric statistics should be employed, since the values are not normally distributed.

4. PROCEDURES RELATED TO THE EVALUATION OF MICTURITION

4.1 Measurement of urinary flow

Urinary flow may be described in terms of *rate* and *pattern* and may be *continuous or intermittent*. *Flow rate* is defined as the volume of fluid expelled via the urethra per unit time. It is expressed in ml/s.

Specify
a) Voided volume.
b) Patient environment and position (supine, sitting or standing).

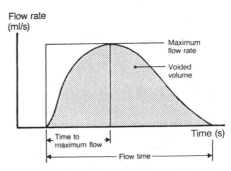

Fig 2. Diagram of a continous urine flow recording with I.C.S. recommended nomenclature.

c) Filling:
   i) by diuresis (spontaneous or forced: specify regimen);
   ii) by catheter (transurethral or suprapubic).
d) Type of fluid.

Technique
a) Measuring equipment.
b) Solitary procedure or combined with other measurements.

Definitions
a) *Continuous flow* (Fig. 2).
   Voided volume is the total volume expelled via the urethra.
   Maximum flow rate is the maximum measured value of the flow rate.
   Average flow rate is voided volume divided by flow time. The calculation of average flow rate is only meaningful if flow is continuous and without terminal dribbling.
   Flow time is the time over which measurable flow actually occurs.
   Time to maximum flow is the elapsed time from onset of flow to maximum flow.
   The flow pattern must be described when flow time and average flow rate are measured.
b) *Intermittent flow* (Fig. 3)
   The same parameters used to characterise continuous flow may be applicable if care is exercised in patients with intermittent flow. In measuring flow time the time intervals between flow episodes are disregarded.
   Voiding time is total duration of micturition, i.e. includes interruptions. When voiding is completed without interruption, voiding time is equal to flow time.

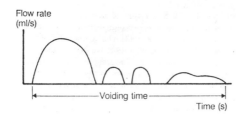

Flow rate
(ml/s)

Voiding time

Time (s)

Fig. 3. Diagram of an interrupted urine flow recording with I.C.S. recommended nomenclature.

4.2 Bladder pressure measurements during micturition

The specifications of patient position, access for pressure measurement, catheter type and measuring equipment are as for cystometry (see 3.1).

Definitions (Fig. 4)
Opening time is the elapsed time from initial rise in detrusor pressure to onset of flow. This is the initial isovolumetric contraction period of micturition. Time lags should be taken into account. In most urodynamic systems a time lag occurs equal to the time taken for the urine to pass from the point of pressure measurement to the uroflow transducer.

The following parameters are applicable to measure-

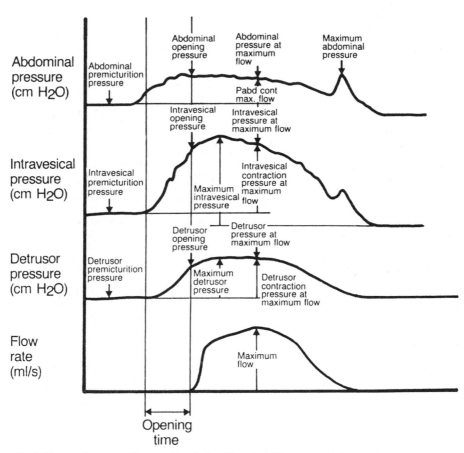

Fig. 4. Diagram of a pressure-flow recording of micturition with I.C.S. recommended nomenclature.

ments of each of the pressure curves: intravesical, abdominal and detrusor pressure.

Premicturition pressure is the pressure recorded immediately before the initial isovolumetric contraction.

Opening pressure is the pressure recorded at the onset of measured flow.

Maximum pressure is the maximum value of the measured pressure.

Pressure at maximum flow is the pressure recorded at maximum measured flow rate.

Contraction pressure at maximum flow is the difference between pressure at maximum flow and premicturition pressure.

Postmicturition events (e.g. after contraction) are not well understood and so cannot be defined as yet.

4.3 Pressure flow relationships

In the early days of urodynamics the flow rate and voiding pressure were related as a 'urethral resistance factor'. The concept of a resistance factor originates from rigid tube hydrodynamics. The urethra does not generally behave as a rigid tube as it is an irregular and distensible conduit whose walls and surroundings have active and passive elements and hence, influence the flow through it. Therefore a resistance factor cannot provide a valid comparison between patients.

There are many ways of displaying the relationships between flow and pressure during micturition, an example is suggested in the I.C.S. 3rd Report (4) (Fig. 5). As yet available data do not permit a standard presentation of pressure/flow parameters.

When data from a group of patients are presented,

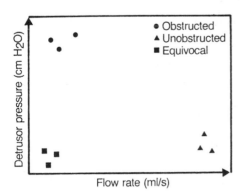

Fig. 5. Diagram illustrating the presentation of pressure flow data on individual patients in three groups of 3 patients: obstructed, equivocal and unobstructed.

pressure-flow relationships may be shown on a graph as illustrated in Fig. 5. This form of presentation allows lines of demarcation to be drawn on the graph to separate the results according to the problem being studied. The points shown in Fig. 5 are purely illustrative to indicate how the data might fall into groups. The group of equivocal results might include either an unrepresentative micturition in an obstructed or an unobstructed patient, or underactive detrusor function with or without obstruction. This is the group which invalidates the use of 'urethral resistance factors'.

4.4 Urethral pressure measurements during voiding (V.U.P.P.)

The V.U.P.P. is used to determine the pressure and site of urethral obstruction.

Pressure is recorded in the urethra during voiding. The technique is similar to that used in the U.P.P. measured during storage (the resting and stress profiles 3.2).

Specify (as for U.P.P. during storage (3.2))

Accurate interpretation of the V.U.P.P. depends on the simultaneous measurement of intravesical pressure and the measurement of pressure at a precisely localised point in the urethra. Localisation may be achieved by radio opaque marker on the catheter which allows the pressure measurement to be related to a visualised point in the urethra.

This technique is not fully developed and a number of technical as well as clinical problems need to be solved before the V.U.P.P. is widely used.

4.5 Residual urine

Residual urine is defined as the volume of fluid remaining in the bladder immediately following the completion of micturition. The measurement of residual urine forms an integral part of the study of micturition. However voiding in unfamiliar surroundings may lead to unrepresentative results, as may voiding on command with a partially filled or overfilled bladder. Residual urine is commonly estimated by the following methods:

a) Catheter or cystoscope (transurethral, suprapubic).
b) Radiography (excretion urography, micturition cystography).
c) Ultrasonics.
d) Radioisotopes (clearance, gamma camera).

When estimating residual urine the measurement of voided volume and the time interval between voiding and residual urine estimation should be recorded: this is particularly important if the patient is in a diuretic phase. In the condition of vesicoureteric reflux, urine may re-enter the bladder after micturition and may falsely be interpreted as residual urine. The presence of urine in bladder diverticula following micturition present special problems of interpretation, since a diverticulum may be regarded either as part of the bladder cavity or as outside the functioning bladder.

The various methods of measurement each have limitations as to their applicability and accuracy in the various conditions associated with residual urine. Therefore it is necessary to choose a method appropriate to the clinical problems. The absence of residual urine is usually an observation of clinical value, but does not exclude infravesical obstruction or bladder dysfunction. An isolated finding of residual urine requires confirmation before being considered significant.

5. PROCEDURES RELATED TO NEUROPHYSIOLOGICAL EVALUATION OF THE URINARY TRACT DURING FILLING AND VOIDING

5.1 Electromyography

Electromyography (E.M.G.) is the study of electrical potentials generated by the depolarization of muscle. The following refers to striated muscle E.M.G. The functional unit in E.M.G. is the motor unit. This is comprised of a single motor neurone and the muscle fibres it innervates. A motor unit action potential is the recorded depolarization of muscle fibres which results from activation of a single anterior horn cell. Muscle action potentials may be detected either by needle electrodes, or by surface electrodes.

Needle electrodes are placed directly into the muscle mass and permit visualization of the individual motor unit action potentials.

Surface electrodes are applied to an epithelial surface as close to the muscle under study as possible. Surface electrodes detect the action potentials from groups of adjacent motor units underlying the recording surface.

E.M.G. potentials may be displayed on an oscilloscope screen or played through audio amplifiers. A permanent record of E.M.G. potentials can only be made using a chart recorder with a high frequency response (in the range of 10 kHz).

E.M.G. should be interpreted in the light of the patients symptoms, physical findings and urological and urodynamic investigations.

General information

Specify
a) E.M.G. (solitary procedure, part of urodynamic or other electrophysiological investigation).
b) Patient position (supine, standing, sitting or other).
c) Electrode placement:

i) sampling site (intrinsic striated muscle of the urethra, periurethral striated muscle, bulbocavernosus muscle, external anal sphincter, pubococcygeus or other). State whether sites are single or multiple, unilateral or bilateral. Also state number of samples per site;

ii) recording electrode: define the precise anatomical location of the electrode. For needle electrodes, include site of needle entry, angle of entry and needle depth. For vaginal or urethral surface electrodes state method of determining position of electrode;

iii) reference electrode position.

Note: ensure that there is no electrical interference with any other machines, e.g. X-ray apparatus.

Technical information

Specify
a) Electrodes:
   i) needle electrodes:
     - design (concentric, bipolar, monopolar, single fibre, other);
     - dimensions (length, diameter, recording area);
     - electrode material (e.g. platinum);
   ii) surface electrodes:
     - type (skin, plug, catheter, other);
     - size and shape;
     - electrode material;
     - mode of fixation to recording surface;
     - conducting medium (e.g. saline, jelly).
b) Amplifier (make and specifications).
c) Signal processing (data: raw, averaged, integrated or other).
d) Display equipment (make and specifications to include method of calibration, time base, full scale deflection in microvolts and polarity):
   i) oscilloscope;
   ii) chart recorder;
   iii) loudspeaker;
   iv) other.
e) Storage (make and specifications):
   i) paper;
   ii) magnetic tape recorder;
   iii) microprocessor;
   iv) other.
f) Hard copy production (make and specifications):
   i) chart recorder;
   ii) photographic/video reproduction of oscilloscope screen;
   iii) other.

E.M.G. findings

a) Individual motor unit action potentials - Normal motor unit potentials have a characteristic configuration, amplitude and duration. Abnormalities of the motor unit may include an increase in the amplitude, duration and complexity of waveform (polyphasicity) of the potentials. A polyphasic potential is defined as one having more than 5 deflections. The E.M.G. findings of fibrillations, positive sharp waves and bizarre high frequency potentials are thought to be abnormal.

b) Recruitment patterns - In normal subjects there is a gradual increase in 'pelvic floor' and 'sphincter' E.M.G. activity during bladder filling. At the onset of micturition there is complete absence of activity. Any sphincter E.M.G. activity during voiding is abnormal unless the patient is attempting to inhibit micturition. The finding of increased sphincter E.M.G. activity, during voiding, accompanied by characteristic simultaneous detrusor pressure and flow changes is described by the term, detrusor-sphincter-dyssynergia. In this condition a detrusor contraction occurs concurrently with an inappropriate contraction of the urethral and or periurethral striated muscle.

5.2 Nerve conduction studies

Nerve conduction studies involve stimulation of a peripheral nerve, and recording the time taken for a response to occur in muscle, innervated by the nerve under study. The time taken from stimulation of the nerve to the response in the muscle is called the "latency". Motor latency is the time taken by the fastest motor fibres in the nerve to conduct impulses to the muscle and depends on conduction distance and the conduction velocity of the fastest fibres.

General information
(also applicable to reflex latencies and evoked potentials - see below).

Specify
a) Type of investigation:
   i) nerve conduction study (e.g. pudendal nerve);
   ii) reflex latency determination (e.g. bulbocavernosus);
   iii) spinal evoked potential;
   iv) cortical evoked potential;
   v) other.
b) Is the study a solitary procedure or part of urodynamic or neurophysiological investigations?
c) Patient position and environmental temperature, noise level and illumination.
d) Electrode placement: define electrode placement in precise anatomical terms. The exact interelectrode distance is required for nerve conduction velocity calculations:
   i) stimulation site (penis, clitoris, urethra, bladder neck, bladder or other);
   ii) recording sites (external anal sphincter, periurethral striated muscle, bulbocavernosus muscle, spinal cord, cerebral cortex or other). When recording spinal evoked responses, the sites of the recording electrodes should be specified according to the bony landmarks (e.g. L4). In cortical evoked responses the sites of the recording electrodes should be specified as in the International 10-20 system (6). The sampling techniques should be specified (single or multiple, unilateral or bilateral, ipsilateral or contralateral or other);
   iii) reference electrode position;
   iv) grounding electrode site: ideally this should be between the stimulation and recording sites to reduce stimulus artefact.

Technical information
(also applicable to reflex latencies and evoked potential - see below)

Specify
a) Eletrodes (make and specifications). Describe separately stimulus and recording electrodes as below:
   i) design (e.g. needle, plate, ring, and configuration of anode and cathode where applicable);
   ii) dimensions;
   iii) electrode material (e.g. platinum);
   iv) contact medium.
b) Stimulator (make and specifications):
   i) stimulus parameters (pulse width, frequency, pattern, current density, electrode impedance in Kohms. Also define in terms of threshold e.g. in case of supramaximal stimulation).
c) Amplifier (make and specifications):
   i) sensitivity (mV-μV);
   ii) filters - low pass (Hz) or high pass (kHz);
   iii) sampling time (ms).
d) Averager (make and specifications):
   i) number of stimuli sampled.
e) Display equipment (make and specifications to include method of calibration, time base, full scale deflection in microvolts and polarity):
   i) oscilloscope.
f) Storage (make and specifications):
   i) paper;
   ii) magnetic tape recorder;
   iii) microprocessor;
   iv) other.
g) Hard copy production (make and specification):
   i) chart recorder;

ii) photographic/video reproduction of oscilloscope screen;

iii) XY recorder;

iv) other.

Description of nerve conduction studies

Recordings are made from muscle and the latency of response of the muscle is measured. The latency is taken as the time to onset, of the earliest response.

a) To ensure that response time can be precisely measured, the gain should be increased to give a clearly defined takeoff point. (Gain setting at least 100 µV/div and using a short time base e.g. 1-2 ms/div).

b) Additional information may be obtained from nerve conduction studies, if, when using surface electrodes to record a compound muscle action potential, the amplitude is measured. The gain setting must be reduced so that the whole response is displayed and a longer time base is recommended (e.g. 1 mV/div and 5 ms/div). Since the amplitude is proportional to the number of motor unit potentials within the vicinity of the recording electrodes, a reduction in amplitude indicates loss of motor units and therefore denervation. (Note: a prolongation of latency is not necessarily indicative of denervation).

5.3 Reflex latencies

Reflex latencies require stimulation of sensory fields and recordings from the muscle which contracts reflexly in response to the stimulation. Such responses are a test of reflex arcs which are comprised of both afferent and efferent limbs and a synaptic region within the central nervous system. The reflex latency expresses the nerve conduction velocity in both limbs of the arc and the integrity of the central nervous system at the level of the synapse(s). Increased reflex latency may occur as a result of slowed afferent or efferent nerve conduction or due to central nervous system conduction delays.

General information and technical information

The same technical and general details apply as discussed above under nerve conduction studies (5.2).

Description of reflex latency measurements

Recordings are made from muscle and the latency of response of the muscle is measured. The latency is taken as the time to onset, of the earliest response.

To ensure that response time can be precisely measured, the gain should be increased to give a clearly defined take-off point. (Gain setting at least 100 µV/div and using a short time base e.g. 1-2 ms/div).

5.4 Evoked responses

Evoked responses are potential changes in central nervous system neurones resulting from distant stimulation usually electrical. They are recorded using averaging techniques. Evoked responses may be used to test the integrity of peripheral, spinal and central nervous pathways. As with nerve conduction studies, the conduction time (latency) may be measured. In addition, information may be gained from the amplitude and configuration of these responses.

General information and technical information

See above under Nerve conduction studies (5.2).

Description of evoked responses

Describe the presence or absence of stimulus evoked responses and their configuration.

Specify

a) Single or multiphasic response.

b) Onset of response: defined as the start of the first reproducible potential. Since the onset of the response may be difficult to ascertain precisely, the criteria used should be stated.

c) Latency to onset: defined as the time (ms) from the onset of stimulus to the onset of response. The central conduction time relates to cortical evoked potentials and is defined as the difference between the latencies of the cortical and the spinal evoked potentials. This parameter may be used to test the integrity of the corticospinal neuraxis.

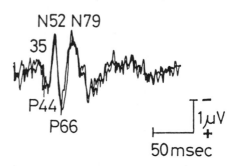

Fig. 6. Multiphasic evoked response recorded from the cerebral cortex after stimulation of the dorsal aspect of the penis. The recording shows the conventional labelling of negative (N) and positive (P) deflections with the latency of each deflection from the point of stimulation in milliseconds.

d) Latencies to peaks of positive and negative deflections in multiphasic responses (Fig. 6). P denotes positive deflections. N denotes negative deflections. In multiphasic responses, the peaks are numbered consecutively (e.g. P1, N1, P2, N2...) or according to the latencies to peaks in milliseconds (e.g. P44, N52, P66 ...).

e) The amplitude of the responses is measured in μV.

5.5 Sensory testing

Limited information, of a subjective nature, may be obtained during cystometry by recording such parameters as the first desire to micturate, urgency or pain. However, sensory function in the lower urinary tract, can be assessed by semi-objective tests by the measurement of urethral and/or vesical sensory thresholds to a standard applied stimulus such as a known electrical current.

General information

Specify

a) Patients position (supine, sitting, standing, other).

b) Bladder volume at time of testing.

c) Site of applied stimulus (intravesical, intraurethral).

d) Number of times the stimulus was applied and the response recorded. Define the sensation recorded, e.g. the first sensation or the sensation of pulsing.

e) Type of applied stimulus:
   i)   electrical current: it is usual to use a constant current stimulator in urethral sensory measurement:
   - state electrode characteristics and placement as in section on E.M.G.;
   - state electrode contact area and distance between electrodes if applicable;
   - state impedance characteristics of the system;
   - state type of conductive medium used for electrode/epithelial contact. *Note: topical anaesthetic agents should not be used;*
   - stimulator make and specifications;
   - stimulation parameters (pulse width, frequency, pattern, duration, current density);
   ii)   other - e.g. mechanical, chemical.

Definition of sensory thresholds

The vesical/urethral sensory threshold is defined as the least current which consistently produces a sensation perceived by the subject during stimulation at the site under investigation. However, the absolute values will vary in relation to the site of the stimulus, the characteristics of the equipment and the stimulation parameters. Normal values should be established for each system.

6. A CLASSIFICATION OF URINARY TRACT DYSFUNCTION

The lower urinary tract is composed of the *bladder* and *urethra*. They form a functional unit and their interaction cannot be ignored. Each has two functions, the bladder to store and void, the urethra to control and convey. When a reference is made to the hydrodynamic function or to the whole anatomical unit as a storage organ - the vesica urinaria - the correct term is the *bladder*. When the smooth muscle structure known as the m.detrusor urinae is being discussed then the correct term is *detrusor*. For simplicity the bladder/detrusor and the urethra will be considered separately so that a classification based on a combination of functional anomalies can be reached. Sensation cannot be precisely evaluated but must be assessed. This classification depends on the results of various objective urodynamic investigations. A complete urodynamic assessment is not necessary in all patients. However, studies of the filling and voiding phases are essential for each patient. As the bladder and urethra may behave differently during the storage and micturition phases of bladder function it is most useful to examine bladder and urethral activity separately in each phase.

Terms used should be objective, definable and ideally should be applicable to the whole range of abnormality. When authors disagree with the classification presented below, or use terms which have not been defined here, their meaning should be made clear.

Assuming the absence of inflammation, infection and neoplasm, *Lower urinary tract dysfunction* may be caused by:

a) Disturbance of the pertinent nervous or psychological control system.

b) Disorders of muscle function.

c) Structural abnormalities.

Urodynamic diagnoses based on this classification should correlate with the patients symptoms and signs. For example the presence of an unstable contraction in an asymptomatic continent patient does not warrant a diagnosis of detrusor overactivity during storage.

6.1 The storage phase

6.1.1 Bladder function during storage
This may be described according to:
6.1.1.1 Detrusor activity.
6.1.1.2 Bladder sensation.
6.1.1.3 Bladder capacity.
6.1.1.4 Compliance.

6.1.1.1 Detrusor activity. In this context detrusor activity is interpreted from the measurement of detrusor pressure (pdet). Detrusor activity may be:
a) Normal.
b) Overactive.

a) Normal detrusor function. During the filling phase the bladder volume increased without a significant rise in pressure (accommodation). No involuntary contractions occur despite provocation. A normal detrusor so defined may be described as "stable".

b) Overactive detrusor function. Overactive detrusor function is characterised by involuntary detrusor contractions during the filling phase, which may be spontaneous or provoked and which the patient cannot completely suppress. Involuntary detrusor contractions may be provoked by rapid filling, alterations of posture, coughing, walking, jumping and other triggering procedures. Various terms have been used to describe these features and they are defined as follows.

The unstable detrusor is one that is shown objectively to contract, spontaneously or on provocation, during the filling phase while the patient is attempting to inhibit micturition. Unstable detrusor contractions may be asymptomatic or may be interpreted as a normal desire to void. The presence of these contractions does not necessarily imply a neurological disorder. Unstable contractions are usually phasic in type (Fig. 7A). A gradual increase in detrusor pressure without subsequent decrease is best regarded as a change of compliance (Fig. 7B).

Detrusor hyperreflexia is defined as overactivity due to disturbance of the nervous control mechanisms. The term detrusor hyperreflexia should only be used when there is objective evidence of a relevant neurological disorder. The use of conceptual and undefined terms such as hypertonic, systolic, uninhibited, spastic and automatic should be avoided.

6.1.1.2 Bladder sensation. Bladder sensation during filling can be classified in qualitative terms (see 3.1) and by objective measurement (see 5.5). Sensation can be classified broadly as follows:
a) Normal.
b) Increased (hypersensitive).
c) Reduced (hyposensitive).
d) Absent.

6.1.1.3 Bladder capacity. See 3.1.

6.1.1.4 Compliance. Compliance is defined as: $\Delta V / \Delta p$ (see 3.1). Compliance may change during the cystometric examination and is variably dependent upon a number of factors including:

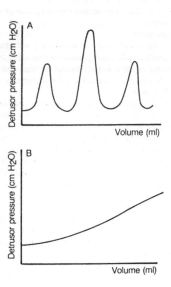

Fig. 7. Diagrams of filling cystometry to illustrate:
A. Typical phasic unstable detrusor contraction.
B. The gradual increase of detrusor pressure with filling characteristic of reduced bladder compliance.

a) Rate of filling.
b) The part of the cystometrogram curve used for compliance calculation.
c) The volume interval over which compliance is calculated.
d) The geometry (shape) of the bladder.
e) The thickness of the bladder wall.
f) The mechanical properties of the bladder wall.
g) The contractile/relaxant properties of the detrusor.
During normal bladder filling little or no pressure change occurs and this is termed 'normal compliance'. However at the present time there is insufficient data to define normal, high and low compliance.

When reporting compliance, *specify*
a) The rate of bladder filling.
b) The bladder volume at which compliance is calculated.
c) The volume increment over which compliance is calculated.
d) The part of the cystometrogram curve used for the calculation of compliance.

6.1.2 Urethral function during storage
The urethral closure mechanism during storage may be:
a) Normal.
b) Incompetent.

a) The *normal urethral closure mechanism* maintains a positive urethral closure pressure during filling even in the presence of increased abdominal pressure. Immediately prior to micturition the normal closure pressure decreases to allow flow.

b) *Incompetent urethral closure mechanism.* An incompetent urethral closure mechanism is defined as one which allows leakage of urine in the absence of a detrusor contraction. Leakage may occur whenever intravesical pressure exceeds intraurethral pressure (Genuine stress incontinence) or when there is an involuntary fall in urethral pressure. Terms such as 'the unstable urethra' await further data and precise definition.

6.1.3 Urinary incontinence
Urinary incontinence is involuntary loss of urine which is objectively demonstrable and a social or hygienic problem. Loss of urine through channels other than the urethra is extraurethral incontinence.

Urinary incontinence denotes:
a) A symptom.
b) A sign.
c) A condition.

The symptom indicates the patients statement of involuntary urine loss.

The sign is the objective demonstration of urine loss.

The condition is the urodynamic demonstration of urine loss.

Symptoms
Urge incontinence is the involuntary loss of urine associated with a strong desire to void (urgency). Urgency may be associated with two types of dysfunction:
a) Overactive detrusor function *(motor urgency).*
b) Hypersensivity *(sensory urgency).*

Stress incontinence: the symptom indicates the patient's statement of involuntary loss of urine during physical exertion.

'Unconscious' incontinence. Incontinence may occur in the absence of urge and without conscious recognition of the urinary loss.

Enuresis means any involuntary loss of urine. If it is used to denote incontinence during sleep, it should always be qualified with the adjective 'nocturnal'.

Post-micturition dribble and *Continuous leakage* denote other symptomatic forms of incontinence.

Signs
The sign stress-incontinence denotes the observation of loss of urine from the urethra synchronous with physical exertion (e.g. coughing). Incontinence may also be observed without physical exercise. Postmicturition dribble and continuous leakage denote other signs of incontinence. Symptoms and signs alone may not disclose the cause of urinary incontinence. Accurate diagnosis often requires urodynamic investigation in addition to careful history and physical examination.

Conditions
Genuine stress incontinence is the involuntary loss of urine occurring when, in the absence of a detrusor contraction, the intravesical pressure exceeds the maximum urethral pressure.

Reflex incontinence is loss of urine due to detrusor hyperreflexia and/or involuntary urethral relaxation in the absence of the sensation usually associated with the desire to micturate. This condition is only seen in patients with neuropathic bladder/urethral disorders.

Overflow incontinence is any involuntary loss of urine associated with over-distension of the bladder.

6.2 The voiding phase

6.2.1 The detrusor during voiding
During micturition the detrusor may be:
a) Acontractile.
b) Underactive.
c) Normal.

a) The *acontractile detrusor* is one that cannot be demonstrated to contract during urodynamic studies. *Detrusor areflexia* is defined as acontractility due to an abnormality of nervous control and denotes the complete absence of centrally coordinated contraction. In detrusor areflexia due to a lesion of the conus medullaris or sacral nerve outflow, the detrusor should be described as *decentralised* - not denervated, since the peripheral neurones remain. In such bladders pressure fluctuations of low amplitude, sometimes known as 'autonomous' waves, may occasionally occur. The use of terms such as atonic, hypotonic, autonomic and flaccid should be avoided.

b) *Detrusor underactivity.* This term should be reserved as an expression describing detrusor activity during micturition. Detrusor underactivity is defined as a detrusor contraction of inadequate magnitude and/or duration to effect bladder emptying with a normal time span. Patients may have underactivity during micturition and detrusor overactivity during filling.

c) *Normal detrusor contractility.* Normal voiding is achieved by a voluntarily initiated detrusor contraction that is sustained and can usually be suppressed voluntarily. A normal detrusor contraction will effect complete bladder emptying in the absence of obstruction. For a given detrusor contraction, the magnitude of the recorded pressure rise will depend on the degree of outlet resistance.

6.2.2 Urethral function during micturition

During voiding urethral function may be:

a) Normal.
b) Obstructive
    - overactivity
    - mechanical.

a) *The normal urethra* opens to allow the bladder to be emptied.

b) *Obstruction due to urethral overactivity:* this occurs when the urethral closure mechanism contracts against a detrusor contraction or fails to open at attempted micturition. Synchronous detrusor and urethral contraction is *detrusor/urethral dyssynergia*.

This diagnosis should be qualified by stating the location and type of the urethral muscles (striated or smooth) which are involved. Despite the confusion surrounding 'sphincter' terminology the use of certain terms is so widespread that they are retained and defined here. The term *detrusor/external sphincter dyssynergia* or *detrusor-sphincter-dyssynergia (D.S.D.)* describes a detrusor contraction concurrent with an involuntary contraction of the urethral and/or periurethral striated muscle. In the adult, detrusor sphincter dyssynergia is a feature of neurological voiding disorders. In the absence of neurological features the validity of this diagnosis should be questioned. The term *detrusor/bladder neck dyssynergia* is used to denote a detrusor contraction concurrent with an objectively demonstrated failure of bladder neck opening. No parallel term has been elaborated for possible detrusor/distal urethral (smooth muscle) dyssynergia.

Overactivity of the striated urethral sphincter may occur in the absence of detrusor contraction, and may prevent voiding. This is not detrusor/sphincter dyssynergia.

Overactivity of the urethral sphincter may occur during voiding in the absence of neurological disease and is termed *dysfunctional voiding*. The use of terms such as 'non-neurogenic' or 'occult neuropathic' should be avoided.

Mechanical obstruction is most commonly anatomical e.g. urethral stricture.

Using the characteristics of detrusor and urethral function during storage and micturition an accurate definition of lower urinary tract behaviour in each patient becomes possible.

7. SYMBOLS AND UNITS OF MEASUREMENT

7.1 Units of measurements

In the urodynamic literature pressure is measured in cm H_2O and *not* in millimeters of mercury. When Laplace's law is used to calculate tension in the bladder wall, it is often found that pressure is then measured in dyne cm^{-2}. This lack of uniformity in the systems used leads to confusion when other parameters, which are a function of pressure, are computed, for instance, 'compliance', contraction force, velocity etc. From these few examples it is evident that standardisation is essential for meaningful communication. Many journals now require that the results be given in SI Units. This section is designed to give guidance in the application of the SI system to urodynamics and defines the units involved. The principal units to be used are listed below (Table 1).

Table 1.

Quantity	Acceptable unit	Symbol
Volume	millilitre	ml
Time	second	s
Flow rate	millilitres/second	ml s^{-1}
Pressure	centimetres of water[1]	cm H_2O
Length	metres or submultiples	m, cm, mm
Velocity	metres/second or submultiples	m s^{-1}, cm s^{-1}
Temperature	degrees Celsius	°C

[1] The SI Unit is the pascal (Pa), but is only practical at present to calibrate our instruments in cm H_2O. One centimetre of water pressure is approximately equal to 100 pascals (1 cm H_2O = 98.07 Pa = 0.098 kPa).

7.2 Symbols

It is often helpful to use symbols in a communication. The system in Table 2 has been devised to standardise a code of symbols for use in urodynamics. The rationale of the system is to have a basic symbol representing the physical quantity with qualifying subscripts. The list of basic symbols largely conforms to international usage. The qualifying subscripts relate to the basic symbols to commonly used urodynamic parameters.

Table 2 . List of symbols.

Basic symbols		Urological qualifiers		Value	
Pressure	p	Bladder	ves	Maximum	max
Volume	V	Urethra	ura	Minimum	min
Flow rate	Q	Ureter	ure	Average	ave
Velocity	v	Detrusor	det	Isovolumetric	isv
Time	t	Abdomen	abd	Isotonic	ist
Temperature	T	Exeternal		Isobaric	isb
Length	l	Stream	ext	Isometric	ism
Area	A				
Diameter	d				
Force	F				
Energy	E				
Power	P				
Compliance	C				
Work	W				
Energy per unit volume	e				

Examples:

pdet.max   =   maximum detrusor pressure;

e.ext   =   kinetic energy per unit volume in the external stream.

8. REFERENCES

1. Abrams P, Blaivas JG, Stanton SL, Andersen JT, Fowler CJ, Gerstenberg T, Murray K. Sixth report on the standardisation of terminology of lower urinary tract function. Procedures related to neurophysiological investigations: Electromyography, nerve conduction studies, reflex latencies, evoked potentials and sensory testing. World J Urol 1986; 4: 2-5. Scand J Urol Nephrol 1986; 20: 161-164.

2. Bates P, Bradley WE, Glen E, Melchior H, Rowan D, Sterling A, Hald T. First report on the standardisation of terminology of lower urinary tract function. Urinary incontinence. Procedures related to the evaluation of urine storage: Cystometry, urethral closure pressure profile, units of measurement. Br J Urol 1976; 48: 39-42. Eur Urol 1976; 2: 274-276. Scand J Urol Nephrol 1976; 11: 193-196. Urol Int 1976; 32: 81-87.

3. Bates P, Glen E, Griffiths D, Melchior H, Rowan D, Sterling A, Zinner NR, Hald T. Second report on the standardisation of terminology of lower urinary tract function. Procedures related to the evaluation of micturition: Flow rate, pressure measurement, symbols. Acta Urol Jpn 1977; 27: 1563-1566. Br J Urol 1977; 49: 207-210. Eur Urol 1977; 3: 168-170. Scand J Urol Nephrol 1977; 11: 197-199.

4. Bates P, Bradley WE, Glen E, Griffiths D, Melchior H, Rowan D, Sterling A, Hald T. Third report on the standardisation of terminology of lower urinary tract function. Procedures related to the evaluation of micturition: Pressure flow relationships, residual urine. Br J Urol 1980; 52: 348-350. Eur Urol 1980; 6: 170-171. Acta Urol Jpn 1980; 27: 1566-1568. Scand J Urol Nephrol 1980; 12: 191-193.

5. Bates P, Bradley WE, Glen E, Melchior H, Rowan D, Sterling A, Sundin T, Thomas D, Torrens M, Turner-Walwick R, Zinner NR, Hald T. Fourth report on the standardisation of terminology of lower urinary tract function. Terminology related to neuromuscular dysfunction of lower urinary tract. Br J Urol 1981; 52: 333-335. Urology 1981; 17: 618-620. Scand J Urol Nephrol 1981; 15: 169-171. Acta Urol Jpn 1981; 27: 1568-1571.

6. Jasper HH. Report to the committee on the methods of clinical examination in electroencephalography. Electroencephal Clin Neurophysiol, 1958; 10: 370-375.

Index